HEALTH DIVIDES

Where you live can kill you

Clare Bambra

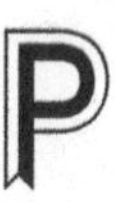

First published in Great Britain in 2016 by

Policy Press
University of Bristol
1-9 Old Park Hill
Bristol BS2 8BB
UK
t: +44 (0)117 954 5940
e: pp-info@bristol.ac.uk
www.policypress.co.uk

North American office:
Policy Press
c/o The University of Chicago Press
1427 East 60th Street
Chicago, IL 60637, USA
t: +1 773 702 7700
f: +1 773-702-9756
e:sales@press.uchicago.edu
www.press.uchicago.edu

Reprinted 2017

British Library Cataloguing in Publication Data
A catalogue record for this book is available from the British Library.

Library of Congress Cataloging-in-Publication Data
A catalog record for this book has been requested.

ISBN 978-1-4473-3035-6 paperback
ISBN 978-1-4473-3036-3 ePub
ISBN 978-1-4473-3037-0 Mobi

Cover design by Soapbox Design
Printed and bound in Great Britain by Clays Ltd, St Ives plc
Policy Press uses environmentally responsible print partners

For Mam, Dad and Ian

Contents

List of figures, tables and boxes

Figures

Tables

Boxes

Acknowledgements

First, I would like to thank Chris Orton of the Durham Cartography Unit for his heroic levels of support with the mapping, tables and visualisations. The book would not have been possible without his skilful support. I would also like to thank my colleagues Peter Henderson and Sinclair Sutherland from the Centre for Health and Inequalities Research, Durham University, for their considerable skill and expertise in developing the interactive book website (www.healthdivides.org). Thanks also to Nasima Akhter and Adetayo Kasim for the statistical analysis presented in Figure 4.3.

I would also like to thank my students Jenni Remnant and Nick Walton for their support with referencing using electronic software, and to Nick for helping substantially with the proofs. Thanks also to David Weeks for typing support in the final stages of manuscript preparation.

The book also benefited from insightful comments from my dear colleagues Professor Ted Schrecker of the Centre for Public Policy and Health, Durham University, and Dr Tim Brown from the Department of Geography, Queen Mary University of London.

Finally, this book was made possible by a generous Research Leadership grant awarded to me by the Leverhulme Trust to investigate health inequalities (reference RL-2012-006).

About the author

Clare Bambra PhD is Professor of Public Health Geography and Director of the Centre for Health and Inequalities Research at Durham University, and Associate Director of Fuse: the Centre for Translational Research in Public Health, Newcastle University. Her research focuses on the health effects of labour markets, health and welfare systems, as well as the role of public policies in reducing health inequalities. She has published extensively in the field of health inequalities including *Work, worklessness and the political economy of health* (Oxford University Press, 2011) and *How politics makes us sick: Neoliberal epidemics* (Palgrave Macmillan, 2015). She contributed to the Marmot Reviews of Health Inequalities in England (2010) and Europe (2013); the US National Research Council Report on US Health in International Perspective (2013); a UK Parliamentary Labour Party Inquiry into International Health Systems (2013); as well as the Public Health England-commissioned report on health equity in the North of England, *Due North* (2014). She can be followed on Twitter @ProfBambra

Foreword: killing you softly

Danny Dorling

Inequality kills slowly, gently, just a small additional effect every day. As this book shows, we can see the effects of inequality in the variations in life expectancy between countries, between the regions of the UK and across every city in the high- income world. We can see it in the past and we can see it in the present – and if nothing changes, we will continue to see it in the future. We can see it in every wealthy country and in every local neighbourhood. We can see it in the differences in average heights between different populations, those places where people tend to be shorter, and where they are taller. We can see it in the diets people are able to afford, in the stress that leads so many to smoke and is so dramatically varied across the country. And we can see it in who is forced to live in the sink estates and sink towns, and in who is showered with all the economic advantages available to the elites today: the good food, well-resourced schools, easy-to-come-by university places and jobs, and the social networks of privilege and family inheritance that protect a few from ever having to consider using a food bank, or even having to use the state education system – they can always go private.

As demonstrated with great clarity in this book, the UK and the USA have much larger inequalities than the countries of Western Europe. In the UK, we have the widest inequalities in income of any European country. We spend less per head on healthcare than any other country in Western Europe. Luckily for us, the NHS is incredibly efficient, but it is starved of resources in comparison with what is normal in Germany and France. Even more importantly, the population is starved of resources to live well. In Germany and France the median family has a far higher income after tax, and far lower housing and other costs to pay. People elsewhere in Europe have choices that most of the British do not have. Nowhere else in Western Europe are so many people so poor. Nowhere else in all of Europe is there such spatial segregation between neighbourhoods, or such high and growing regional divides. And these have been growing for so long that many of us have become almost immune to them, failing to recognise them as fundamentally unjust. We have grown used to inequality.

In this book Clare Bambra describes the brutal effects that such inequalities have on public health, providing a detailed and passionate analysis of the links between our health and where we live. She examines some of the key health divides of our age – the US health disadvantage, the Scottish health effect, the North–South divide in England and the vast inequalities in life chances between local neighbourhoods in our towns and cities. She provides a strong overview of what they are like today, their historical development and how the key aspects of where we live connect to how long we live. Most significantly, she outlines how these health divides are related to our politics and policies and therefore how they can be altered for good forever.

The current crisis of inequality was decades in the making and it is a crisis which need not happen again – there are alternatives, although, as Clare Bambra explains in what follows, it is only possible to reduce health inequalities if radical steps are taken. In this compelling and compassionate book, she outlines evidence-based solutions to all our health divides and she gives many real-world examples of where – and how – such divides have been reduced, such as the closing of the East–West health gap in Germany following reunification, and the reduction in health inequalities in Britain from the 1950s to the 1970s. She shows that health inequalities are not inevitable or insurmountable. And the lives of both the poor and the rich would be greatly improved if they were drastically narrowed. Ultimately, as this book very clearly articulates, it is our choice – where we live should not determine how long we live.

Danny Dorling is Halford Mackinder Professor of Geography at the University of Oxford. Danny's book *Unequal Health: The Scandal of Our Times* was published in March 2013 by Policy Press.

Preface

My mother was born in the North East of England in the 1950s. She spent her childhood in Newcastle upon Tyne, where her father worked at a shipyard. She moved to the West Midlands city of Coventry, by way of Australia (as a 'Ten Pound Pom'), in the 1970s. This was where she met my father – born and raised in Kent, where his father owned a chain of butcher shops, before he, too, made his way to Coventry as a student. My brother and I were also born in Kent but spent most of our school years in the East Anglian fens of Lincolnshire. My undergraduate years were spent in Birmingham before working across the North in Manchester, Liverpool, Sheffield and Durham. So this book on health divides is in part inspired by this personal experience of England's 'North–South divide'. But it is also a product of my work as a university researcher, based in the North of England, having examined international, national, regional and local inequalities in health for well over a decade.

This book examines geographical health divides between high-income countries (with a focus on the US health disadvantage), between the countries of the UK (particularly the 'Scottish health effect'), between the English regions (the North–South divide) and between deprived and affluent areas of the towns and cities of high-income countries (with a case study of the town of Stockton-on-Tees in the North East of England). The book examines the historical and contemporary nature of these health divides: when they emerged and how they have developed over time, what they are like today, what explains them and what the future might hold. It shows that these geographical inequalities in health are longstanding and universal – present to a greater or lesser extent across both space and time. It examines the multiple causes of these health inequalities and argues that the fundamental drivers are the political and economic choices we make as a society, and the way they shape the places in which we live, work and play. This book *places* inequalities in health and examines how geography is a matter of life and death – *where you live can kill you.*

CHAPTER 1

Health divides

Today, Americans live three years less than their counterparts in France or Sweden. Scottish men live more than two years less than English men, and Northerners in England live two years less than Southerners. Londoners living in Canning Town at one end of the Jubilee tube line live seven years less than those living eight stops along in Westminster. There is a 25-year gap in life expectancy between residents of the Iberville and Naverre suburbs of the US city of New Orleans, although they are just 3 miles apart. This book examines these inequalities in life and death, showing that geographical health divides are longstanding and universal – present to a greater or lesser extent across both time and space.

Drawing on case studies of the US health disadvantage, the 'Scottish health effect', the North–South health divide in England and local health inequalities across the towns and cities of wealthy countries, this book explores the historical and contemporary nature of geographical inequalities in health. It looks at how they have evolved over time, what they are like today, and their social, environmental, economic and – ultimately – political causes. It examines what has and what could be done by governments to reduce these inequalities, and how health divides might develop in the future. The book presents a wealth of international, historical and contemporary data, to demonstrate how and why geography is a matter of life and death.

This introductory chapter introduces the four case study health divides. It provides a general introduction to the themes of the book, outlining the scales of contemporary health divides internationally, nationally, regionally and locally. The chapter concludes by reflecting on the relationship between health and place.

On the health of nations

It is well known that health varies between countries. Most notably, there are considerable differences between the wealthy countries of Western Europe, North America, Australia and New Zealand and those in Africa and Asia. For example, average life expectancy for men and women in countries like Nigeria is as low as 50 years while in countries like the UK, the US, France or Sweden it is over 75. Populations in wealthy countries can more easily access adequate nutrition, medical care, safe drinking water and sanitation, and adequate incomes. These all have considerable population health benefits. However, there are also important health divides *between* as well as *within* wealthy countries. For example, as Table 1.1 shows, in 2010, among the 19 wealthy countries, the UK is ranked 14th for life expectancy and 16th for infant mortality (deaths of children aged under one), with around 2.5 years less average life expectancy than Japan, the best performing country, and an infant mortality rate (IMR) that is almost double that of Iceland. The US, the richest country in the world, was ranked bottom for both outcomes with more than four years less life expectancy than Japan and an infant mortality rate that is three times that of Iceland.[1] This has led to discussions of a 'US health disadvantage' whereby the US has worse outcomes across a number of key health outcomes (such as obesity or heart disease) than other comparable wealthy countries.[2]

This *US health disadvantage* was investigated in a report by the US Institute of Medicine[3] – it found that the US did worse than comparator countries across at least nine health domains: (1) adverse birth outcomes – the US has the worst infant mortality rates, worst rates of low birth weight (LBW) babies, and US children are less likely to live to age five than children in other wealthy countries; (2) injuries and homicide – deaths from motor vehicle crashes, injuries and violence occur at a much higher rate than in other countries, particularly among under-18s; (3) the US has the highest rate of teenage pregnancies, and

Table 1.1: International rankings for life expectancy at birth (men and women) and infant mortality rates, 2010[4]

Rank	Life Expectancy at birth (men and women, years)	
1	Japan	83.0
2	Switzerland	82.6
3	Italy	82.0
4	Australia	81.8
5	Iceland	81.5
6	Sweden	81.5
7	France	81.3
8	Norway	81.2
9	Ireland	81.0
10	New Zealand	81.0
11	Canada	80.8
12	Netherlands	80.8
13	Austria	80.7
14	UK	80.6
15	Germany	80.5
16	Belgium	80.3
17	Finland	80.2
18	Denmark	79.3
19	USA	78.7
Average		**81.0**

Rank	Infant Mortality Rates (deaths under age 1, per 1000 live births)	
1	Iceland	2.2
2	Japan	2.3
3	Finland	2.3
4	Sweden	2.5
5	Norway	2.8
6	Italy	3.4
7	Germany	3.4
8	Denmark	3.4
9	Belgium	3.5
10	France	3.6
11	Switzerland	80.8
12	Netherlands	3.8
13	Ireland	3.8
14	Austria	3.9
15	Australia	4.1
16	UK	4.2
17	Canada	5.1
18	New Zealand	5.2
19	USA	6.1
Average		**3.7**

young people are more likely to acquire sexually transmitted diseases; (4) the US has the highest incidence of AIDS among high-income countries; (5) US adults lost more years of life to alcohol or drugs; (6) obesity and diabetes rates are the highest in the world for those aged over 20; (7) US adults aged over 50 are more likely to die from heart disease than those in other countries; (8) lung disease is more common in the US; and (9) disability rates are higher than most other wealthy nations. This health deficit is despite the wealth and expenditure on healthcare of the US – which are both the highest in the world. However, it should not be ignored that there are also important differences across the countries of Western Europe too, with some countries performing much better in terms of key health outcomes than others. For example, among Western European countries, the UK has the worst all-cause mortality rate and the highest prevalence of obesity among women. The UK does, however, have the smallest diabetes-related death rate. France performs very well in terms of obesity while the Netherlands performs comparatively poorly in terms of both cardiovascular disease (CVD) and cancer deaths. Sweden is arguably the best performer with the lowest rates of CVD and cancer mortality and the lowest prevalence of diabetes among adults and some of the lowest rates of obesity for both men and women. These inequalities in health across Europe can be examined further through the lens of a 'European Health Championship'.

In 2016, the European Championship Finals were held in France between the top footballing nations of Europe. The European Health Championship geocodes these national football teams to their respective country health data using male life expectancy at birth for 2013.[5,6] In the European Championship Finals, teams are initially placed in six groups of four, whereby all teams play each other once, and the top two teams and the four best-placed third teams then go through to the knock-out rounds. Using male life expectancy at birth as the way of scoring, Figure 1.1 shows the results of these groups if health were the determining factor, with:

P (played)	number of matches played
W (won)	number of matches won
D (drawn)	number of matches drawn
L (lost)	number of matches lost
F (for)	'goals' scored – positive gap in life expectancy compared to opponents
A (against)	'goals' conceded – negative gap in life expectancy compared to opponents
GD (goal difference)	difference between F and A
Pts (points)	3 points per win, 1 per draw, 0 for a loss

So, by way of example, England is the winner of Group B by way of beating Russia 16-0 (as there is a gap of 16 years in male life expectancy between the two countries), beating Slovakia 7-0 and Wales (only just) 1-0. This gives them 9 points from

Figure 1.1: European Health Championship Group results

Group A									
	Team	P	W	D	L	F	A	GD	Pts
1	Switzerland (81)	3	3	0	0	20	0	20	9
2	France (79)	3	2	0	1	14	2	12	6
3	Albania (73)	3	1	0	2	2	14	-12	3
4	Romania (71)	3	0	0	3	0	20	-20	0

Group B									
	Team	P	W	D	L	F	A	GD	Pts
1	England (79)	3	3	0	0	24	0	24	9
2	Wales (78)	3	2	0	1	21	1	20	6
3	Slovakia (72)	3	1	0	2	9	13	4	3
4	Russia (63)	3	0	0	3	0	40	-40	0

Group C									
	Team	P	W	D	L	F	A	GD	Pts
1	Germany (79)	3	3	0	0	20	0	20	9
2	Northern Ireland (78)	3	2	0	1	17	1	16	6
3	Poland (73)	3	1	0	2	7	11	-4	3
4	Ukraine (66)	3	0	0	3	0	32	-32	0

Group D									
	Team	P	W	D	L	F	A	GD	Pts
1	Spain (80)	3	3	0	0	18	0	18	9
2	Croatia (75)	3	1	1	1	3	5	-2	4
3	Czech Republic (75)	3	1	1	1	3	5	-2	4
4	Turkey (72)	3	0	0	3	0	14	-14	0

Group E

	Team	P	W	D	L	F	A	GD	Pts
1	Italy (80)	3	2	1	0	3	0	3	7
2	Sweden (80)	3	2	1	0	3	0	3	7
3	Republic of Ireland (79)	3	1	0	2	1	2	-1	3
4	Belgium (78)	3	0	0	3	0	5	-5	0

Group F

	Team	P	W	D	L	F	A	GD	Pts
1	Iceland (81)	3	3	0	0	15	0	15	9
2	Austria (79)	3	2	0	1	9	2	7	6
3	Portugal (78)	3	1	0	2	7	4	3	3
4	Hungary (71)	3	0	0	3	0	25	-25	0

three wins. Wales are the runners-up in the group. From a health perspective, the results of the groups really highlight the immense differences in male life expectancy across Europe, and particularly between the West and East of Europe. In Switzerland (winners of Group A) and Iceland (winners of Group F), baby boys born in 2013 have an average life expectancy of 81, while in Russia (bottom of Group B) it is only 63. There is a West–East gap of 18 years in average life expectancy at birth for men across Europe today.

Figure 1.2 shows the results of the knock-out rounds, with Switzerland emerging as the European Health Championship winner of 2016. While Iceland and Switzerland both have average male life expectancies at birth of 81, female life expectancy in Switzerland is 85 compared to 84 in Iceland – hence Switzerland win ('on penalties', as it were).

Figure 1.2: European Health Championship knock-out rounds and winner

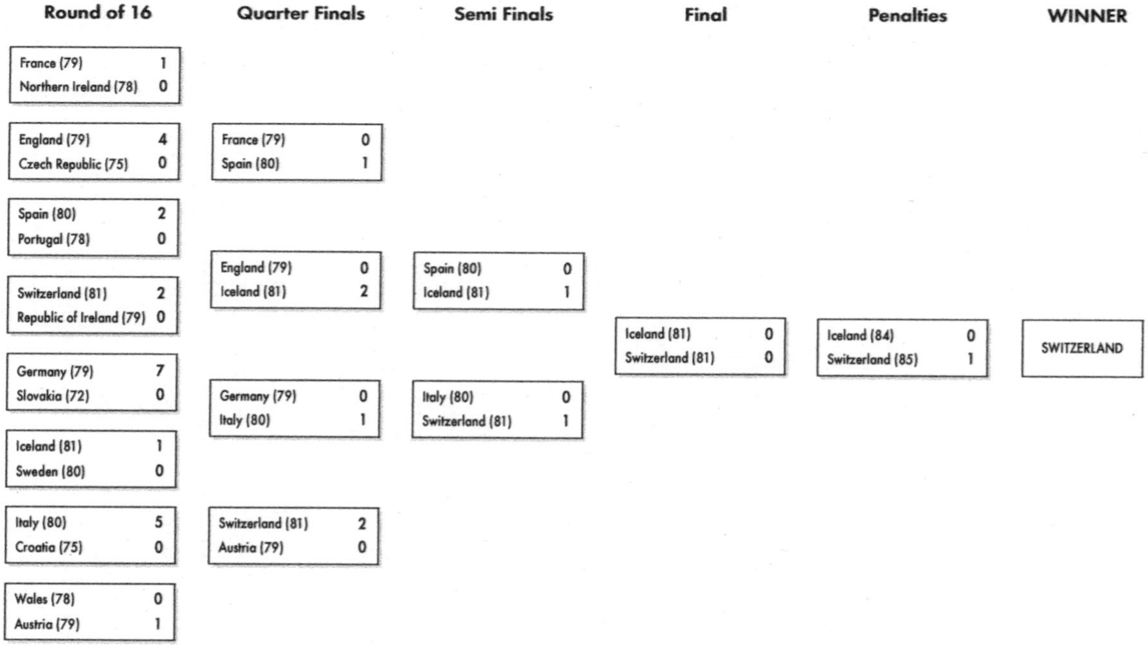

Round of 16

Team	Score
France (79)	1
Northern Ireland (78)	0
England (79)	4
Czech Republic (75)	0
Spain (80)	2
Portugal (78)	0
Switzerland (81)	2
Republic of Ireland (79)	0
Germany (79)	7
Slovakia (72)	0
Iceland (81)	1
Sweden (80)	0
Italy (80)	5
Croatia (75)	0
Wales (78)	0
Austria (79)	1

Quarter Finals

Team	Score
France (79)	0
Spain (80)	1
England (79)	0
Iceland (81)	2
Germany (79)	0
Italy (80)	1
Switzerland (81)	2
Austria (79)	0

Semi Finals

Team	Score
Spain (80)	0
Iceland (81)	1
Italy (80)	0
Switzerland (81)	1

Final

Team	Score
Iceland (81)	0
Switzerland (81)	0

Penalties

Team	Score
Iceland (84)	0
Switzerland (85)	1

WINNER

SWITZERLAND

Disunited Kingdom

There are also substantial differences in health between the constituent countries of the UK, with England (as a whole) faring much better than Scotland, Wales or Northern Ireland. The UK is made up of the three nations within the island of Britain (England, Scotland and Wales), plus Northern Ireland. Until recently, most legislative decisions were made by the government in London (England) for the UK as a whole, and Northern Ireland, Scotland and Wales had only limited powers to shape the interpretation and implementation of these policies. However, in the late 1990s, significant political powers were devolved to these three countries, and health policy was one of the most significant areas to be devolved.[7] However, many other health-relevant policy issues, notably fiscal and welfare policy, continued to be largely determined by the UK (and, to some extent, the European Union [EU]). Since 1997 the Scottish Parliament, the Welsh Assembly (since 2006) and the Northern Ireland Assembly (since 2007) have had full powers over a number of areas including health and education. The Scottish Parliament also has the ability to increase or decrease Income Tax by up to 3p in the pound, although to date this power has never been exercised.

Furthermore, in the early years of devolution, the Labour Party dominated all four political contexts, creating a relatively consistent political context. However, following the 2010 and 2015 UK general elections and the devolved government elections, different political parties now govern in each of the four countries of the UK for the first time, with a Conservative government leading the UK and England, a Labour administration governing in Wales, a coalition including the Democratic Unionist Party and Sinn Féin sharing power in Northern Ireland, and the Scottish National Party (SNP) (left-leaning) governing Scotland (see Figure 1.3 for the political geography of the UK). This is also reflected in the breakdown of Westminster seats for the UK Parliament in the 2015 general election. Devolution and the political differences that have emerged have led to different policies in healthcare and in other areas that might have an impact on health. For example, in contrast to England, there are currently no NHS prescription charges in Scotland, no university tuition fees and far greater provision of free personal care for the elderly. There is also some consensus that a 'natural experiment' is occurring in UK healthcare policy, as England pursues a series of radical, market-orientated reforms to the NHS

Figure 1.3: The political geography of the UK since the 2015 general election[9]

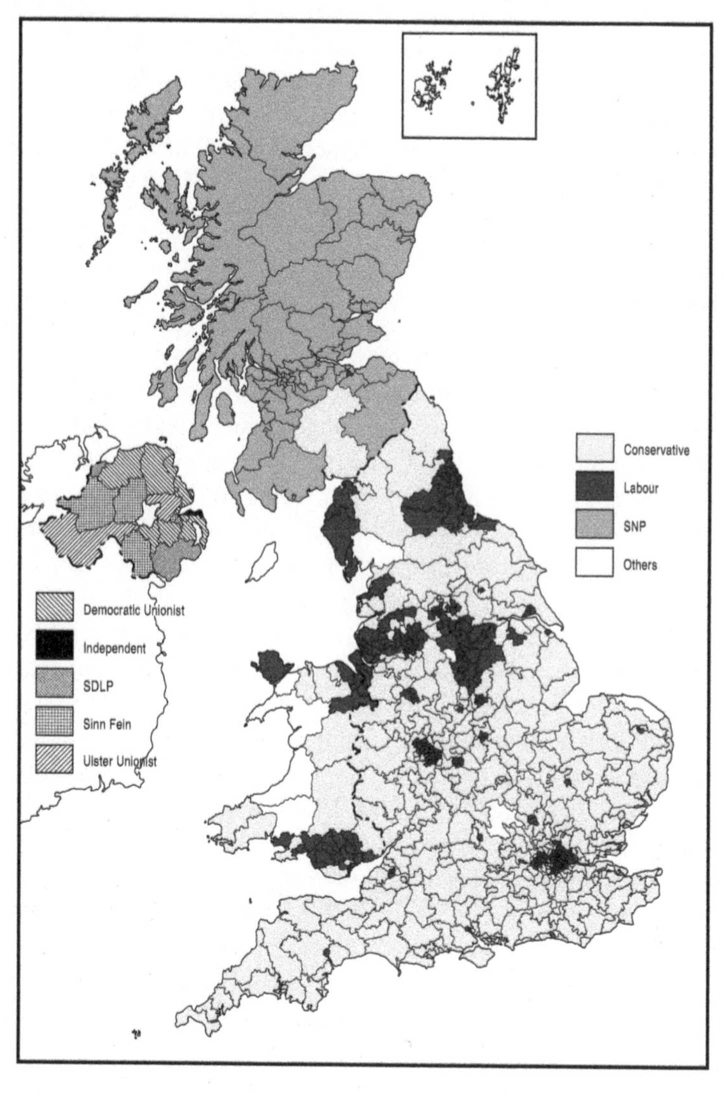

while the devolved regions maintain a more social democratic approach to healthcare.[8]

Scottish men and women have the lowest life expectancy in the UK, at 76.9 and 81.0 years respectively. This is 2.5 and 2.1 years respectively less than the English averages for men and women of 79.4 and 83.1 years.[10, 11] The gap between Scottish and English life expectancy for both men and women widened in the 1950s and then again in the 1980s.[12] This is known as the 'Scottish health effect' and forms another case study in the rest of this book.[13] More widely within the UK, men and women in Wales also live on average one year less than their English counterparts – with Welsh averages for men of 78.3 and women of 82.3 years.[14] Likewise, in Northern Ireland men and women have lower average life expectancies than England – 78.1 and 82.4 years respectively.[15]

A divided land

As noted in the Preface, my mother grew up in Newcastle in the North East of England. In contrast, my father was born and raised in Kent in the South East of England. These places represent the two extremes within the longstanding English divide between the North and the South. Within England, health outcomes are best in the South East and worst in the North East. A baby born today in the North East will live on average six years less in good health than one born in the South East.[16] Likewise, the life expectancy gap (how long someone is expected to live on average based on contemporary mortality rates) between the two regions is over two years for both men and women. These spatial inequalities in health between North and South have been documented since the mid-18th century and have fluctuated over time.[17, 18] In the 1950s, when my parents were children, the health gap between areas of England were smaller, they continued to decrease through to the 1970s, before rising from the 1980s onwards.[19] Indeed, health inequalities between the North and the South, and between affluent and deprived areas more generally, are now at levels only previously seen in the 19th century – the Victorian age.[20] Since 1965, the 'health

Figure 1.4: Regional inequalities in mortality rates in Europe in 2008–10[21]

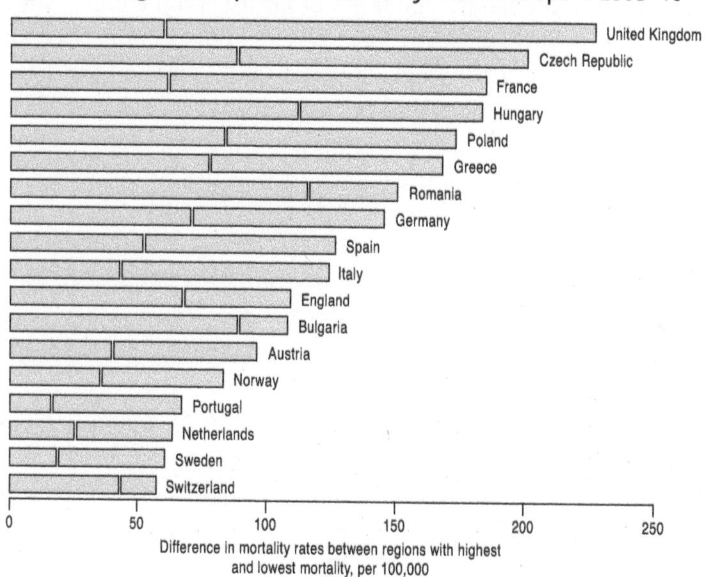

penalty' paid by the North has amounted to 1.5 million excess premature deaths.[22]

While all countries experience regional inequalities in health, today the English health divide is the largest in Europe (see Figure 1.4). England is a very small country (130,000 km^2 or 50,000 square miles), but the scale of the divide is such that the life expectancy gap for women between the North East and North West of England and London in the South East is now greater than the gap between the former West Germany and post-communist East Germany in the mid-1990s.[23] After reunification in 1990, life expectancy for women in East Germany caught up with that of women in West Germany in little more than a decade, whereas the gap between the North East and North West of England and London has persisted for women. East German women now have a higher life expectancy than North Eastern English women. For men, the German life expectancy gap is now smaller than the English one.

These inequalities between North and South are also part of a more extensive regional gradient in health – which encompasses all of England including the Midlands and Coventry, where my parents met, and Lincolnshire, where I grew up – whereby, generally speaking, average levels of health and life expectancy decline the further north you travel.[24] This is illustrated in Figures 1.5 and 1.6, which show life expectancy at birth for men and women in England by region. The maps show a clear spatial patterning, with the areas of lower life expectancy falling towards the North and the higher areas in the South, with the East and West falling between these two extremes.

There are also, however, areas of the North that do better than the national average and areas in the South that fare worse. This is demonstrated in Figures 1.7 and 1.8, which present average life expectancy at birth for both men and women[25] for the stops

Figure 1.5: Map of life expectancy by region for men in England, 2011[26]

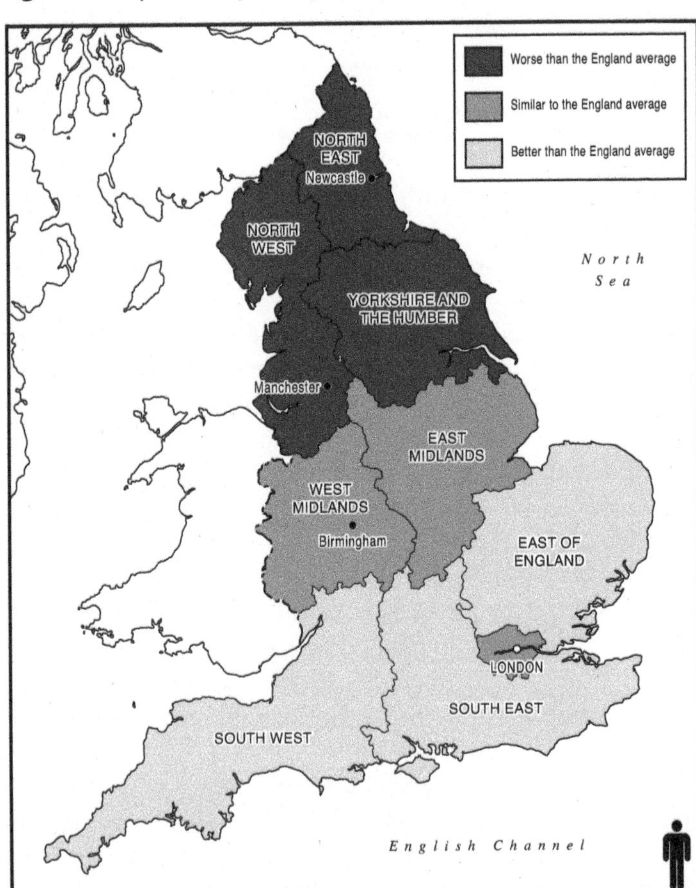

along some of the major train lines in England: the West Coast Mainline (WCM, a route of 300 miles from London Euston to Carlisle in the North West), the East Coast Mainline (ECM, a route of 335 miles from London Kings Cross to Berwick in the North East) and the Great Western Mainline (GWM, a route of 300 miles from London Paddington to Penzance in the South West). The data is geo-referenced to each of the main stations along the routes using the relevant local authority (for example, the data for Newark is for Nottinghamshire). The circles represent values above, around or below the English average of 79.4 years for men and 83.1 years for women.

Figure 1.6: Map of life expectancy by region for women in England, 2011[27]

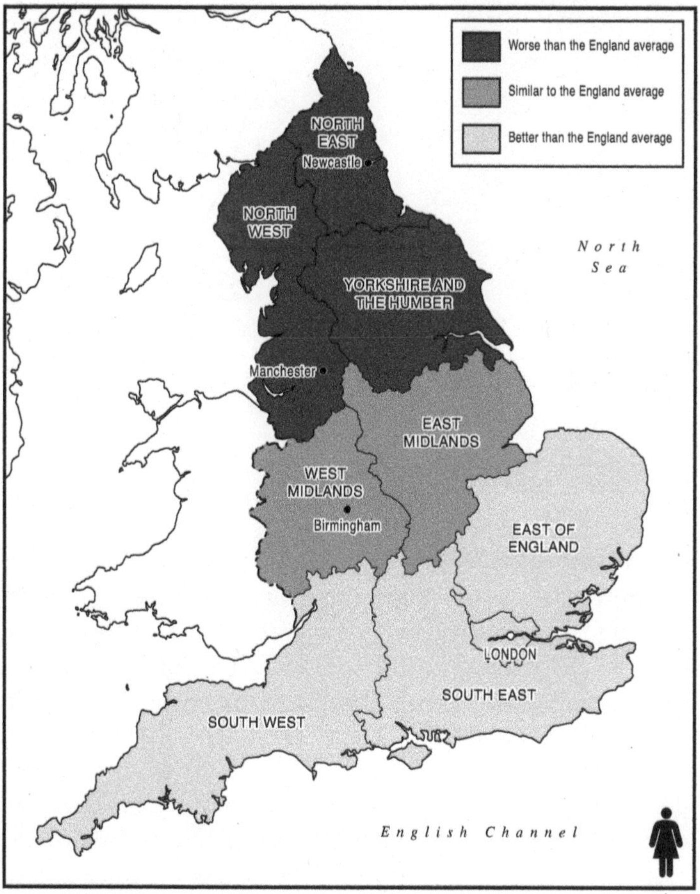

Figure 1.7: An English journey – life expectancy for men along the East Coast, Great Western and West Coast Mainlines, 2011[28]

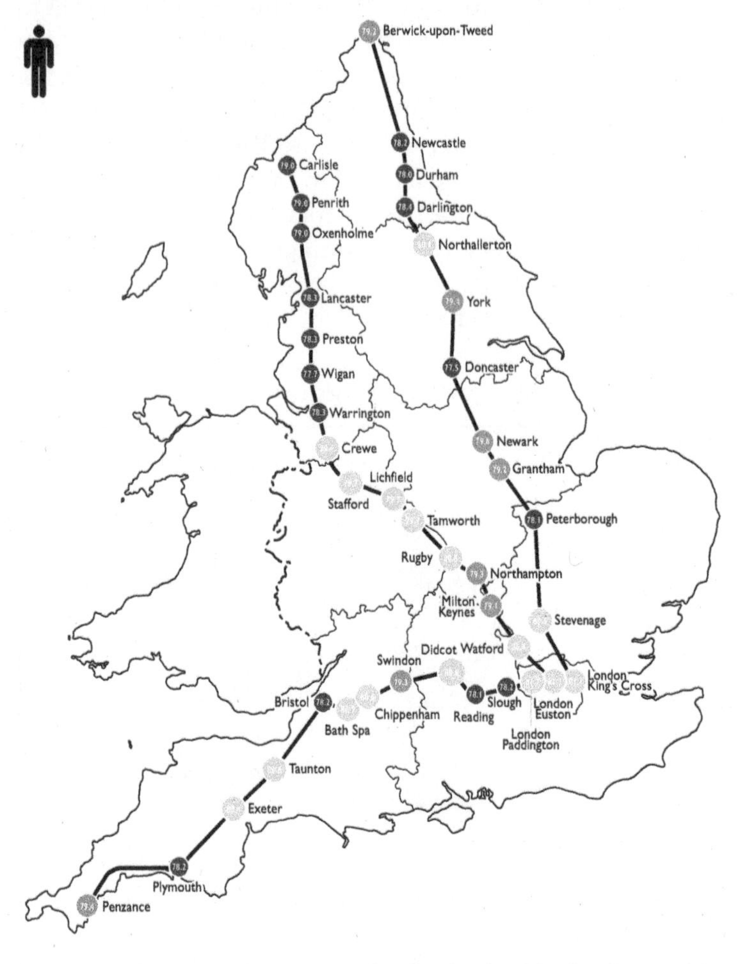

The visualisations show very clearly the health divides within a comparatively small country, particularly between the North East and South East regions that have the lowest and highest life expectancies respectively for both men and women. There are gaps of four years for men and five years for women between the best Southern and worst Northern areas. They also demonstrate a socio-spatial gradient with average life expectancy at birth decreasing the further north the journey takes. There are exceptions to this with some areas that, while 'Northern' (for example, Cheshire or North Yorkshire), have above-average

Figure 1.8: An English journey – life expectancy for women along the East Coast, Great Western and West Coast Mainlines, 2011[29]

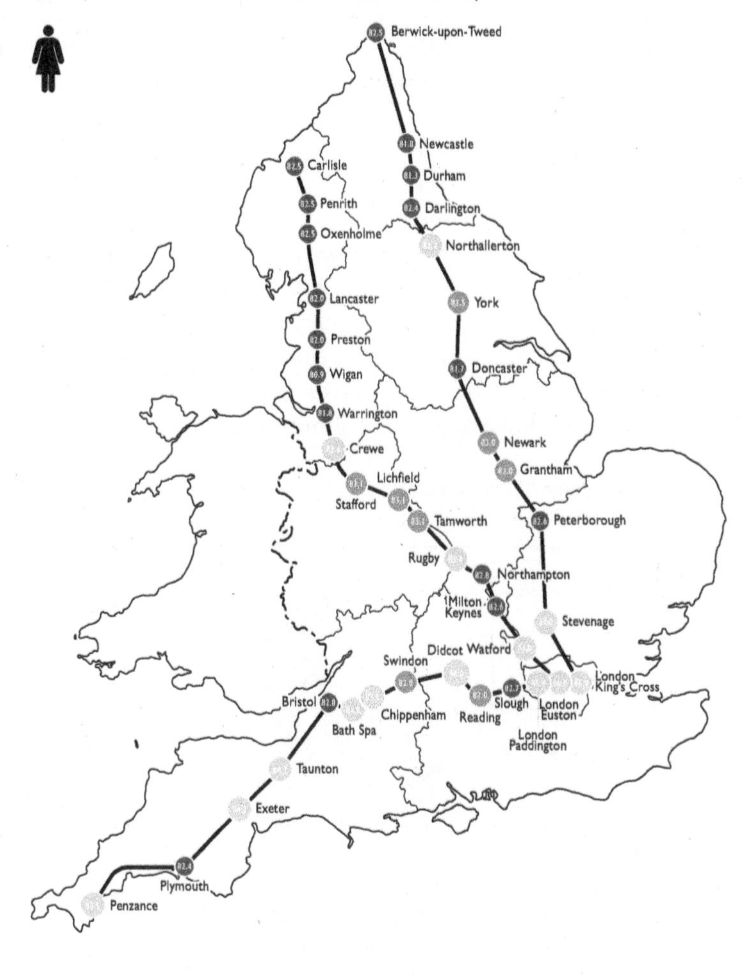

health outcomes, and others that while 'Southern' have below-average health outcomes (for example, Bristol or Peterborough). The graphics therefore also 'problematise' the consistency of the English health divide and expose inequalities *within* the North and the South as well as *between* them.[30]

All countries have a 'North'

In the globally popular BBC TV series 'Dr Who', there is an exchange between Rose Tyler and the Doctor: "If you're an alien, how come you sound like you come from the North", asks Rose. "Lots of planets have a North", replies the Doctor, in a Northern English accent.[31] Indeed, England is not alone in experiencing health inequalities between its regions. The English health divide is replicated to a greater or lesser extent in all other countries. By way of example, Figure 1.9 shows regional inequalities in life expectancy across Europe for men and women combined. As with the previous maps, these divide areas into those below the national average life expectancy, similar to average and above average. It shows that across Europe, all

Figure 1.9: Average life expectancy by European region for men and women, 2012[32]

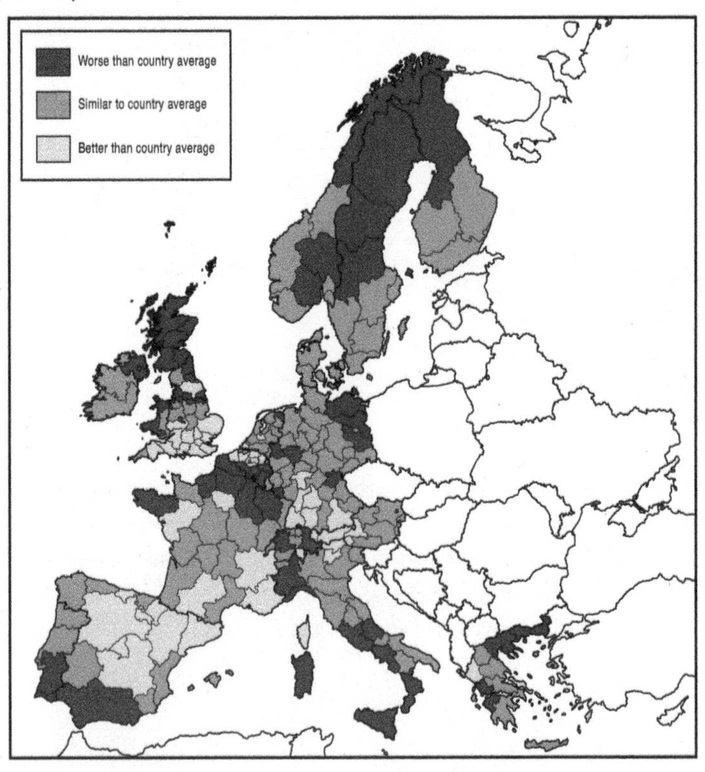

countries experience unequal health – in many countries this divide is the same as England, with poorer health outcomes in the North (for example, France), but others experience the inverse whereby health outcomes are worse in the Southern regions (for example, Italy).

In Scotland, there is an West–East divide with, for example, men in the City of Glasgow in the West of Scotland having an average life expectancy of 73.0 (the lowest in the UK), while those in East Dunbartonshire in the East live an average of 80.5 years – more than seven years longer.[33] Likewise, the Valley areas of South Wales such as Blaenau Gwent have worse life expectancy than the rest of the country, and four to five years less than men and women living in Monmouthshire or Powys. Likewise in Northern Ireland, men and women in Belfast and Derry live four years less on average than their compatriots in North Down or Ballymoney.

These patterns also exist outside Europe as, for example, in China average life expectancy is over five years less in the Northern provinces than in the Southern ones.[34] The most prominent South–North health divide is within the US, as Figure 1.10 shows for life expectancy in 2010. As with the European map, areas are divided into those below the national average life expectancy, similar to average and above average. The states with some of the lowest average life expectancies are clustered within the South East of the US – including a number of the old Southern Confederacy states. Inequalities within the US are examined further later in the book.

For richer or poorer

So, as demonstrated earlier, it is not universally 'grim up North' or 'pleasant down South'. These patterns arise because the North–South health divide is supplemented by a second, more widespread divide in health within regions and within towns and cities – a divide between affluent and deprived areas. By way of example, Table 1.2 shows the relationship between life expectancy and healthy life expectancy (how long someone can be expected to live on average in good or very health) for

Figure 1.10: Average life expectancy by US state for men and women, 2010[35]

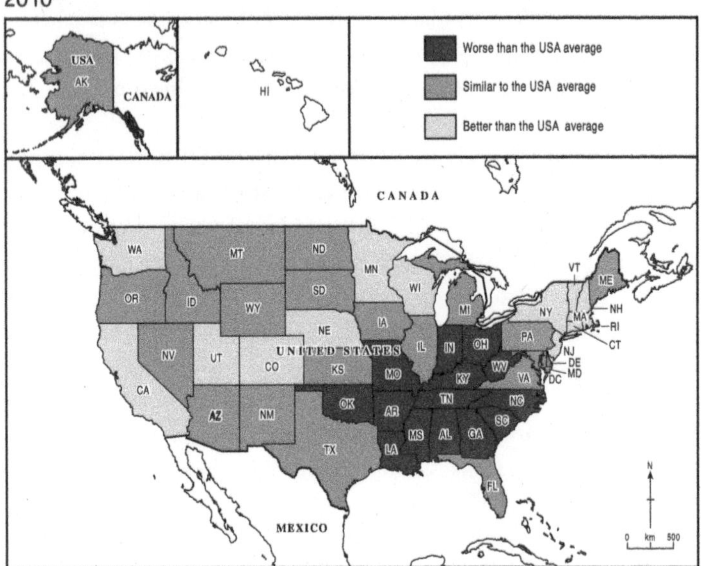

men and women by neighbourhood deprivation decile (bands of 10%) in England.

Table 1.2 uses the most common measure of area-level deprivation, the Index of Multiple Deprivation (IMD). This produces a ranking of areas in England based on relative local scores for income, employment, health, education, crime, access to services and living environment.[36] Neighbourhood is the smallest scale of geographical data (see Figure 1.11), and is defined here by the rather Orwellian sounding 'lower super output areas' (LSOAs) (see Box 1.1). Neighbourhoods that are the most deprived have worse health than those that are less deprived – and this follows a spatial gradient, with each increase in deprivation resulting in a decrease in average health.

In England, the gap between the most and least deprived areas is 9 years average life expectancy and 18 years average healthy life expectancy for men, and around 7 and 19 years respectively for women. Deaths from CVD are almost three times higher in the 20% most deprived areas compared to the 20% least deprived, and alcohol-related hospital admissions were more than twice as high among men and among women in the 20% most deprived

Table 1.2: Life expectancy and healthy life expectancy for men and women by neighbourhood, England, 2011–13[37]

Deprivation Decile*	Life Expectancy (LE), at birth, years	
	Male	Female
1 *Most deprived*	74.1	79.1
2	76.2	80.7
3	77.3	81.5
4	78.5	82.3
5	79.5	83.2
6	80.1	83.6
7	81.0	84.2
8	81.5	84.5
9	82.0	85.1
10 *Least deprived*	83.1	86.0
Gap	**9.0**	**6.9**

Deprivation Decile*	Health Life Expectancy (HLE), at birth, years	
	Male	Female
1 *Most deprived*	52.2	52.4
2	56.2	56.3
3	58.4	59.6
4	61.6	61.6
5	62.8	64.2
6	65.5	65.7
7	66.5	67.0
8	67.5	68.0
9	68.5	69.4
10 *Least deprived*	70.5	71.3
Gap	**18.3**	**18.9**

Figure 1.11: Scaling place

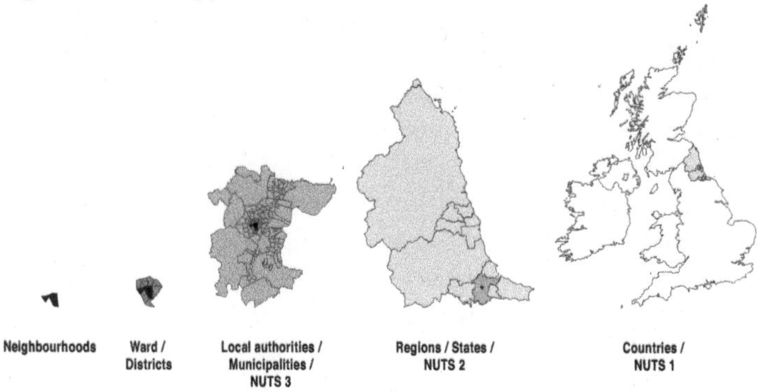

Neighbourhoods
Ward / Districts
Local authorities / Municipalities / NUTS 3
Regions / States / NUTS 2
Countries / NUTS 1

Box 1.1: Definitions of different geographical areas

Neighbourhoods: lower super output areas (LSOAs) that constitute areas (several streets) with an average of 1,500 residents in the UK. For the US the equivalent is census tracts.

Wards: sub-local authority units in the UK with elected representatives (councillors); the equivalent in the US is municipal or county districts. Average population size of a UK ward is around 6,600 people.

Local authorities: in the UK these are the local administrative and democratic units including county councils, unitary authorities, borough or city councils. They have fairly limited powers in terms of the delivery of local services and regulations including education, social work, environmental protection and most highways. In England they also have public health responsibilities. There are 150 in England, 32 in Scotland and 22 in Wales. Northern Ireland has 22 district councils. The equivalents in the US and Europe are municipalities or city/county authorities (although the levels of devolved power are typically higher here).

Regions: in the UK, regions have no administrative or democratic existence – they are currently used for statistical purposes only. In the US the equivalent is states, while in European terms these would include provinces (for example, France) or Lander (for example, Germany). The federal states of the US, and to a lesser extent the Lander and provinces, are democratic and administrative units with a range of powers and responsibilities.

NUTS: the Eurostat Nomenclature of Territorial Units for Statistics (NUTS) are statistical sub-national regional territories divided into areas of approximately the same population size across the EU. They are also used in terms of distributing EU structural funds. There are three levels of NUTS of descending size: NUTS 1, 2 and 3. The nine English regions, Scotland, Northern Ireland and Wales are each a distinct NUTS 1, while there are 30 NUTS 2 regions in England (groupings of local authorities), four in Scotland, one for all of Northern Ireland and two in Wales. There are 133 NUTS 3 areas (largely synonymous with local authorities) in the UK.

Countries: distinct geopolitical and territorial units.

areas compared to the 20% least deprived areas.[38] Deprived and affluent areas with such differences in health outcomes can be located very closely together – indeed, just a few miles apart. By way of example, Figure 1.12 presents a visualisation of how life expectancy varies by stations on the London Underground (tube) system – with every stop east of Westminster (where the Houses of Parliament are situated) on the Jubilee tube line, average life expectancy decreases by a year. There are eight stops between Westminster and Canning Town on the Jubilee Line – so as the tube travels east, each stop, on average, marks nearly a year of shortened lifespan, from 82 years for men living in the ward closest to Westminster tube station to 75 years for men living in the ward closest to Canning Town tube station.[39]

These smaller-scale local health inequalities related to deprivation are also particularly large within Northern towns and cities. The town of Stockton-on-Tees in the North East region, for example, has a 17-year gap in life expectancy for men and 11 years for women between its most and least deprived areas. This is the largest gap in life expectancy within a single local authority in England. Localised and small-scale health inequalities also exist within the towns and cities of the other countries of the UK; for example, the Scottish City of Glasgow has some of the highest urban health inequalities in Europe. Men in the city's more affluent southern neighbourhood of Cathcart are expected to live to almost 82, that is 16 years longer than those in the northern Glasgow areas of Possilpark and Ruchill, where

Figure 1.12: Life expectancy along the Jubilee tube line[40]

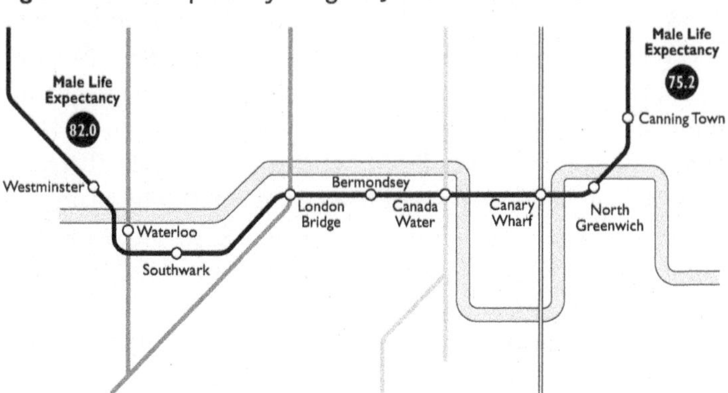

the average life expectancy for men is just 66.[41] The health divide in Glasgow for women is also very high, with women living in Cathcart or Kelvinside in the west end of the city expected to live 11 years longer than those in northern areas of Possilpark and Ruchill. These two areas are just 4.5 miles apart.

Similarly, other high-income countries also experience localised health inequalities with, for example, the US capital Washington DC having a gap in life expectancy of 20 years between the low-income inner-city neighbourhoods and the affluent, leafy suburbs of Maryland.[42] This is equivalent to the gap in average life expectancy between the US (75 years) and Nigeria (55 years). Even newly developing economies, such as China, also experience substantial health divides – say, between rural and urban areas – as well as high inequalities within emerging international cities such as Beijing.[43] However, as mentioned earlier in this chapter, there are counter-cases such as Germany, which show that spatial inequalities in health can be reduced.[44] This book contextualises the English and UK experience within this wider international context throughout the rest of the book by examining the universality of spatial inequalities in health. The next section starts to look at why it is that where you live matters so much for your health.

Place matters

The etymological roots of the term 'health' lie in the Old English for 'whole', implying that a person who is healthy is 'whole'.[45] This is encompassed in the World Health Organization's (WHO) 1948 definition of health as 'a state of complete physical, mental and social well-being, and not merely the absence of disease or infirmity.' Health is therefore a holistic term encapsulating biomedical, social and psychosocial aspects. This chapter has already demonstrated that health varies spatially: locally (between deprived and affluent parts of towns and cities), regionally (for example, between the North and South of England), nationally within the UK, and internationally (for example, between the US and Japan). However, it is *place* that helps in terms of thinking why these spatial variations arise and how our health is inextricably linked to our geographies.[46] 'Space' and 'place' are key overlapping concepts in geography. In a strict sense, space is used to refer to 'a dimension within which matter is located or a grid within which substantial items are contained'.[47] It is concerned with distance and proximity. Place can be seen either in simple geometric terms as 'a portion of space in which people dwell together' (for example, latitude, longitude, elevation, etc), or in a more experiential (phenomenological) sense, as 'a milieu that exercises a mediating role on physical, social and economic processes and which effects how such process operate', or, put more concisely, 'a distinctive coming together in space'.[48] Places are not, however, bounded and static (as is often assumed within statistical spatial analysis), but fluid and relational – nodes within social, economic and political networks.[49] Place does, however, require membership, for example, of communities, cities or states. Place both creates and contains social, economic and political relations as well as physical resources. Spatial inequalities in health are therefore a result of a complex mix of economic, social, environmental and political processes – coming together in particular places. Places can be health-promoting (*salutogenic*) or health-damaging (*pathogenic*).

The academic sub-discipline of health geography has conventionally presented two main explanations as to why these health inequalities exist: compositional and contextual.[50] The compositional explanation argues that the health of a given area, such as a town, region or country, is a result of the individual characteristics of the people who live there, whereas the contextual explanation argues that area-level health is also, in part, determined by the nature of the place itself in terms of its economic, social and physical environmental – the nature of the neighbourhood. The relationship between health and place has therefore been thought of in terms of 'who lives here?' (compositional/individual) and 'what is this place like?' (contextual/neighbourhood). More recently, however, drawing on political economy and political geography, the political determinants of health (the macro/societal context) have also been examined – how our *political choices* shape the relationship between health and place, although it should be noted that the contextual, compositional and political explanations for how place relates to health are not mutually exclusive.[51] The characteristics of individuals are influenced by the characteristics of the area, for example, education level can be determined by local school quality and employment status by the availability of jobs in the local labour market, while these contextual factors are, in turn, influenced by the wider political and economic environment. Health is influenced by individual (compositional), collective (contextual) and political-economic (macro) factors.

Who lives here?

The compositional view argues that 'who you are', the demographic (age, sex and ethnicity/race), risky health behaviours (smoking, alcohol, physical activity, diet, drugs) and socioeconomic (income, education, occupation) profile of the people within a community, determines its health outcomes. Generally speaking, health deteriorates with age and health also varies by ethnicity/race.[52] For example, in the UK, all-cause mortality rates are more than 25% higher among men and women of West/South/East African descent, even after adjusting for other factors.[53] Racial inequalities in health are particularly high in the US.[54] Smoking, alcohol, physical activity, diet and drugs – the five so-called 'lifestyle factors' or health behaviours – all influence health significantly. For example, smoking remains the most important preventable cause of mortality in the wealthy world.[55] Alcohol-related deaths and diseases, as well as obesity, are on the increase, while exercise rates are in decline, and drugs are an increasingly important determinant of death among the young.[56] The socioeconomic status of people living in an area is of huge health significance. Socioeconomic status – or social class in 'old money' – is a term that refers to occupational class, income or educational level.[57] People with higher occupational status (for example, professionals such as teachers or lawyers) have better health outcomes than non-professional workers (for example, manual workers). By way of example, English data shows that infant mortality rates were 16% higher in children of routine and manual workers compared to professional and managerial workers.[58] On average, people with higher income levels or a university degree have better health than those with a low income or no qualifications. The poorer someone is, the less likely they are to live in good quality housing, have time and money for leisure activities, feel secure at home or work, have good quality work or a job at all, or afford to eat healthy food. These socioeconomic inequalities in health are not restricted to differences between the most privileged groups and the most disadvantaged; health inequalities exist across the entire social gradient that runs from the top to the bottom of society, and 'even comfortably off people somewhere in the middle tend to have poorer health than those above them'.[59]

What is this place like?

So, while the compositional view argues that it is 'who you are' that matters for health – and that 'poor people make poor health' – the contextual approach suggests that 'where you live' also matters, and that the economic, social, physical and political environment of a place contributes to area-level health – that *poor places* lead to *poor health.* More salutogenic (health-giving) environments are more likely to be found in affluent compared to deprived areas. Area-economic factors that influence health are often summarised in terms of 'area-level deprivation'; these include area poverty rates, unemployment rates, wages and types of employment in the area. Low poverty rates, low unemployment rates, high wages and non-manual work are all associated with better health outcomes.[60] Social place-based factors include opportunity structures and collective social functioning and practices. Opportunity structures are the socially constructed and patterned features of the area that may promote health through the possibilities they provide.[61] These include the services provided, publicly or privately, to support people in their daily lives such as childcare or transport, food availability or access to a general practitioner (GP) or hospital, as well as the availability of health-promoting environments at home (for example, good housing quality, access and affordability), work (good quality work) and play (such as high quality schools). Collective social functioning and practices that are beneficial to health include high levels of social cohesion and social capital; more negative effects can come from the reputation (for example, stigmatised places can result in discrimination against people living in such areas) and history of an area (for example, if there has been a history of racial oppression). Local attitudes, say, around smoking, can also influence health and health behaviours either negatively or positively.

The physical environment is widely recognised as an important determinant of health and health inequalities.[62] There is a sizeable literature on the positive health effects of access to green space,[63] as well as the negative health effects of waste facilities,[64] brownfield or contaminated land,[65] as well as air pollution.[66] For example, a recent report found that up to 10,000 deaths per year in London were as a result of air pollution, and the five-year gap in life expectancy between the North and South of China is largely due to the higher pollution levels in the North.[67] This has led to the development of the concept of 'environmental deprivation' to be considered alongside economic deprivation.[68]

Politics of health and place

It is increasingly being acknowledged that compositional and contextual determinants of health are themselves shaped by political factors, and that health inequalities between people and places are thereby politically determined.[69] In this sense, patterns of health and disease are produced by the structures, values and priorities of political and economic systems.[70] Area-level health divides – local, regional, national or international – are determined in part by the wider political system and the actions of the state (government) and international level actors (supra-national government bodies such as the EU, inter-state trade agreements such as the Transatlantic Trade and Investment Partnership (TTIP), as well as the actions of large corporations): politics can make us sick – or healthy.[71, 72] Understanding how place relates to health therefore also requires insights from political science and political geography to think about the more fundamental causes of health divides: *the politics of health and place*.

The political approach to explaining health divides focuses on the 'social, political and economic structures and relations' that may be, and often are, outside the control of the individuals or the local areas they affect. Compositional and collective factors such as income levels, public services and employment rates –

indeed, many of the issues that dominate political life – are key determinants of health and wellbeing.[73] Why some places and people are consistently privileged while others are consistently marginalised is a political choice – political choices can thereby be seen as the fundamental causes of health divides.

Let's take heart disease as an example. An immediate clinical 'cause' could be hypertension (high blood pressure). The 'proximal cause' of the hypertension itself could be 'compositional' lifestyle factors such as poor diet, of which the 'contextual cause' could be living in a low-income neighbourhood. The causes of the latter are arguably political – low incomes and low-income neighbourhoods exist because the political and economic system *allows* them to exist. Wages could be regulated so that they are higher (an example being the living wage), or food prices could be controlled/subsidised (for example, in the US it is meat and corn oil that receive government subsidies, not fruit and vegetables, and likewise in the EU, farmers are encouraged to produce dairy), and neighbourhood food provision does not have to be left to the vagaries of the market (which leads to clustering of poor food availability in poor neighbourhoods).Another way to think about this is to imagine a river – downstream are the individual clinical and proximal lifestyle factors (composition), mid-stream are the contextual factors, and upstream are the macro economic and political factors.[74] The latter are largely national level government actions – but also increasingly international and global ones such as those of the EU or the International Monetary Fund (IMF).[75] If something polluting is put in the river upstream, it will contaminate all the water in the river – mid-stream and downstream. In terms of health, our political choices result in particular economic and social policies being pursued – these can be either salutogenic or pathogenic to the people and areas they effect as they have an impact on all the other 'downstream' determinants of health. The river analogy is demonstrated in Figure 1.13. In this sense, patterns of health and disease are produced by the structures, values and priorities of political and economic systems.[76]

Figure 1.13: Going upstream – the political determinants of health

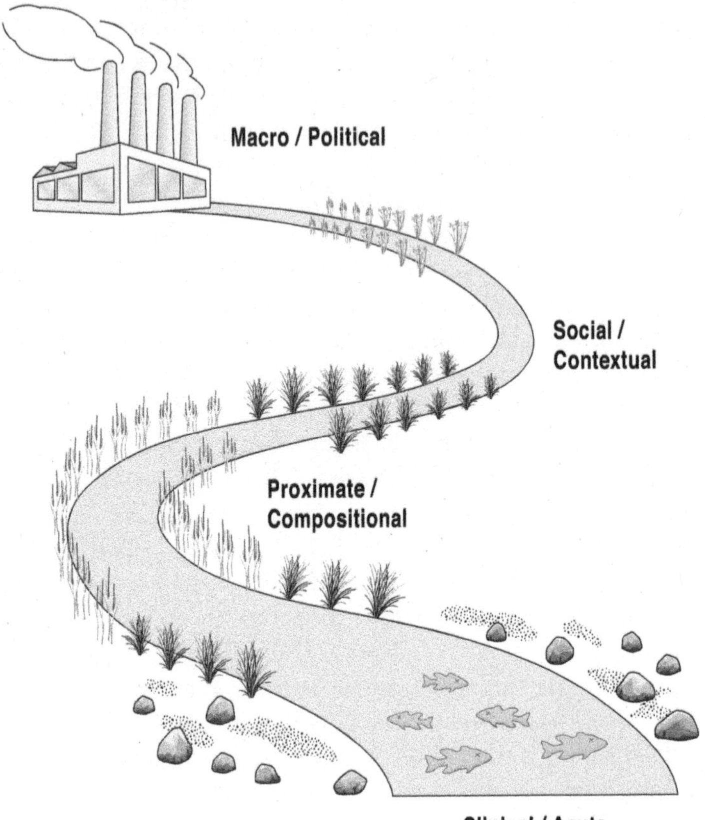

Macro / Political

Social / Contextual

Proximate / Compositional

Clinical / Acute

Outline of the book

This book examines geographical health divides between high-income countries (with a focus on the US health disadvantage), between the countries of the UK (particularly the 'Scottish health effect'), between the English regions (the North–South divide) and between deprived and affluent areas of the towns and cities of high-income countries (with a case study of the town of Stockton-on-Tees in the North East of England). The book examines the historical and contemporary nature of these health divides: when they emerged and how they have developed over time, what they are like today, what explains them and what the future might hold. It shows that these geographical inequalities in health are longstanding and universal – present to a greater of lesser extent across both space and time. It examines the multiple causes of these health inequalities and argues that the fundamental drivers are the political and economic choices we make as a society and the way they shape the places in which we live, work and play. This book *places* inequalities in health and examines how geography is a matter of life and death: *where you live can kill you.*

Chapter 2 outlines the historical patterns of health and disease in wealthy countries from the 19th century, through the epidemiological transition and into the modern era. It examines the key health divides of the industrial past.

Chapter 3 examines the contemporary causes of death and disease in wealthy countries and how where you live still matters for your health. It demonstrates the consistent nature of health divides and their starkness, proximity and universality today.

Chapter 4 draws on traditional geographical theories of how place effects health and starts to explain *why* health divides exist. It provides a detailed overview of the role of different compositional (*who lives here*) and contextual (*what this place is like*) factors in creating healthy or unhealthy places. Using the case studies, it shows that health divides are a combination of both *poor people* and *poor places.*

Building on this, Chapter 5 argues that while place matters for health, politics matters for place. So *placing health inequalities* therefore requires analysis to focus *further upstream* on the fundamental causes of such inequalities – the politics of health. It shows how political ideologies, the exercise of power, and the resulting policy decisions shape the composition and context of places resulting in health inequalities. It concludes that the nature and extent of geographical health divides are a result of political and economic choices.

Chapter 6 follows on from this by examining how public policies have (or have not) addressed health inequalities. Using the UK as an example, health inequalities policy since the 1980s is examined within the wider context of the social and spatial determinants of health. The chapter shows the contradictions and inadequacies of such policies in the face of the wider political and economic context of neoliberalism.

The concluding Chapter 7 examines the lessons from the past in terms of the waxing and waning of health divides, the challenges of the present, and speculates about the future, considering what *could* and *should* be done to reduce health divides. The rest of the book examines how and why it is that *where you live can kill you.*

CHAPTER 2

King Cholera to the 'c' word

Life was cheap in the 19th century – in the 1840s, the average age of death in England, France and the US was 45. There were huge health divides within countries, however, as, for example, the average age of death for working-class men in urban, industrial Manchester, was just 17, while it was 38 in rural areas such as Rutland. The middle classes fared much better than labourers in both town and country, although there were still large inequalities, with average life expectancies for men of 38 in Manchester and 52 in Rutland.[1] These divides were similar in other industrial countries like the US where life expectancies were 15 years higher in rural areas of New England than in the large cities of Boston, New York, and Philadelphia.[2] Compare that to average life expectancies in wealthy countries today, where most people can expect to exceed 75 years. So, in the 19th and early 20th century, it was remarkably easy to die – indeed, surviving childhood was quite an achievement, as over a third of children died before the age of nine. Life was 'nasty, brutish and short'.[3]

This chapter provides the historical context to health divides by examining life and death in the 19th century. It starts by examining the industrial revolution and how it shaped the disease environment in the 19th century, the time of Queen Victoria, Napoleon and Abraham Lincoln. It then examines the main causes of death and disease in wealthy countries in the industrial age – the time of epidemics when infectious diseases such as cholera, typhus, smallpox, typhoid or tuberculosis claimed millions of lives. It then outlines the key health divides of the period: between the North and South of England, between rural and urban areas and between rich and poor areas of towns and cities. It also examines the changing nature of death and disease from the end of the 19th century onwards, including the emergence of the welfare state in the 20th century.

In the court of King Cholera

This section examines death and disease during the industrial revolution of the 19th century, outlining the nature of the industrial revolution itself, its impact on the population and on public health.

Dark Satanic mills

From the late 18th century onwards, wealthy countries like the UK and the US experienced significant and very rapid economic change: the industrial revolution. Before this period, manufacturing was conducted within the home (for example, weaving) or in small artisan workshops. The mechanisation of production made possible by inventions such as steam engines and power looms saw a huge shift in production spaces to large factories and industrial mills. Industrialisation meant that goods such as textiles could be produced in much higher quantities, at a quicker pace and at a lower cost. Older forms of 'cottage industries' could not compete, and so people were compelled to work in the new industries. Also, these new forms of workplace employed hundreds (and later thousands) of workers (the 'industrial proletariat') in one place – concentrated around ports, rivers or the raw materials required for specific products.

There were mass migrations from the countryside and small towns into the new urban cities as workers needed to live near to the factories. New conurbations developed almost overnight with, for example, the population of Manchester in the North West of England (often called the birthplace of the industrial revolution) increasing three-fold from when it was a village in 1700 to being the centre of the world cotton industry in 1800. Likewise, in older towns like Leeds in Yorkshire the population also increased three-fold between 1801 and 1851, from 53,000 to 170,000.[4] In Middlesbrough in the North East of England the population went from 25 in 1801 to 91,000 in 1901. The rural/urban share of the population reversed over the 19th century in England: in 1801, 70% of the population lived in rural areas; by 1881, 70% lived in towns and cities.[5] In the short term, the industrial revolution had negative impacts on people's livelihoods – no longer were they independent, skilled and highly sought-after artisans; they were merely unskilled machine operatives and as such, easily replaced. This meant that they had little bargaining power in the new economy, and were forced by circumstance to accept the low wages and insecurity that the employers offered. Indeed, while even before the industrial revolution average wages had seldom been sufficient for maintaining health, the average wage of workers actually declined significantly in the early part of the 19th century such that even those who were fully employed were unable to adequately feed, house and clothe themselves or their families, resulting in destitution.[6]

Not only were wages low, but also the working conditions in the new industrial centres were extremely dangerous. First, factory workers, including very young children (and earning only 10–20% of an adult man's wage), were expected to work extremely long hours – averaging around 12–16 hours per day with little by way of breaks – so that machines could be used for as long as possible.[7] Miners regularly worked similar long hours underground, manually digging coal (paid by weight of coal, not hours worked), and yet still had insufficient funds to adequately feed and clothe themselves and their families. An example of a typical working day of a child factory worker in Manchester in the early 1800s is provided in Figure 2.1.

Second, cramped, hot and humid workplaces, an exhausted workforce, the speed of the mechanised work and the failure of employers to make any safety precautions (for example, the cleaning of machines was conducted while they were running, as stopping the machines for cleaning would have lowered profits) meant that fatal accidents or loss of limbs were commonplace. Friedrich Engels (1820–95) in his book *The conditions of the working class in England*[8] described these accidents as follows:

> The work between the machinery gives rise to multitudes of accidents of a more or less serious

> nature, which have for the operative the secondary effect of unfitting him for his work more or less completely. The most common accident is the squeezing off of a single joint of a finger, somewhat less common is the loss of a whole finger, half or a whole hand, an arm etc, in the machinery.

Figure 2.1: A child's working day in the early 19th century

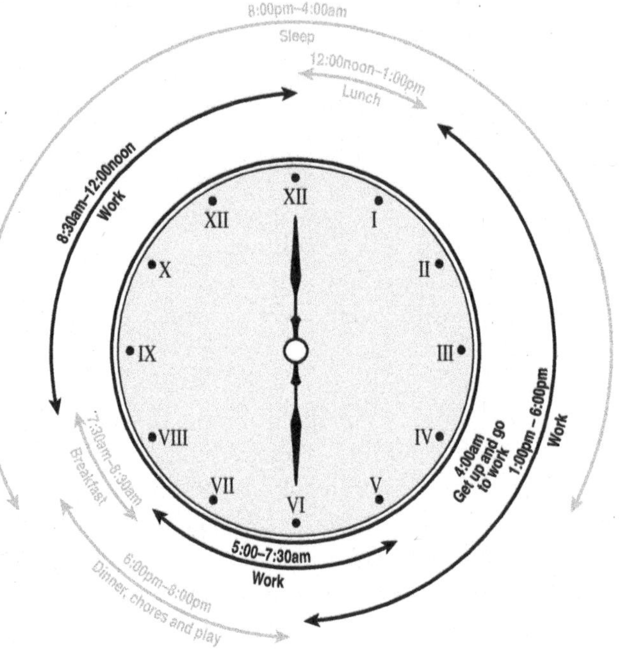

Such industrial 'accidents' were commonplace with, for example, over 330 miners per 100,000 dying each year on the job in the US in the early 1900s.[9]

Third, the nature of production also exposed workers to longer-term occupational illnesses – respiratory conditions were common among cotton workers from breathing in the fibrous dust or miners from the coal dust, including pneumoconiosis (black lung), eye disease and blindness among weavers, or lead and arsenic poisoning among pottery makers.[10] The respiratory effects of work in the cotton mills were noted in Gaskell's contemporary novel *North and South*[11] as follows:

> They say it winds round the lungs, and tightens them up. Anyhow, there's many a one works in the carding-room., that falls into a waste, coughing and spitting blood, because they've just been poisoned by the fluff.

Work-related musculoskeletal deformities were also common and developed rapidly with, for example, shoulder deformities among flax workers, one-sided muscular development among miners or pelvic deformities among women factory workers.[12] Again, Engels'[13] contemporary account provides vivid descriptions:

> Protracted work frequently causes deformities of the pelvis, partly in the shape and abnormal position and development of the hip bones, partly of malformation of the lower portion of the spinal column ... that factory operatives undergo more difficult confinements [pregnancies] than other women is testified to by midwives.

For those without work, times were even harder. Even in the burgeoning industrial economy, there were those without work – often because they were too ill, too old or injured. In England and Wales, this was the time of the workhouses. Established by the Poor Law Amendment Act 1834, these institutions provided 'indoor relief' for those without work. They provided a prison-like setting with the bare minimum by way of food (think of Oliver Twist's experiences), families were separated into men and women's sections, inmates were put to work doing menial but demanding tasks such as sewing coarse sacks, and conditions were deliberately harsh so that the workhouse would not be a disincentive to work in the real economy. Workhouses were understandably feared.

Alongside destitute wage levels, unemployment and workhouses, poor working conditions and job insecurity, the urban population was also subject to extremely hazardous environmental and housing conditions. This was the time of urban slums as the rapidly expanding towns and cities suffered from acute housing shortages, remedied in part by the building of quick, cheap and sub-standard accommodation ('jerry built'), often 'back to back', which meant that houses literally backed onto one another. Cellars with no light or ventilation and usually very damp and vermin-infested were also used for accommodation.[14] These were particularly common in the North of England, while in Scotland, tenement flats dominated – where an existing house was divided up into several small rooms separately rented with up to 12 occupants per room.[15] Few such houses had any access to water or sanitation. However, due to the increasing demand for housing arising from the rapid expansion of the urban populations, rents were high. Sir Edwin Chadwick, in his 1842 *Report on the sanitary conditions of the labouring population of Great* Britain,[16] described the typical housing in poor urban areas as follows:

> Families were attracted from all parts for the benefit of employment and obliged as a temporary resort to crowd together into such dwellings as the neighbourhood afforded: often two families into one house; others into cellars or very small dwellings; eventually, as the works became established, either the proprietor or some neighbour would probably see it as advantageous to build a few cottages; these were often of the worst description; in such cases the prevailing consideration was not how to promote the health and comfort of the occupants, but how many cottages could be built upon the smallest space of ground and at the least possible cost.

Similarly, in New York's 10th ward, as many as 12 families would live on one floor of a small tenement block.[17] In Liverpool, the medical officer for health, Dr William Duncan, reported that 40,000 of the population lived in damp, unventilated cellars.[18] The streets in the poorest areas of towns and cities were likewise awash with effluence and waste. The highly unhygienic living conditions of working-class areas of towns and cities, inhabited by exhausted, low-paid and malnourished workers, were ideal

Figure 2.2: A court for King Cholera[19]

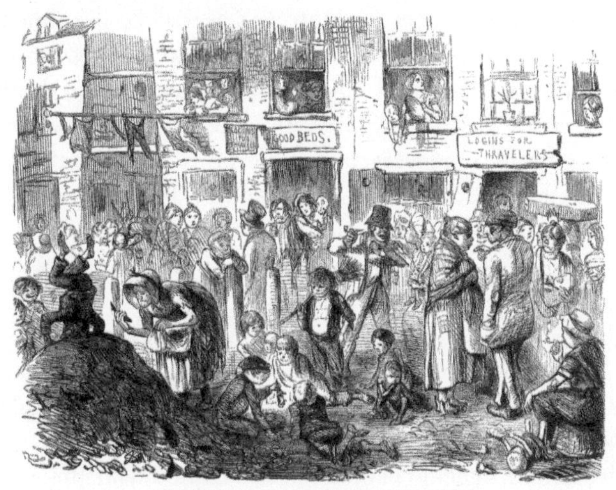

A COURT FOR KING CHOLERA.

for the infectious disease killers of the day to thrive and spread – as a cartoon from 1852 shows (see Figure 2.2).

Nasty, brutish and short

This section outlines the key causes of death and disease in the 19th century: dysentery, typhoid, typhus, small pox, tuberculosis, and the most infamous of the era, cholera. These infectious diseases were responsible for over 50% of deaths over the course of the 19th century.[20] Tuberculosis – also called the white plague or consumption at the time – and typhus were responsible for the majority of these deaths, leading historians to call it the 'century of fever and consumption'.[21] However, it was the new disease – cholera – with its recurrent epidemics that was the most feared at the time, leading to the popular moniker 'King Cholera'.[22] The environmental conditions of the new urban industrial centres in countries like England and the US allowed such diseases to spread rapidly – through contaminated water supplies, lack of basic hygiene (for example, hand washing), through to the population's close proximity to raw sewage, and through overcrowded homes, neighbourhoods and workplaces.

Infectious diseases claimed lives across the rich–poor divide, in both urban and rural areas. However, as shall be examined in a later section of this chapter, it was those in the poorest urban areas who were the most vulnerable to infection and death.[23]

Dysentery, the 'bloody flux', inflames the intestine causing diarrhoea with blood, fever and abdominal pain. It results from viral, bacterial or parasitic infestations.[24] Typhoid is a disease that inflames the intestines leading to death from dehydration, intestinal haemorrhage, perforation or infection.[25] It is caused by the Salmonella Typhi bacterium.[26] Typhus – another form of fever – is caused by infection with the Rickettsia bacteria.[27] Typhoid means 'typhus-like', as for both typhoid and typhus, high fever is the main symptom, alongside weakness, abdominal pain, rashes, constipation or diarrhoea and headaches. Additionally, with typhoid, infected people can also exhibit delirium – giving it the name of 'nervous fever'. However, it can also be carried by someone not exhibiting symptoms and thereby passed on to others. The most famous of such cases was Mary Mallon, an Irish immigrant in the US, 'Typhoid Mary', a cook who, it was estimated, infected over 50 people. Dysentery and typhoid are spread through contact between people, as well as via contaminated water or food. Typhus is spread by body lice and fleas infected with the bacteria and transmitted by bites.[28] It is estimated that in the 19th century, typhoid, typhus and dysentery killed more soldiers and sailors than combat. For example, they decimated Napoleon's army in Russia,[29] and more than 80,000 Union soldiers died of dysentery and typhoid during the American Civil War.[30]

Smallpox is caused by the variola virus and is transmitted via breathing in infected droplets during close (usually face-to-face) contact with infected symptomatic people.[31] It can also spread through direct contact with infected bodily fluids or contaminated objects such as bedding or clothing. The classic symptoms are raised bumps/pustules (hence 'pox') that appear on the face and body of an infected person.[32] Recorded cases of small pox date back to at least the 10th century BC. It was seen as the 'scourge of mankind' with rapid contamination, and 30% of cases were fatal.[33] Smallpox has a special place in the history of public health, as the British medical scientist

Edward Jenner noted that people infected with a similar (but less dangerous disease) 'cowpox' were immune to smallpox. In 1796, he conducted a series of experiments with dairy maids and volunteers that showed that cowpox could be transmitted from one person to another as a way of protecting against small pox infection. By 1800, Jenner's cowpox vaccination was being used across Europe, and by 1870 vaccination against small pox was compulsory in England and Germany.[34] It was the first vaccine to be developed against any disease, making Jenner the founding father of immunology.

Tuberculosis, known also as TB, 'the white plague' or consumption, is a respiratory disease. It is estimated that it accounted for a third of deaths in the 19th century,[35] when mortality rates from acute TB were as high as 500 per 100,000 as 80% of cases were fatal.[36] It was an ever-present disease, a chronic epidemic. For example, in 1870 alone, acute TB was responsible for 54,000 deaths – 10% of the total of all deaths that year, and higher than the 53,000 deaths caused by the most fatal cholera epidemic of 1849.[37] TB can also be dormant, and infected people may not develop symptoms of acute TB, greatly increasing the likely number of people with TB in the 19th century. TB attacks the lungs and is transmitted through the air when infected people cough or sneeze, or pass respiratory fluids.[38] TB symptoms include a chronic cough, coughing up blood, fever, night sweats and weight loss (hence 'consumption', as it *consumes* the patient). In the early 19th century, it was assumed that TB was caused by having a predisposition to it, and it was stigmatised as a result.[39] However, in 1882, Robert Koch, a German scientist, identified that TB was, in fact, caused by the Mycobacterium Tuberculosis, and was transmitted between people (see Table 2.1). Koch attempted to create a vaccination but with little effect. Sanatoriums instead were developed so that consumptive patients, or 'lungers' as they became known, could be quarantined from others and removed from the 'unclean' airs and overcrowding of the cities, which were, rightly, thought to be harmful.[40]

Cholera was new to Europe in the 19th century, and as such was one of the most feared diseases of the industrial age. It arrived suddenly in Britain in 1832, arriving on ships from Asia into port towns like Sunderland, Liverpool and Manchester, spreading north into Scotland and south down to London. Within the course of 1832, the epidemic had killed around 30,000 people. Death rates were high with, for example, over half of the people who contracted cholera in Manchester dying.[41] Further epidemics occurred in 1848, 1853 and 1866 (see Table 2.1). Cholera struck victims with little warning – 'the unfortunate individual was gripped by a sudden bout of vomiting and severe diarrhoea, and within only a few hours severe dehydration caused the body's tissues to collapse, the blood to coagulate, the skin to turn blue, and the internal organs to fail.'[42] The suddenness of the disease, the severity of symptoms, the relatively quick and

Table 2.1: Timeline of landmarks in 19th century public health (UK)

1786	Mechanisation introduced to textile factories
1800	Small pox vaccination available
1830-36	Typhoid epidemics (four outbreaks)
1832	First cholera epidemic 30,000 deaths
1834	Poor Law Amendment Act establishes workhouses
1842	Edwin Chadwick's Report on the Sanitary Condition of the Labouring Classes in Great Britain published
1848	Second cholera epidemic 70,000 deaths
1848	First Public Health Act introduces urban sanitation reform
1853	Third cholera epidemic 30,000 deaths
1854	John Snow's research on cholera published
1860	Government food inspections started
1865	Louis Pastuer's germ theory published
1866	Fourth cholera epidemic 18,000 deaths
1867	Second Reform Act gave working class men the vote
1867	Factory Act put restrictions on child labour and hours of work
1869	Local Government Board Act placed responsibility for public health local authorities
1870	National vaccination programmes for small pox
1872	Second Public Health Act - local medical officers for health responsible for sanitation
1875	Trade unions and strikes legalised
1875	Third Public Health Act - local authorities responsible for lighting, water supply, sewage disposal, parks, toilets and housing
1882	Robert Koch identifies the germ that causes tuberculosis
1883	Robert Koch identifies the germ that causes cholera

high death rates, and its Asiatic origins led to it being the most feared disease of the 19th century.

Cholera was feared by rich and poor alike, the latter because they were more at risk and the former because they thought they were at risk and also because they feared the political effects of the epidemics. Indeed, across Europe and even in the US there were a series of 'cholera riots'.[43] In Britain there were over 30 such riots in 1832 alone. Fear of cholera combined with existing social tensions over the division between rich and poor, the poor conditions of the working class as well as fears of the medical profession (cholera bodies were dissected) and the increasing role of the state in disease control (isolation in hospitals was fiercely resisted). In France, cholera was seen as a conspiracy by the richer classes against the poorer classes.[44] Many richer people, especially in continental Europe, fled urban areas for the comparative safety of the countryside to avoid both the disease and political unrest. Indeed, the conditions of urban areas in the industrial revolution meant that cholera (and other infectious diseases) claimed more lives in urban areas than rural ones. This political context provided the impetus for the early, modest Victorian sanitation reforms such as those of the Public Health Act 1848 in England that made local authorities responsible for water supplies and drainage.

There were several theories at the time for the causes of cholera, ranging from it being divine punishment for the decadence and degradation of industrial society, to being a result of unemployment or a miasma.[45] Ultimately the correct one was Dr John Snow's theory that cholera was spread by contaminated water. In the early 1850s, John Snow (1813–58) studied the incidences of cholera in Soho, London. He mapped where cholera victims lived, and found that there was a very high correlation with a specific water pump (the Broad Street pump). Writing at the time, Snow commented on the case of a woman cholera victim:

> I was informed by this lady's son that she had not been in the neighbourhood of Broad Street for many months. A cart went from Broad Street to West End every day and it was the custom to take out a large

> bottle of the water from the pump in Broad Street, as she preferred it. The water was taken on Thursday 31st August and she drank of it in the evening, and also on Friday. She was seized with cholera on the evening of the latter day, and died on Saturday.[46]

John Snow's map is shown in Figure 2.3, in which the dark bars represent cholera deaths and the circles represent water pumps. There is a clear clustering of deaths around the Broad Street pump. He famously got the pump handle removed to stop the spread of the disease. At the time, this was considered to have dramatically reduced the incidence of cholera in the neighbourhood, although later analysis has shown that cases were already in decline.[47] Nonetheless, in 1883, Snow's hypothesis was confirmed when the cholera germ (bacterium Vibrio Cholera) was finally identified by Robert Koch and its waterborne nature

Figure 2.3: John Snow's map of the distribution of cholera cases in 1850s London[48]

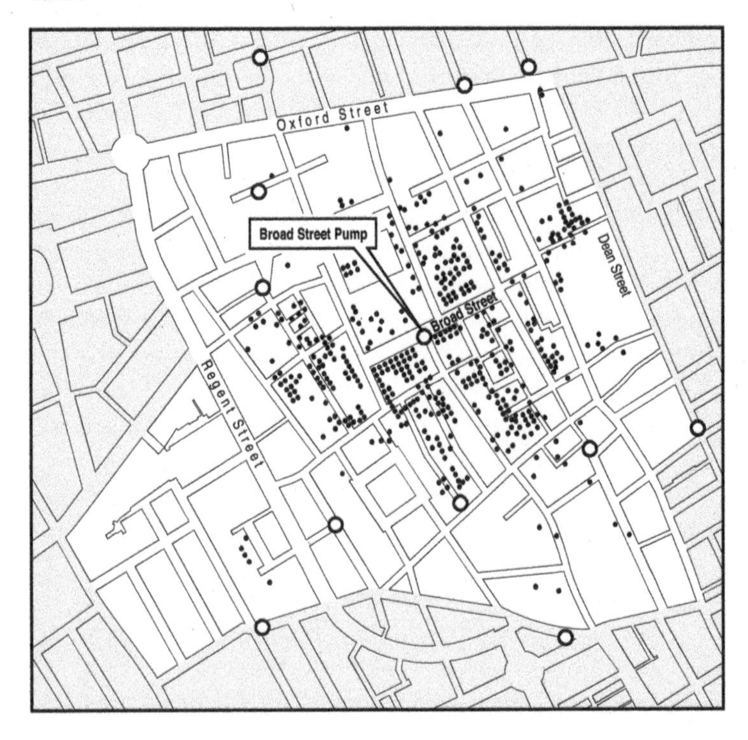

was proved (see Table 2.1). John Snow's work was also some of the first to overtly identify the importance of *place* for health, so he is often claimed to be the first health geographer.

Old sores

So death and disease were widespread in the 19th century, but not everyone or everywhere was at equal risk. This section examines the main health divides in the epidemic age: between the North and the South of England, between urban and rural areas, and between rich and poor areas of towns and cities.

Coketown and Darkshire

The North–South divide occupies a particular place within the English imagination, and the term itself dates back to the 1920s.[49] It came to prominence in the 19th century as the process of industrialisation started (and was more intense) in the North of England. The North therefore typified the problems (and benefits) of industrialisation while the South became associated with rurality and the 'rural idyll'. This is apparent in the literary works of the times, particularly those of Charles Dickens (for example, *Hard Times*, 1854[50] or *A Tale of Two Cities*, 1859[51]) and Elizabeth Gaskell (for example, *North and South*, 1855[52]). These authors contrasted the horrors of the newly industrialised North with the implicit tranquillity of the still largely rural South. Dickens' *Hard times* portrays the social and working conditions of the North in the industrial revolution, where the location is named *Coketown* (a fictional location, but widely believed to be Manchester). Similarly, in *North and South*, life in the idyllic southern village of *Helstone* is contrasted unfavourably with the oppressive and dangerous industrial conditions of *Milton-Northern* in *Darkshire*, a fictional Northern cotton town (believed to be based on Preston in Lancashire). It is not a pleasant place: 'For several miles before they reached Milton, they saw a deep lead-coloured cloud hanging over the horizon in the direction in which it lay.'

From a public health perspective, these contemporary novels were right to contrast the North with the South, and to do so in terms of an urban versus rural divide. The North experienced rapid urbanisation and industrialisation in the early 19th century while the South remained predominantly rural and agricultural. In 1842, the social reformer Edwin Chadwick (later associated with the creation of the Public Health Act 1848) published his government commissioned *Report on the sanitary conditions of the labouring population of Great Britain* in which he described and contrasted living and working conditions across the country. It highlighted how the death rate in England, which had been falling during the 18th century, had risen rapidly between 1831 and 1841 in places like Birmingham (where it increased from 14.6 to 27.2 per 1,000), Leeds (from 20.7 to 27.2 per 1,000) and Liverpool (from 21 to 34.8 per 1,000). Chadwick's report also presented contemporary mortality and life expectancy data that showed that the mortality rate in rural areas was 18.2 per 1,000 in 1831–39 while in urban areas it was 26.2 per 1,000.[53] Some of this data is presented in Table 2.2, which shows the average life expectancy in years of men by occupation and location. Men living in urban areas fared worse – in all occupational classes –

Table 2.2: Average life expectancy in years (men) by occupation and location, England, 1840s[54]

	Gentry and Professionals	Tradesmen	Labourers
Rural / Agricultural			
Bath	55	37	25
Kendall	45	39	34
Rutland	52	41	38
Wiltshire	50	48	33
Urban / Industrial			
Bolton	34	23	18
Bethnal Green (London)	45	26	16
Leeds	44	27	19
Liverpool	35	22	15
Manchester	38	20	17
Whitechapel (London)	45	27	22

than those living in the rural areas. Indeed, as Chadwick himself noted, labourers in the rural area of Rutland did almost as well as gentry in Liverpool or Manchester.

In his report, Chadwick reported comments from the Army Medical Board, to the effect that in the 1840s, soldiers from the agricultural districts were in far better health than those from the manufacturing towns. Chadwick, however, blamed filth, dirt, lack of hygiene and insanitary conditions for the health problems of the urban North rather than the poverty and dangerous working conditions of industrialisation itself. His main recommendations were therefore that the local authorities should provide better urban environments, specifically improving drainage, ventilation and water supplies. This eventually resulted in the Public Health Act 1848. The urban/rural divide was also evident in the 19th-century US with, for example, life expectancies 15 years higher in rural areas of New England than in the large cities of Boston, New York and Philadelphia.[55]

Chadwick's 19th-century data (which was not collected to the same standards as today) is also supported by more recent research that retrospectively examined the differences in mortality across cities in 19th-century England. This found that in the 1860s, the life expectancies of Northern industrial cities (including Sheffield, Leeds, Newcastle, Manchester and Liverpool) had fallen behind those of Southern industrial cities such as Bristol or Birmingham.[56] For example, in the period 1861 to 1870, life expectancy in Bristol was 40 years and in Birmingham it was 37. In contrast, in Leeds, Sheffield and Newcastle, it was 35, and in Liverpool and Manchester, it was 34. The national average for England and Wales at this time was 41 years. This North–South gap between cities continued throughout the 19th century. So the North–South health divide dates back to at least the 19th century. This was, in part, a reflection of the wider rural–urban divide, but it was also due to the particular speed, intensity and nature of industrialisation in the North (for example, the Cotton Mills).

Death and the city

Health inequalities between rich and poor areas were officially 'discovered' in the 19th century, although modern research suggests that they date back to at least Roman times.[57] The collection of mortality data became more standardised and comprehensive in the 19th century, and the earliest statistical evidence of spatial health inequalities in urban areas comes from the work of Louis René Villermé in Paris in the 1820s. He examined differences in mortality rates by arrondissement (districts or neighbourhoods), finding that areas with lower-income households (indicated by the proportion of houses for which no tax was levied) had significantly higher mortality rates than more well-to-do neighbourhoods.[58] By the 1890s, life expectancy differences between richer and poorer areas of Paris amounted to 12 years.[59] Chadwick's data (see Table 2.2) also revealed great local health divides between the rich and poor in 19th-century England – middle-class residents of Manchester or Liverpool, for example, lived more than twice as long on average as working-class ones. These differences in life expectancy reflected the great divide in infant mortality rates by occupational class, with 10% of children born to professionals dying within the first year of birth compared to 15% among those working in trade and 25% among the working classes.[60] In the US there were similarly stark 19th-century health divides between rich and poor – professionals were over 2cm taller than labourers in the latter half of the 19th century, and in the areas where labourers lived, the infant mortality rates were 157 in every 1,000 (almost 16%), while in areas where professionals lived, it was 37 in 1,000 (less than 4%).[61]

More recent research has also shown spatial patterning in the 19th century with the inner-city suburbs of English cities faring worse than the outer suburbs. For example, life expectancy in the outer, more wealthy Bristol suburb of Clifton in 1850 was 42, which was 7 years higher than in the neighbouring inner-city suburbs, where it was 35.[62] The gap between the outer suburb of Chorlton and the inner-city areas of Manchester also stood at 7 years (30 years compared to 37 years), and between inner-city Liverpool areas and the nearby suburb of West Derby it was 11 years (27 years compared to 38 years). This was largely a result of the fact that a third more infants died in the poorest areas (inner city) than in the richest areas (outer suburbs).[63] These socio-spatial inequalities between richer and poorer areas continued throughout the 19th century, and were noted at the time.[64] In his 1842 report, for example, Chadwick noted that, when he asked for two maps of Aberdeen, one marked with the prevalence of fever and one with the location of the different social orders: 'They returned a map so marked as to disease, but stated that it had been thought unnecessary to distinguish the streets inhabited by the different orders of society, as that was done with sufficient accuracy by the different tints representing the degrees of the prevalence of fever.'[65]

These health inequalities across 19th-century cities were a reflection of the different social, economic, working and environmental circumstances in which different parts of the urban population lived. The spatial patterning of poverty, for example, was shown at the time in London by the maps of Charles Booth that found great concentrations of poverty and poor environmental conditions in some areas, while other neighbourhoods – predominantly inhabited by the wealthy – fared much better in terms of housing, sanitation, etc, and, of course, health.[66] Similar socio-spatial patterns existed in 19th-century Paris, as data from the 1876 housing census shows: across the city 10% of households were rich while 68% were poor. However, these two groups inhabited different parts of the city – there were 12 Eastern arrondissements in which more than 90% of the households were categorised as poor (and in which less than 1% of households were rich), and five arrondissements (all in the North East of the City) in which more than 40% of households were rich and less than 30% poor.[67] In the richer areas such as the Champs Elysées, rents were 20 times those in the poorest areas such as Charonne. These differences in rents reflected huge differences in housing quality, size, amenities, sanitation and air quality – key determinants of health. Rich and poor inhabited completely different parts of the city.[68] The living conditions of the poorest areas of 19th-century industrial cities are captured vividly by contemporary British accounts, as noted in Box 2.1.

Box 2.1: Nineteenth-century descriptions of living conditions in poor areas

From a *Report on the sanitary conditions of the labouring population of Great Britain,* Edwin Chadwick (1842):

> In Liverpool (which is a commercial and not a manufacturing town) where, however, the condition of the dwellings are reported to be the worst, where, according to the report of Dr Duncan, 40,000 of the population live in cellars, where 1 in 25 of the population are annually attacked with fever, there the mean chances of life appear from the returns to the Registrar-general to be still lower than in Manchester, Leeds, or amongst the silk weavers in Bethnal Green.

From *An inquiry into the state and condition of Leeds*, Robert Baker (1842):

> Courts and cul-de-sacs exist everywhere.... In one cul-de-sac in Leeds there are 34 houses, and in ordinary times there dwell in these houses 340 persons, or ten to every house. The name of this place is Boot and Shoe Yard, from whence the commissioners removed, in the days of Cholera, 75 cartloads of manure which had been untouched for years. For the most part these houses are built back-to-back.... A house of this description will contain a cellar, a house and chamber.... To build the largest number of cottages on the smallest possible space seems to have been the original view of the speculators. Thus neighbourhoods have arisen in which there is neither water nor privies.

From a *Report on the state of Newcastle-upon-Tyne and other towns*, Dr David B. Reid (1845):

> The streets most densely populated by the humbler classes are a mass of filth [excrement] where the direct rays of the sun never reach. In some of the courts, I have seen heaps of filth, amounting to 20 or 50 tons, which, when it rains penetrate into some of the cellar dwellings. A few public necessaries have been built, but too few to serve the population.... Stagnant ditches may be seen in the vicinity of most of these houses and part of the ground in the lowest districts is apt to be flooded after heavy rains, and long

> open sewers cross the public paths.... In numerous dwellings a whole family shares one room.

From Friedrich Engels, *The condition of the working class in England* (1845):

> Such is the Old Town of Manchester ... filth, ruin, and uninhabitableness, the defiance of all considerations of cleanliness, ventilation, and health which characterise the construction of this single district, containing at least twenty to thirty thousand inhabitants. And such a district exists in the heart of the second city of England, the first manufacturing city of the world. If any one wishes to see in how little space a human being can move, how little air – and such air! – he can breathe, how little of civilisation he may share and yet live, it is only necessary to travel hither.

From a *Report on the sanitary conditions of the labouring population of Great Britain*, Edwin Chadwick (1842):

> The pernicious effects resulting from the vitiation of the atmosphere by the congregation of many persons in a confined space are lamentably illustrated in the common lodging-houses of the poor; the crowded, dirty, and ill ventilated state of which is, I conceive, without doubt one of the most prolific sources of fever in Manchester. To those who have not visited them, no description can convey anything like an accurate idea of the abominable state of these dens of filth, disease, and wretchedness.

The social, working and environmental conditions of the urban poor in the US were similarly harsh. Child labour was common with, for example, in the 1830s, a third of the New England workforce aged less than 16. Unemployment was common – in the late 1800s, around a quarter of the US workforce experienced unemployment on an annual basis. Average incomes were also low while working weeks were long, with average weekly hours in manufacturing of 69 hours in the 1850s. Working conditions were also as hazardous as in Britain or France with, for example, the steel mills of Pittsburgh reporting 195 fatalities a year.[69]

The wider urban environment for the poor also resembled the European industrial experience, with New York's 10th ward said to be the most crowded place on earth at the time with little by way of sanitation and filth filling the streets: 'filth everywhere, trampled into sidewalks, lying in windows, collected in the eddies of doorsteps'.[70] The links between these conditions and health were made at the time with a New York City public health report of 1858 linking the high mortality rates in poorer areas with the overcrowded tenement housing, poor lighting, bad ventilation, filthy streets and insufficient sewers.[71]

From King Cholera to the 'c' word

So in the 19th century, in all areas, it was remarkably easy to die – indeed, surviving childhood was quite an achievement. Death rates were far higher than today, and life expectancy correspondingly lower – at less than 45 years on average. Infectious diseases were the main killer, claiming millions of lives, especially during epidemic outbreaks: in 1850s England, infectious disease accounted for almost 50% of deaths, higher even than that in poor urban areas of London or Liverpool, the urban penalty.[72] In contrast, today, the main causes of death and disease in wealthy countries are chronic diseases (such as cancer, the 'c' word) as people now live long enough (over 75 years on average in wealthy countries) to succumb to these. This section examines explanations for this transformation in death and disease – the *epidemiological transition*.

The epidemiological transition started at around 1890 in England and at around 1900 in France and the US, when life expectancies began to rapidly increase.[73] Mortality declined at such a rapid rate that in some countries life expectancy increased by over 10 years in just three decades.[74] This decline in mortality in wealthy countries has, with the exceptions of the two World Wars and the 1918–19 flu pandemic, continued until today. The 'mortality revolution' was most pronounced among children aged 1–14 years, and death rates fell quicker in urban than rural areas – a reversal of the urban health penalty.[75] Mortality declined although there was a corresponding increase in sickness as people lived longer with their illnesses. These improvements were largely a result of the declining impact on public health of infectious disease. There are various explanations as to why infectious diseases started to be less important at this time.

Conventionally, medical historians tended to view the increase in life expectancy at around the turn of the 20th century to be a result of improvements in medicine, healthcare and public health: as scientists started to identify the germs responsible for specific diseases, they were able to develop drugs to combat or prevent them, and the subsequent vaccination and antibiotic treatment programmes then effectively wiped the diseases out.[76] The 'medical thesis' is supported by the fact that by the outbreak of the First World War (1914), scientists had discovered the causes of diseases such as smallpox, tuberculosis, cholera and typhoid.[77] Vaccination programmes for smallpox had been implemented as early as the 1870s in England and Germany and 1901 in France, while vaccines for tuberculosis, influenza and typhoid were developed in the 1940s. A related perspective argued that these changes occurred as a result of the public health regulations and improvements of the late 19th century. This 'public health thesis' argued that the sanitation reforms such as the Public Health Act 1848 in England (implemented by a Liberal government and which, it is argued, led to immediate reductions in mortality rates such as in Macclesfield, where the death rate fell from 42 per 1,000 in 1847 to 26 per 1,000 in 1858; see Box 2.2), quarantine procedures, workplace health regulations, for example, restrictions on child labour or hours of work (Factory Act 1867), and regulations to prevent the adulteration of food (which had been a common practice, with a *Lancet* inquiry in the 1850s finding all bread, butter and most of the milk and oatmeal tested to be adulterated).[78] This explanation helps to explain why urban areas did better as they were the first to have sewage systems, for example.

Box 2.2: Public Health Act 1848

The main features of the Public Health Act 1848 were:

- The establishment of a Central Board of Health.
- Responsibility for water supplies and drainage given to local authorities.
- Local taxes would pay for the improvements.
- Where the death rate exceeded 23 in every 1,000, a Local Board of Health could be imposed by the Central Board of Health.

The medical and public health views were challenged, however, in the 1970s by Professor Thomas McKeown. He asserted that the epidemiological transition was not due to advances in sanitation or vaccination practices, but as a result of better nutrition – which itself was a result of increases in the incomes of industrial workers. McKeown's 'social thesis'[79] showed how the majority of the decline in infectious disease mortality occurred before medical vaccination programmes had been developed (the only exception being smallpox). For example, in England, over two-thirds of the reduction in deaths from tuberculosis and from pneumonia, bronchitis and influenza occurred *before* the introduction of treatment in the 1930s and 1940s.[80] This was also the case in other countries such as the US.[81] Indeed, it has since been claimed that less than 10% of the mortality decline was actually due to medical advances.[82] McKeown also argued that the public health explanation also suffers from a timing problem in that the major advances – such as the introduction of sanitation systems in cities – were also *after* the decline in mortality had started. He also asserted that sanitation reforms would only have an impact on water-borne diseases such as cholera and not on airborne diseases such as tuberculosis or influenza. Other factors must be at work, chief among them increased resistance to disease from better nutrition, itself a product of wage increases from the late 19th century onwards.[83] Indeed, the consumption of fruit and meat increased from around 1870.[84] Again, this helps explain the reversal of the urban health penalty as, by the latter 19th century, wages for industrial workers were higher than for agricultural workers. It also fits in with the increase in sickness that was observed alongside a decrease in infectious disease mortality as more nourished workers could live longer with an illness that might otherwise kill them (for example, TB).

A third explanation comes from what can be called the 'political economy thesis'. Drawing on the seminal work of Karl Polanyi,[85] Professors Robert Chernomas and Ian Hudson of the University of Manitoba, Canada[86] argue that while there is evidence to support both the public health thesis and McKeown's social thesis, there is still a need to look 'further upstream' as to why these two contextual and proximate factors – the public health reforms and income increases for industrial workers – occurred in the late 19th century. They assert that a political conjunction of working-class (for example, trade unions campaigning for better wages, shorter hours and safer working conditions) and middle-class movements (for example, the sanitary reform movement that campaigned for better sanitation and conditions for the poor), especially after a widening of who could vote, led to considerable gains in the latter part of the 19th century in Britain and from the 1900s onwards (the so-called 'Progressive Era') in the US. For example, in Britain, the Factory Act 1867 limited the working day for women and children to 10 hours; trade unions were legalised in 1875; government food inspections started in 1860; and sewers were built in most conurbations from 1870 onwards (see Table 2.1). Wider state welfare also emerged from the late 19th century onwards alongside the slum clearances and sanitation reforms. In the early 20th century, continued political pressure as a result of the rise of working-class political movements led to more social reform as, for example, basic state pensions were introduced in 1908 in the UK for those aged over 70; in 1911 unemployment benefits (the 'dole') and some access to medical care were provided under the National Insurance Act; 1919 saw the first wave of state house building to replace slums; and from 1918 onwards an evolving system of 'outdoor relief' was provided for the poor. These changes – implemented despite considerable opposition from business owners – meant that conditions, particularly in industrial urban areas, improved, and workers had higher incomes so they could obtain better nutrition. So, it was political change that led to public health legislation, higher living standards, better nutrition and ultimately a population better equipped to withstand infectious disease. Indeed, it can be argued that it was 'economic policy in support of private sector profits that caused epidemic disease' – it was liberal, laissez-faire capitalism rather than industrialisation itself that was the root issue.[87] Political reforms that regulated the workplace, alongside political pressures from trade unions that increased wages, reduced the health impacts of industrialisation. The epidemiological transition was a political transition.

These beneficial reforms were subsequently strengthened and institutionalised in the inter-war period with the advent of the welfare state and a more regulatory and interventionist approach to the economy. Outdoor relief finally replaced the workhouse in England in the 1930s (low level welfare payments were made available to the destitute, for example, but only after all other means were exhausted as determined by the much resented 'household means test'). Likewise, in the US, the 1930s saw the introduction of pensions and welfare benefits for the unemployed and single mothers (Aid to Dependent Children, white mothers only), as part of Roosevelt's 'New Deal' programmes. The welfare provided in this period, however, was minimal, and research by the British Medical Association at the time showed that the benefits received by those without work (and many on low wages in work) were not sufficient to maintain good health.[88]

These welfare reforms were largely responses to the 'Great Depression' – the worldwide economic collapse that saw mass unemployment in most wealthy countries, with more than 50% of men out of work in most industrial areas for a five-year period. The most famous example of a depression-hit town in England is that of Jarrow in the North East of England where, in 1936, a group of over 200 men marched the 300 miles to London to petition Parliament to highlight the extent of the problems in their area, where unemployment rates were in excess of 70% as a result of the closure of the local shipyard. This mass unemployment exacerbated the existing problems in the town – poverty, overcrowding, poor housing and high mortality rates particularly from consumption. The local MP Ellen Wilkinson commented that the town was 'utterly stagnant. There was no work. No one had a job except a few railwaymen, officials, the workers in the co-operative stores, and a few workmen who went out of the town ... the plain fact [is] that if people have to live and bear and bring up their children in bad houses on too little food, their resistance to disease is lowered and they die before they should.'[89] Healthcare provision also improved in the inter-war period and, as medical science continued to advance, more vaccinations were developed (for example, the TB, influenza and scarlet fever vaccines were all developed in the 1940s),[90] although access to healthcare was still largely the preserve of the wealthy who could afford private doctors and medicine.

The real expansion of welfare and healthcare came in the immediate post-war period (after 1945), when most Western European countries established full 'welfare states' providing unprecedented levels of support in terms of welfare, education and healthcare for all, across the life course, from 'cradle to grave'.

Again, as a result of political change (such as the election of a social democratic Labour government in 1945), in the UK, the National Health Service (NHS) was established in 1948, providing healthcare free at the point of need and accessible to all, funded from general taxation. Likewise, unemployment benefits, as well as support for those who could not work due to ill health, were improved, mandatory state-funded education for all children to the age of 16 was provided, health and safety in the workplace was more regulated, the state committed to taking an active role in economic policy and promoting full employment, wages increased, there was an increase in public house building (council houses), and the state even took over ownership of some key industries (for example, coal mining was nationalised in the UK in 1946). This was the age of the Keynesian welfare state.

Similar reforms were enacted in some other wealthy countries in the immediate post-war period including France, Germany and Sweden, while in other countries the expansion did not occur until later. For example, Finland's welfare state was not established until the 1960s due to later industrialisation. Spain and Portugal were dictatorships until the 1970s, and expansion in the US only really occurred during the 'war on poverty' in the 1960s when, for example, the Medicare and Medicaid systems were established and the 1930s welfare programmes were improved on (for example, Aid to Dependent Children was extended to also include black mothers). The welfare states of wealthy countries also varied in this period in terms of the levels of support they provided – some were more generous (for example, the Scandinavian ones) than others (for example, the UK and US) in terms of the payments that unemployed workers received, or in respect of how much healthcare support could be accessed without personal cost. However, significant reductions to the size and scale of the welfare states of *all* wealthy countries occurred from the 1980s onwards as a result of political and economic changes – the rise of neoliberalism.

The importance for death, disease and health divides of this expansion and contraction of welfare states over the course of the 20th and 21st centuries will be returned to at various points in later parts of this book. There is first a need to understand what death, disease and health divides are like today, more than a hundred years after the *epidemiological transition*. This is the subject of the next chapter.

CHAPTER 3

In sickness and in health

The previous chapter provided an overview of public health and health divides in the 19th and early 20th century, and outlined the epidemiological shift from infectious to chronic disease. This chapter now examines what geographical inequalities in health are like today, providing an overview of the main contemporary causes of death and disease in wealthy countries. It demonstrates the consistent nature of health divides across the major causes of death and disease, that internationally, health is worse in the US; within the UK, that Scotland fares worse; regionally, that the North of England does worse than the South; and that deprived neighbourhoods in the major towns and cities of wealthy countries experience a health penalty. The starkness, proximity and universality of contemporary health divides are demonstrated.

Death and disease today

Since the 'epidemiological transition' the main causes of death in the UK, the US and other wealthy countries are chronic diseases such as cancer and CVD that now account for over 50% of deaths. Chronic diseases are characterised by slow development, long morbidity period and multiple causes. Table 3.1 shows the average proportion of deaths accounted for by communicable (infectious) diseases compared to non-communicable diseases (including CVD and cancer) for the World Health Organisation's (WHO) wealthy countries in 2012.[1] These data illustrate the scale of the epidemiological shift in wealthy countries as communicable diseases now account for less than 3% of all deaths, while in contrast, cancers account for 25% and CVD accounts for 38%. Likewise, the significant contemporary causes of ill health and disease (or morbidity) are largely chronic in nature such as diabetes, obesity, mental health or musculoskeletal problems. This section provides a general overview of the leading causes of death and disease in wealthy countries today to aid understanding of the spatial data that is presented later in the chapter.

Table 3.1: Causes of death in wealthy countries, 2012[2]

	Number of deaths (000s)			Percentage of all deaths*		
	Total	Men	Women	Total	Men	Women
All causes	11,483,576	5,863,412	5,620,164	100	100	100
Communicable (infectious) diseases	301,019	172,690	128,329	2.6	2.9	2.3
Non-communicable diseases	10,000,586	4,967,538	5,033,048	87.1	84.7	89.6
Cancer	2,847,634	1,582,329	1,265,305	24.8	27.0	22.5
Cardiovascular disease	4,379,335	2,042,055	2,337,280	38.1	34.8	41.6

*Author calculation from number of deaths

CVD is the leading cause of death in the majority of wealthy countries, accounting for over 300,000 deaths every year in the UK, over a third of total deaths. CVD is a general term that describes a disease of the heart or blood vessels.[3] The two most common types are coronary heart disease and stroke. Coronary heart disease occurs when the flow of oxygen-rich blood to the heart is blocked or reduced by a build-up of fatty material in the two major blood vessels (coronary arteries) that supply blood to the heart. This restricts blood supply to the heart and if completely blocked, a heart attack results. Heart failure occurs when the heart's ability to pump blood is reduced. Stroke occurs when a blood vessel to the brain bursts or is blocked by a blood clot.[4]

Cancer is the second most common cause of death today, accounting for 31% of deaths among men and 26% among women.[5] More than a third of people will develop some form of cancer during their lifetime.[6] Cancer is a condition where cells in a specific part of the body grow and reproduce uncontrollably, destroying surrounding healthy tissue, including organs, and spreading from one part of the body to other areas – metastasis.[7] The four most common types of cancer, accounting for over half (54%) of all new cases, are: breast cancer, lung cancer, prostate cancer and bowel cancer.[8]

Diabetes is a progressive, chronic metabolic condition that causes blood glucose (sugar) levels to become too high.[9] There are two types of diabetes: type 1, which occurs when the body does not produce any insulin at all (this usually develops by age 40); and type 2, which is when the body does not produce enough insulin or the body does not process it properly (this insulin resistance usually develops later in life).[10] In England in 2010 there were over 2 million people adults with diagnosed diabetes (6% of the population).[11] In the US, the lifetime risk of 20-year-olds developing diabetes is now 40% for both men and women (more than a one in three chance of getting diabetes), and among Hispanic men and women, and non-Hispanic black women, the lifetime risk is over 50% (more than one in two will develop diabetes).[12]

The rapid rise in type 2 diabetes in wealthy countries is in part due to increasing levels of obesity. Obesity is a condition in which a person has an abnormally high and unhealthy proportion of body fat, and it is measured using BMI (see Box 3.1). Obesity leads to other chronic diseases such as diabetes, CVD, osteoarthritis, back pain and certain forms of cancer.[13] Rates of obesity have been growing rapidly throughout the wealthy world, and particularly in countries like the UK and the US:[14] in the UK in the late 1970s obesity was 6% among men and 8% among women; by the early 2000s, this had almost tripled to 23% of men and 25% women.[15] Among children (aged 2–15) in England, the prevalence of obesity is estimated to have increased from 11% among boys and 12% of girls in 1995 to 18-19% for both sexes in 2005.[16]

Mental health is a key component within the WHO's definition of health, as 'A state of complete physical, mental and social well-being, and not merely the absence of disease'.[17] It is therefore a wide-ranging and positive term relating to wellbeing,

Box 3.1: Definition of obesity

Among adults, 'obesity' and 'overweight' are usually defined with reference to the Body Mass Index (BMI). BMI is calculated by dividing a person's weight in kilogrammes divided by the square of his or her height in metres (kg/m^2). In adults, the WHO defines overweight as having a BMI greater than or equal to 25, and obesity as a BMI greater than or equal to 30.

although it is more commonly used to refer to mental health disorders. The most common mental health disorders in wealthy countries are anxiety and depression with, for example, around one-fifth of UK adults reporting these conditions.[18] Mental health problems are the biggest source of health-related disability and suffering in wealthy countries, accounting for 26% of the total disease burden and over 40% of 'years lost due to disability'.[19] Depression alone accounts for 8% of the disease burden – more than any other condition.[20] Mortality and physical morbidity are also higher among people with poor mental health.[21] Suicide – the act of deliberately killing oneself[22] – is strongly associated with poor mental health, and around 90% of the 4,400 people who end their own lives in England each year suffer from a psychiatric disorder at the time of their death.[23]

Musculoskeletal disorders are the second leading cause of disability in wealthy countries, with up to a third of people experiencing some form of the condition. Musculoskeletal conditions are defined as 'inflammatory and degenerative conditions affecting the muscles, tendons, ligaments, joints, peripheral nerves, and supporting blood vessels'.[24] Disorders of the back (including lower back pain, disc degeneration and herniation) are the most common form of musculoskeletal disorder, accounting for up to 60% of complaints, while neck and upper limb pain followed by knee and hip disorders make up the remainder.[25]

Where you live can kill you

This section examines how these chronic causes of death and disease vary spatially today, starting with the health divides between wealthy countries and the emergence of the US disadvantage.

From the tallest to the fattest

The key health issues outlined above are common to all wealthy countries today. However, as noted in Chapter 1, some countries do better and some do worse than others. This is demonstrated in Table 3.2, which shows some of the key health outcomes across 10 wealthy countries. It shows some important differences across the countries of Western Europe with some countries performing much better in terms of key health outcomes than others. For example, among Western European countries, the UK has the worst all-cause mortality rate and the highest prevalence of obesity among women. The UK does, however, have the smallest diabetes-related death rate. France performs very well in terms of obesity while the Netherlands performs comparatively poorly in terms of both CVD and cancer deaths. Sweden is arguably the best performer, with the lowest rates of CVD and cancer mortality and the lowest prevalence of diabetes among adults and some of the lowest rates of obesity for both men and women.

However, the key finding of Table 3.2 is the relative underperformance of the world's richest country, the US. The US does the worst for six of the eight health outcomes – with the highest rates of all-cause mortality, CVD mortality, deaths from injuries and violence, and deaths as a result of diabetes. In terms of morbidity, the US fares the worst for rates of depression and rates of obesity. It is second worst for the prevalence of diabetes, and only for cancer mortality does it do comparatively well. Further, the US also does comparatively poorly in terms of life expectancy (Americans can expect to live two years less on average than UK citizens) and infant mortality rates (50% higher than the UK). These issues are common across the social/spatial gradient, with the poorest areas and social groups faring worse than the poorest areas or social groups of other countries. Likewise, even more affluent areas and higher income groups in the US fare worse than their comparators in other countries.

Table 3.2: Key health outcomes for 10 wealthy countries[26, 27, 28, 29]

	Mortality					Morbidity			
	All-cause mortality per 100,000	CVD deaths per 100,000	Cancer deaths per 100,000	Deaths and injuries from violence per 100,000	Deaths from diabetes per 100,000	Diabetes (adult) %	Obese adults (BMI >30) %		Depression (adults) %
							Men	Women	
USA	505	156	124	53	15	11	30	33	8
Australia	378	117	119	30	10	10	25	25	·
Canada	401	119	126	32	13	10	25	24	·
France	398	138	138	38	8	8	17	15	6
Germany	440	128	128	25	11	12	23	19	3
Italy	383	124	124	25	12	8	19	15	3
Netherlands	427	147	147	22	10	8	17	17	5
Spain	398	122	122	23	9	11	25	23	4
Sweden	410	116	116	32	9	6	18	15	·
UK	462	137	137	26	5	7	24	25	·

In historical terms, the relatively poor health performance of the US has been a relatively recent phenomenon, largely dating back to the 1980s (and paralleling the escalation of the 'Scottish health effect', as examined later in this chapter).[30] Through to the 1940s the US had one of the healthiest populations in the world. In the 19th century, for example, it was not a case of a US health disadvantage so much as a health *advantage*: Americans were taller and had longer life expectancies than their European counterparts. In the mid-19th century, Americans were between 3cm and 9cm taller than Europeans, and even during the 17th century, American men averaged around 173cm, something that Europeans did not achieve until the post-war era.[31] Likewise, life expectancies were higher in the US than Western European countries from the 1700s to the turn of the 19th century. Americans have, however, gone – in a short epidemiological time frame – from being the tallest and healthiest population in the immediate post-war period to being the fattest and least healthy of all wealthy countries today.[32]

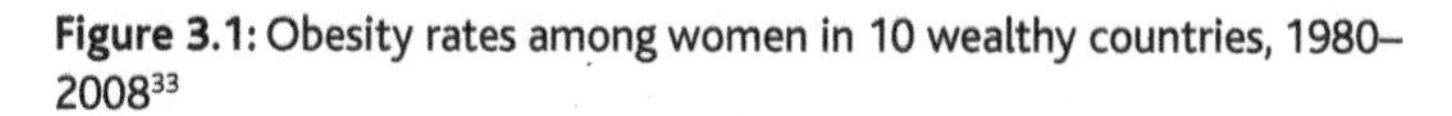

Figure 3.1: Obesity rates among women in 10 wealthy countries, 1980–2008[33]

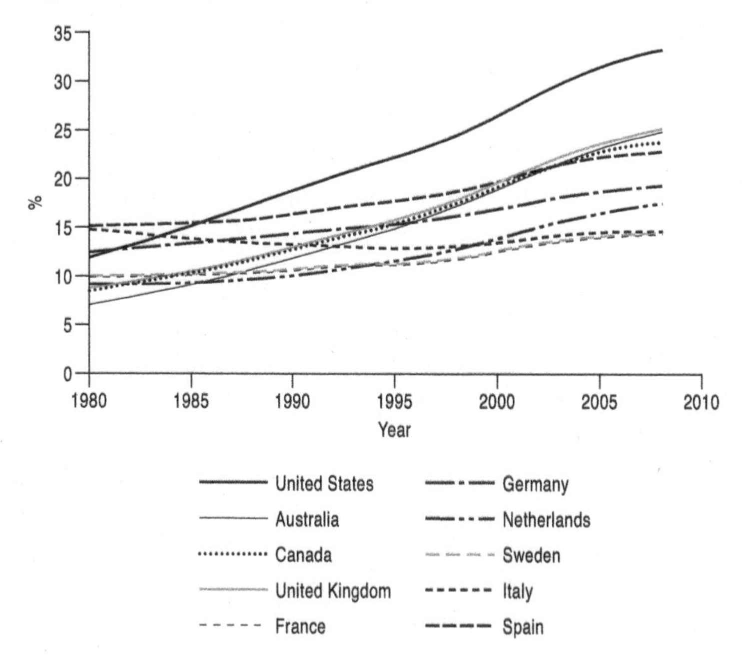

Americans are now considerably shorter than Europeans: the Dutch, Swedes and Norwegians are now the tallest, although the Danes, British, Germans and even the East Germans are also taller than Americans, between 2cm and 6cm taller in fact.[34] In terms of obesity, this is demonstrated in Figures 3.1 and 3.2, which show trends across 10 wealthy countries for 1980 to 2008. The US has by far the highest rates, and they have increased at a much more rapid pace than in other comparable countries. For women, the US obesity rate (33%) is twice that of France, Italy and Sweden (all 15%), and more than 30% higher than the UK (25%). Likewise for men, the US obesity rate (30%) is almost twice that of France and the Netherlands (both 17%), and 25% more than the UK (24%).

There are also striking regional inequalities in obesity within the US. Figure 3.3 shows the spatial patterning of the obesity epidemic within the US from 1990 to 2010. In 1990, there were 10 states where 10% or less of the population were obese (BMI >30), and none of the states had obesity levels higher

Figure 3.2: Obesity rates among men in 10 wealthy countries, 1980–2008[35]

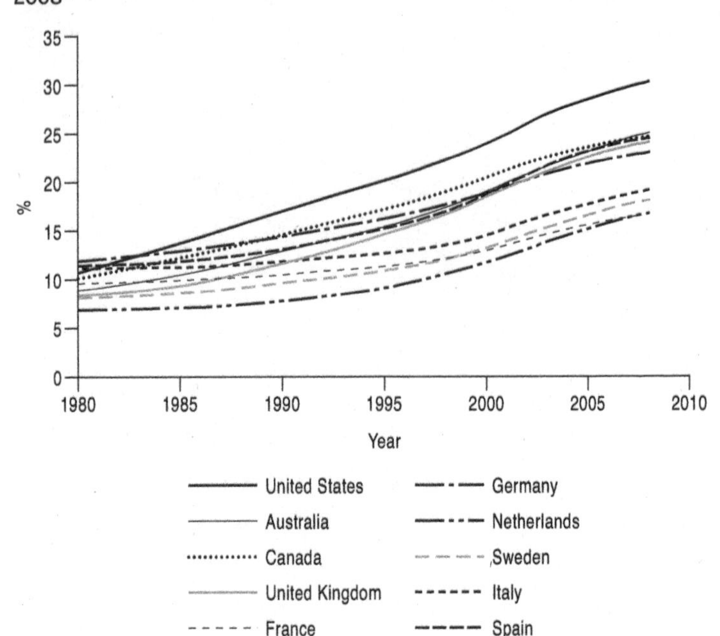

than 15%. However, only 10 years later in 2000, no state had obesity rates that were under 10%, while 23 states were 20-25%. By 2010, no state had less than 20% obesity prevalence, 36 had a prevalence greater than 25%, of which 12 Southern states (Alabama, Arkansas, Kentucky, Louisiana, Michigan, Mississippi, Missouri, Oklahoma, South Carolina, Tennessee, Texas and West Virginia) had rates of over 30%.[36] So, in a 20-year period, obesity rates had doubled in all states, but some states did much worse than others.

Another way of looking at health divides within the US is to return to the use of sports metaphors, looking at how health varies when the Major League Baseball (MLB) teams are used as the geo-reference point, the *Health League Baseball* (HLB). In 2014 the San Francisco Giants won the World Series crown, but which team would win if health data were used?

MLB has two main leagues, the American League and the National League, each of which has three regional sub-leagues of East, Central and West. In the main season, the teams play several series of home and away matches against each of their regional sub-league opponents as well as inter-league games against the teams in the closest regional sub-leagues of the other national league (for example, American League West teams play National League West teams). The winners of each regional league as well as two wildcards for each national league go through to the

Figure 3.3: Emergence of the obesity epidemic in the US, 1990–2010[37]

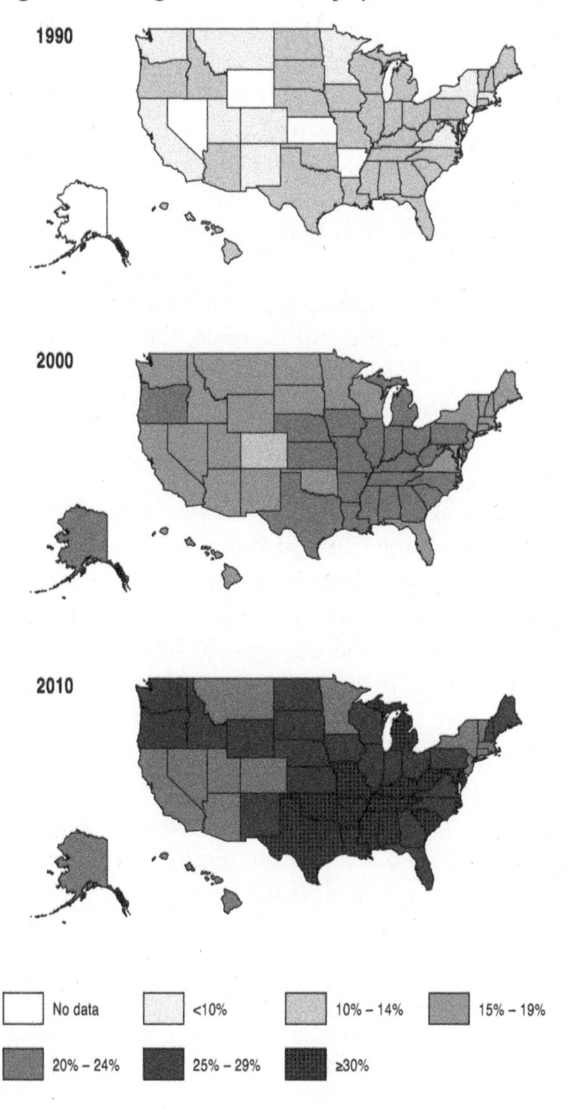

play-off season, a knock-out system between the best teams of the American League and the National League. The ultimate game of this is the World Series between the best American League team and the best National League team. Regional league winners and wildcard teams are determined in terms of their win percentage (as there are no draws/ties in baseball).

The HLB uses US county-level life expectancy data for men and women obtained from the Robert Woods Johnson Foundation[38] and Statistics Canada[39] for the areas local to the 30 2014–15 MLB clubs (Toronto data is for the province of Ontario, Canada). For the HLB, a simplified version of the MLB structure is used whereby each team plays a total of 18 games in the main season as follows: a series of two games against each of their regional sub-league rivals, one at home (male life expectancy) and one away (female life expectancy) (8 games), and a series of two inter-league home and away games against all the teams in the corresponding regional sub-league of the other national league (10 games, for example, San Francisco of the League 2 West would play the teams in the League 1 West). The team with the highest local life expectancy (using the zip code of their stadium as the geo-reference) wins the game. In the event of a tied game, each team is given half a win (0.50) and half a loss (0.50), as there are no ties/draws in baseball (for example, Chicago W against Chicago C is a tie in terms of life expectancy as the health data for each team is for Cook County). As with the real MLB, the six regional league winners (highest win percentages for each of the six regional sub-leagues) and four wildcards (the two teams in each of the two national leagues with the highest percentage win of all the teams that did not win their own leagues) go through to the play-offs. For the play-offs only female life expectancy is used in the head-to-head games.

Table 3.3 shows the outcomes of the main season games for each league, while Figure 3.4 shows the results of the play-off season. In the main season in the HLB League 1, Toronto wins the East Regional League (win rate 97.2%) with life expectancies of 79.0 (men) and 84.0 (women); Minnesota wins the Central Regional League (win rate 100%) with life expectancies of 78.6 (men) and 82.6 (women); Los Angeles A wins the West Regional League (win rate 94.4%) with life expectancies of 80.1 (men)

Table 3.3: Health League Baseball main season leagues 1 and 2

HLB League 1			
Team	Home	Away	Win %
EAST			
Toronto	79.0	84.0	0.972
New York Y	75.0	81.2	0.555
Boston	76.4	80.7	0.527
Tampa Bay	74.7	80.5	0.277
Baltimore	68.9	76.0	0.000
CENTRAL			
Minnesota	78.6	82.6	1.00
Chicago W	75.8	81.0	0.833
Cleveland	74.8	79.9	0.527
Kansas City	73.9	78.9	0.222
Detroit	72.2	78.0	0.055
WEST			
Los Angeles A	80.1	83.8	0.944
Seattle	79.3	83.3	0.833
Oakland	79.2	83.1	0.666
Houston	76.1	80.7	0.222
Texas	76.0	80.2	0.055

HLB League 2			
Team	Home	Away	Win %
EAST			
New York M	79.0	83.8	0.916
Miami	77.5	83.4	0.777
Washington	76.9	80.7	0.583
Atlanta	74.8	79.6	0.277
Philadelphia	71.5	78.4	0.055
CENTRAL			
Chicago C	75.8	81.0	0.833
Pitsburgh	75.3	80.6	0.666
Cincinnati	74.8	79.0	0.416
Milwaukee	74.2	79.6	0.333
St Louis	69.7	78.4	0.000
WEST			
San Francisco	78.8	84.4	0.777
San Diego	78.9	82.9	0.555
Los Angeles D	78.4	83.0	0.500
Arizona	77.6	82.2	0.333
Colorado	75.1	80.5	0.055

and 83.8 (women). The two League 1 wildcards are Seattle (win rate 83.3%, life expectancies of 79.3 and 83.3) and Chicago W (win rate 83.3%, life expectancies of 75.8 and 81.0). For the HLB League 2, New York M win the East Regional League (win rate 91.6%) with life expectancies of 79.0 (men) and 83.8 (women); Chicago C win the Central Regional League (win rate 83.3%) with life expectancies of 75.8 (men) and 81.0 (women); and San Francisco win the West Regional League (win rate 77.7%) with life expectancies of 78.8 (men) and 84.4 (women). The two wildcards are Miami (win rate 77.7%, life expectancies of 77.5 and 83.4) and Pittsburgh (win rate 66.6%, life expectancies of 75.3 and 80.6).

These 10 teams go through to the play-off season, which, for simplicity, only uses female life expectancy (see Figure 3.4). The World Series final game is played between Toronto and San Francisco, and, just as in the real 2014 MLB World Series, San Francisco emerge as the champions of the HLB with life expectancy of 84.4 for women. In terms of famous baseball rivalries, Boston beat New York Y in terms of male life expectancy

(76.4 vs 75.0) but New York Y win on female life expectancy (81.2 vs 80.7) while San Francisco beat Los Angeles D in both male (78.8 vs 78.4) and female (84.4 vs 83.0) life expectancies.

As with the European Health Championship, HLB has a serious purpose as it demonstrates the stark differences in health across a single country – in this case, the US. Life expectancy varies for women, from 76.0 for Baltimore City County to 84.4 in San Francisco County, a gap of over eight years. The health divide for men in the HLB is even greater as there is an 11-year life expectancy gap between men in Baltimore City County (where the Orioles play, 68.9 years) and the men in Orange County where the LA Dodgers play (80.1 years). In Chapters 4 and 5 the underpinning reasons for such stark differences in life and death are examined.

Figure 3.4: Health League Baseball play-off season

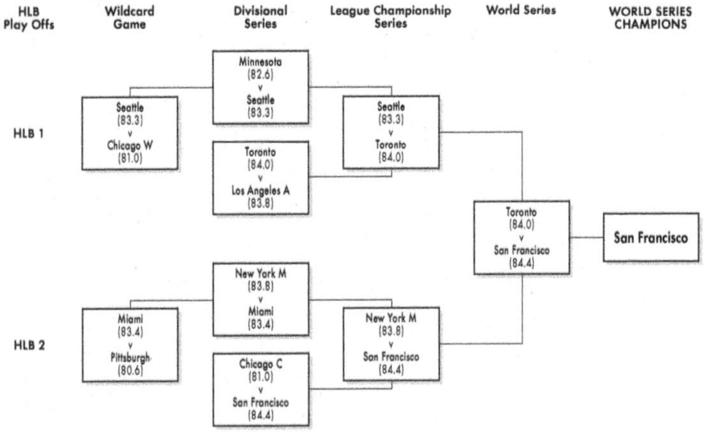

The sick man of Europe

This section examines how health varies between the countries of the UK, with a particular focus on the 'Scottish health effect'. It also examines differences between the East and West of Scotland. Table 3.4 shows differences between the four countries of the UK for the main contemporary causes of death and disease today.

Table 3.4: Key health outcomes for men and women across the countries of the UK[40-49]

	England			Scotland			Wales			Northern Ireland		
	Men	Women	All	Men	Women	All	Men	Women	All	Men	Women	All
Cardiovascular disease deaths (per 100,000)[a]	350.0	240.2	289.4	416.6	292.4	347.3	389.2	265.6	320.6	374.0	254.6	307.0
Cancer deaths (per 100,000)[b]	200.8	145.7	-	235.1	171.8	-	209.3	153.1	-	212.0	150.1	-
Suicide rate (per 100,000)[c]	-	-	10.7	-	-	14.0	-	-	15.6	-	-	17.0
Life expectancy at birth (years)[d]	78.7	82.7	-	76.2	80.6	-	77.8	82.0	-	77.4	81.8	-
Obesity prevalence (percentage)[e]	-	-	25.0	-	-	27.1	-	-	22.0	-	-	25.0
Disability Free Life expectancy at birth (years)[f]	64.5	65.0	-	60.6	64.0	-	61.7	62.9	-	59.9	61.0	-

[a] Age standardised 2014
[b] Age standardised 2010
[c] Age standardised 2013, except for Northern Ireland (crude rate)
[d] 2011
[e] BMI >25, 2013
[f] 2011

This demonstrates a clear Scottish effect, with Scotland performing worst on all health counts. For example, in terms of obesity, over 27% of Scottish adults are obese compared to 25% in England and Northern Ireland and 22% in Wales. Likewise in terms of the leading causes of death – cancer and CVD – rates are much higher in Scotland, and particularly for men. Death rates from CVD and cancer are almost 20% higher among Scottish men compared to English men; life expectancy is two years less and disability free life expectancy is almost five years less. Suicide rates are substantially higher in Scotland (14/100,000) compared to England (11/100,000), although Scotland fares better here than Wales or Northern Ireland. Indeed, overall Scotland has one of the worst health profiles in Europe, and has been characterised by a slower rate of improvement in life expectancy compared with other Western European nations since the 1950s (see Table 3.5).[50] This has been called the 'Scottish health effect'.

During the 19th century and in the early 20th century, the health of Scots was equivalent to that of the citizens of other wealthy countries. However, since 1950, and particularly since 1980, mortality rates in Scotland have become worse than those of similar countries such as England, Wales and Northern Ireland (see Figure 3.5).[51] The 'Scottish effect' is most marked among working-age Scots, more among men than women, and is more pronounced in the West than across Scotland as a whole.[52] This has led to descriptions of Scotland as being the 'sick man of Europe'.

Health divides are also present within Scotland, as demonstrated in Figure 3.6, which maps life expectancy differences for men and women across Scotland. These maps show stark regional inequalities in health with an East–West divide: life expectancy is worse in the West of Scotland than in the East. Indeed, the West Central region of Scotland (the Greater Glasgow area) has some of the worst health outcomes in Western Europe, with particularly high rates of premature mortality among men.[53] It also has some of the towns and cities with the lowest life expectancies in Europe, with men in Glasgow City living an average of 73 years and women 78 years. This is 7.5 years less than men and 5 years less than women living in East Dunbartonshire, the area of Scotland with the highest life expectancies for both men and women. This has led to discussions of a 'Glasgow health effect' in addition to the 'Scottish health effect'. (Local inequalities in health in Scotland are looked at in more detail in a later section of this chapter.)

Table 3.5: Life expectancy in Scotland compared to 14 European countries, 2011[54, 55]

Country	Women	Men	All
Scotland	80.9	76.4	78.7
England and Wales	82.9	79.1	81.0
Germany	82.9	78.2	80.5
France	85.0	78.5	81.8
Portugal	83.5	77.2	80.4
Ireland	83.0	78.0	80.8
Spain	85.1	79.3	82.2
Belgium	82.9	77.8	80.4
Austria	83.4	78.1	80.8
Denmark	81.8	77.7	79.8
Finland	83.5	77.2	80.4
Netherlands	82.9	79.2	81.1
Italy	84.8	79.7	82.6
Sweden	83.7	79.8	81.6
Norway	83.4	79.0	81.2

Figure 3.5: Trends in life expectancy – Scotland compared to England and Wales and Northern Ireland, 1940–2010[56]

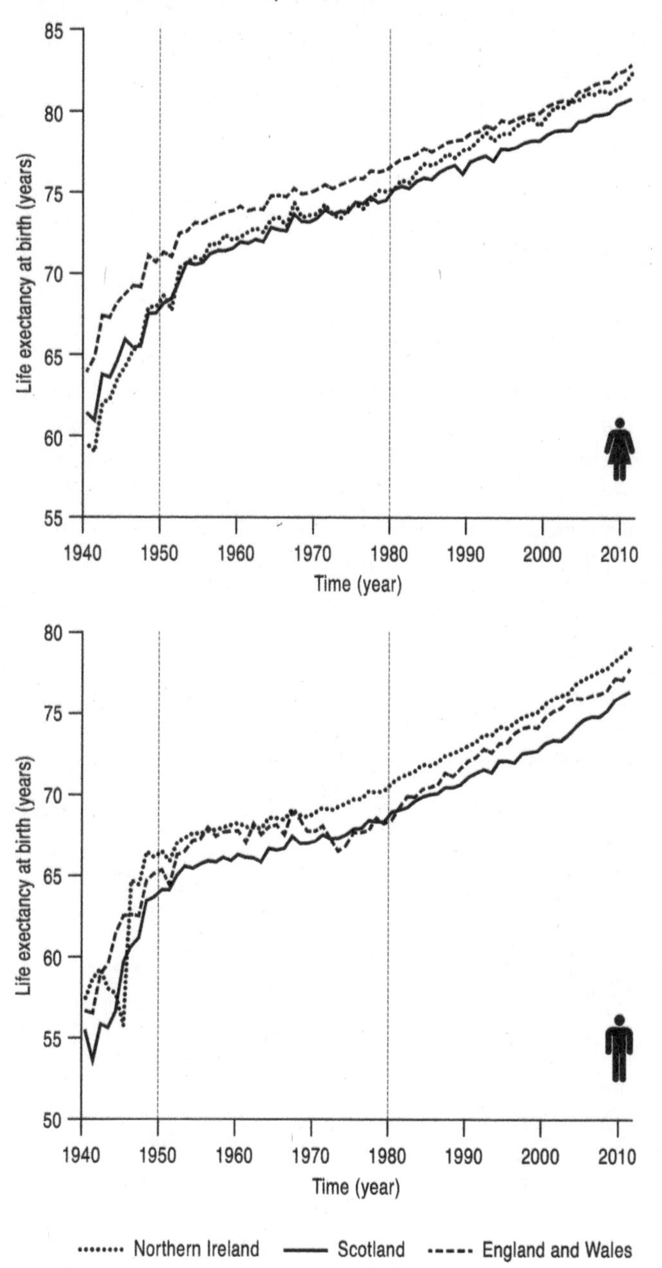

This England

In the previous section, we examined the 'Scottish effect', whereby health in Scotland is worse than that in the other countries of the UK, and England in particular. In this section, we examine in more detail the contemporary nature of the North–South health divide in England, and see the extent of the 'Northern health effect' today. Chapter 2 noted the historical aspects of the North–South divide – the industrial North compared to the rural South. It also discussed its cultural presence within Victorian literature. Today, perceptions of a North and a South still hold a special place within the English imagination, with regular references in popular culture. By way of example, the popular novel and TV series 'Game of Thrones'[57] replicates longstanding English cultural tropes[58] that contrast the stoic, loyal and hardworking Northerners (the Stark family, all with Northern English accents) with the hedonistic, deceitful and immoral Southerners (the Lannister family of Kings Landing). Linking all this, across the 19th to 21st centuries, is a portrayal

Figure 3.6: Life expectancy for men and women by Scottish local authority[59]

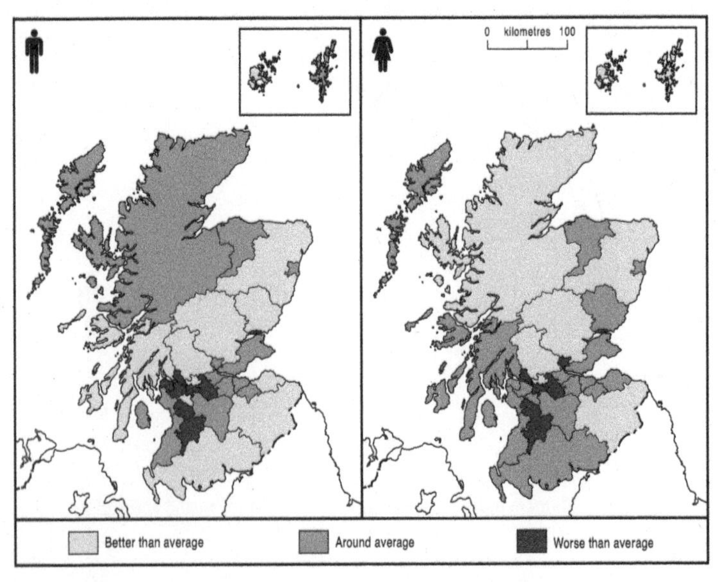

of the North and the South as two different countries, two different types of England.[60] But is this true today?

Before answering this question, there is a need to establish where the dividing line falls between these two regions. But this is not a simple task, as underpinning our conceptions of North and South are longstanding and sometimes controversial historical, cultural, economic, social and political factors. The map in Figure 3.7 demonstrates some of the different ways in which the North has been conceptualised: the Humber-Mersey line, the Severn–Wash line, the historical seven counties of the North, the administrative North, as well as the Lowry line. Perhaps inevitably within a debate that splits England into two

Figure 3.7: Dividing lines between North and South

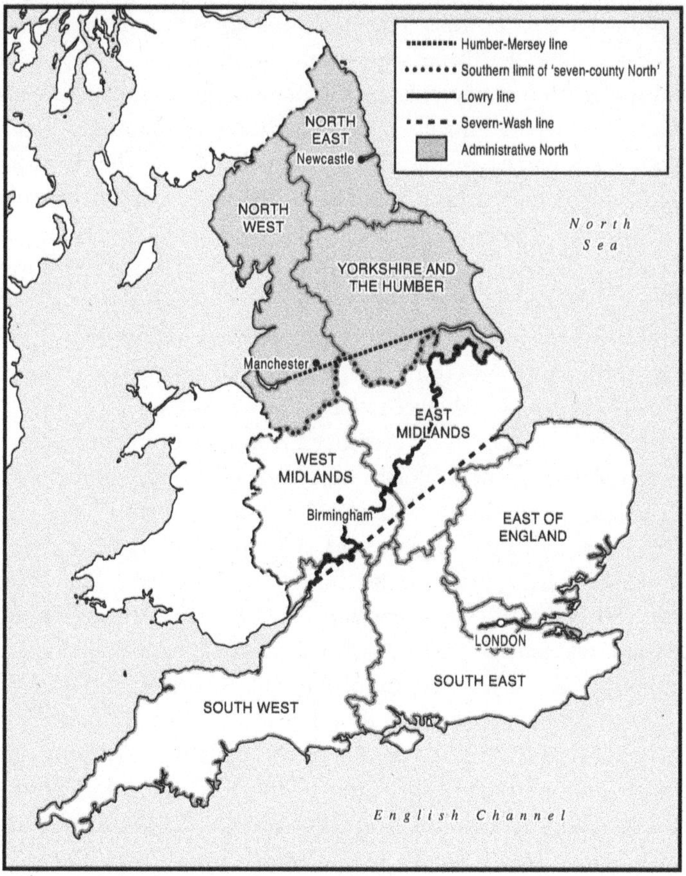

halves, the Midlands (both East and West) are carved up and parts subsumed into either the North or the South.

Historically, the North has existed as a distinct region within England for many centuries, dating back to the ancient Anglo-Saxon kingdom of Northumbria. This existed from the 7th to 10th centuries and stretched from the Scottish borders to just south of the River Humber (today the boundary between the counties of Yorkshire and Lincolnshire) and the River Mersey (just below Manchester and Liverpool), with the southern boundary broadly following the Humber-Mersey line (see Figure 3.7). Some historical researchers have claimed that as early as the 13th century, at least in administrative terms, the southern boundary of the North stretched down to the river Trent (which flows through Nottinghamshire) or the Wash (Lincolnshire and Cambridgeshire border). This generous bounding of the North has been extended by more recent commentators to go as far south as the River Severn, near Gloucester, the so-called Severn-Wash line.[61] This line sits fairly closely to the infamous claim often made in the media that the North starts at the 'Watford Gap' (Northamptonshire). The administrative North (which dates back to the 1994 establishment of Government Offices for the Regions) encompasses three regions: the North East, the North West and Yorkshire and Humber. It encompasses the southern hinterland around the Humber (for example, Grimsby) in the East through to Cheshire in the West. All official data that is available at a regional level reflects these borders.

Russell,[62] in examining Northern arts and culture, identifies a historical seven-county North comprising Cheshire, Cumberland, Durham, Lancashire, Northumberland, Westmorland and Yorkshire. A more recent, and perhaps most controversial, drawing of the North–South border is the Lowry line. This was devised by the social geographer Professor Danny Dorling of the University of Oxford, who used social, economic, health and political data to determine an empirical divide: those living below this line, on average, have better life chances than those living above it (for example, the health penalty of living below the line is one year in life expectancy).[63] This resulted in the Northern border running from Worcester in the West Midlands up to Grimsby in the East Midlands. However, as Russell[64] points out, these broader approaches to the North 'colonise large numbers of people who have no meaningful connection with the region', and it ignores the cultural – and political – nature of Northern identity. The North, it can be argued, is 'as much a state of mind as a place'.[65]

So, while there is a general consensus around the existence of some kind of North–South divide in England,[66] the actual border is contested, and so it needs to be seen as soft and porous rather than hard and clear. There are also divisions within the North, of course, between the 'Far North' of the North East and the 'Near North' of Leeds and Manchester.[67] However, for a book on this topic, especially one that will be presenting data geographically, a clear North–South delineation is required. So this book uses the administrative North of the regions of the North East, North West and Yorkshire and Humber as 'the North'. This is partly a pragmatic decision, so that this book can make use of official regional level data. However, this administrative definition of the North also forms quite a close approximation to the more cultural and historical conceptualisations of the North. For example, the only difference from Russell's[68] cultural-historical seven-county North is the minor addition of two small parts of Lincolnshire that border the Humber (the local authorities of North and North East Lincolnshire, which, from 1974 to 1996, constituted the county of Humberside), and the only major difference with the historic Kingdom of Northumbria is the inclusion of Cheshire. So it can be argued that these three regions are a fair representation of the North as understood in more historical-cultural terms.

Taking the Northern regions of England as the North East, the North West and Yorkshire and Humber, what are they like today?[69] The North East has suffered from sustained economic decline as industries such as coal mining and ship building have virtually disappeared. There has been very little by way of new economic activities to replace these old, high employment industries. It has the highest proportion of workless households and deprivation in any English region. The North West regional economy went through a major period of restructuring and underperformance during the 1980s and 1990s, but since then has grown faster than the England average. The region's employment rate, however, is lower than every other English region except the North East. Yorkshire and the Humber has also experienced significant economic change – in the 1980s and 1990s the region suffered from decline in its traditional industries in coal mining, steel, engineering and textiles. However, in recent years, the region has done relatively well economically, at least in comparison to the North East and North West.

The Southern regions of England are the South East, the East and West Midlands, the East of England, the South West and London. The South East is the most economically successful of England's regions, regularly achieving high growth rates, high economic activity rates and low unemployment. It is the 22nd largest economy in the world. The South East economy is advanced, high income, broadly based and service oriented. In the East Midlands, manufacturing represents around a fifth of economic output, but labour market sectors, such as agriculture, that involve a high percentage of low-skilled jobs, are more dominant in the region. While the economy has relatively high employment and relatively high levels of economic growth, it performs less well than the UK average on productivity. The West Midlands has undergone significant economic changes over the last three decades with the service sector replacing manufacturing as the principal source of employment. The region contributes 8% of the UK's Gross Domestic Product (GDP). However, despite recent improvements, income per head is around 11% lower than the UK average. The East of England has one of the highest long-term economic growth rates in England, benefiting from its proximity to the South East and London. The East of England is the most research and development-intensive region in the UK. Levels of economic growth vary across the region. The South West is a relatively productive and wealthy region, yet there are some persistent pockets of disadvantage. The region is characterised by a largely rural landscape. Over 80% of jobs are in the service sector and tourism is an important part of the local economy. London has the highest productivity rate, and is the world's fourth largest sub-economy. Employment is dominated by the financial, business and creative industries. A third of residents are from minority ethnic groups, and the region contains some areas with high levels of deprivation and unemployment.

Table 3.6 shows a regional breakdown of some key health indicators. It demonstrates that the North–South health divide in life expectancy discussed in Chapter 1 is replicated in other leading causes of death and disease: the Southern regions outperform the Northern ones on all indicators.

Table 3.6: Key health outcomes by English region[70, 71]

	Population (millions)	Life expectancy at birth (LE, years)		CVD deaths (<75 years per 100, 000)	Cancer deaths (<75 years per 100, 000)	Diabetes % (> 17 years)	% Obese or overweight (> 16 years)
		Men	Women				
NORTH[a]	**15**	**78**	**81.9**	**89.6**	**161.4**	**6.5**	**66.5**
North East	2.6	78	81.7	88.8	169.5	6.5	68.0
North West	7.1	78	81.8	92.8	159.8	6.5	66.0
Yorkshire and Humber	5.3	78.5	82.2	87.3	155.0	6.4	65.4
SOUTH[b]	**38**	**79.8**	**83.6**	**74.3**	**138.7**	**6.2**	**63.3**
East Midlands	4.5	79.3	83.0	80.0	143.8	6.6	65.6
West Midlands	5.6	78.8	82.8	82.1	147.8	7.1	65.7
East of England	5.8	80.3	83.8	70.0	136.0	6.0	65.1
South West	5.3	80.1	83.8	80.1	136.5	6.0	57.3
London	8.2	80.0	84.1	66.4	134.0	5.6	63.1
South East	8.6	80.4	83.9	67.1	134.3	5.9	62.7
ENGLAND	**53**	**79.4**	**83.1**	**78.2**	**144.4**	**6.2**	**63.8**

[a] Author calculated mean of NE, NW, YH; [b] Author calculated mean of EE, EM, L, WM, SE. SW.

The North East of England (where I currently live) is one of the worst performers on all health outcomes, while the South East (where I was born) is one of the top performers. By way of example, cancer mortality rates are 25% higher in the North East than the South East. However, other Southern regions are the best performers on other health outcomes. For example, in the North East of England, 7 out of 10 adults are obese or overweight compared to 6 out of 10 in the South West (this is still, of course, very high by historical standards).

Beyond the regional averages, the Northern health effect can also be demonstrated by looking at data by local authority. Figures 3.8 and 3.9 show life expectancy at birth for men and women in England by local authority. The maps show that the North–South divide, at least in terms of life expectancy, is more evident among women than men. They also show that there are areas of lower than average life expectancy in the South (such as Portsmouth on the south coast) and areas of above-average life expectancy in the North (such as North Yorkshire), but these are very evidently exceptions.

We can also look at which English local authorities perform the best and the worst in terms of our key health indicators. This is demonstrated in Tables 3.7 and 3.8, which show the top five and bottom five of English local authorities. In each case, the top five local authorities are in the South, and the bottom five are predominantly in the North. The notable exception

Figure 3.8: Map of life expectancy for men in England by local authority, 2011[72]

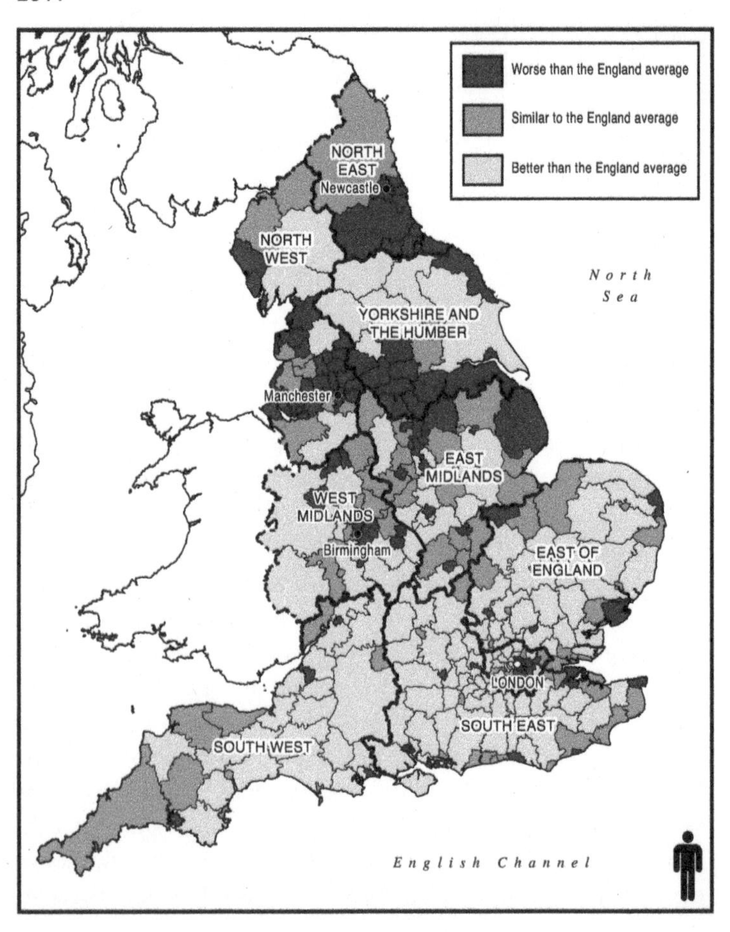

to the latter is the dominance of Southern local authorities in terms of the worst places for diabetes (which could be a result of older populations as the data is not adjusted for age; there is more on this in Chapter 4). The obesity/overweight 'hotspots' are predominantly (although not exclusively) in the North. This is further demonstrated in Figure 3.10, which maps obesity and overweight by local authority in England.

The Northern face of obesity is something that is regularly commented on in the popular media, as the headline in Figure 3.11 demonstrates.

Figure 3.9: Map of life expectancy for women in England by local authority, 2011[73]

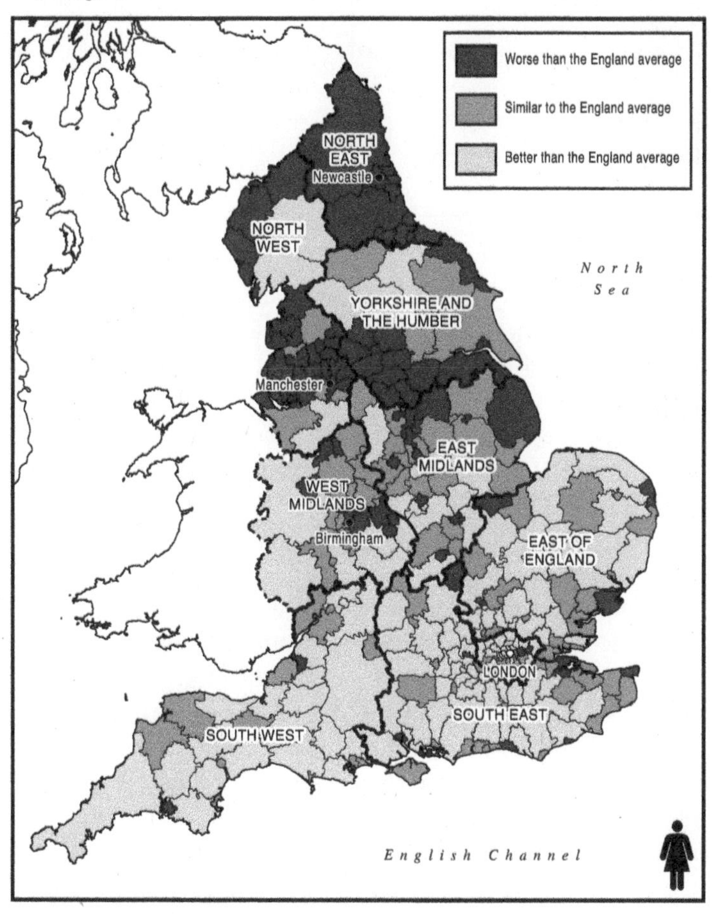

Table 3.7: Top five English local authorities for key health indicators[74]

CVD deaths (<75 years per 100,000)[a]		Cancer deaths (<75 years per 100,000)[a]		Diabetes % (> 17 years)[a]		% Obese or overweight (> 16 years)[b]	
Dorset	52.1	Harrow	104.0	City of London	2.6	Kensington and Chelsea	46.0
Surrey	54.4	Kensington and Chelsea	116.3	Richmond upon Thames	3.7	Tower Hamlets	47.2
Wokingham	54.9	Barnet	118.0	Isles of Scilly	3.8	Richmond upon Thames	47.6
Kensington and Chelsea	54.9	Rutland	119.3	Camden	3.9	Hackney	48.7
Richmond upon Thames	55.9	Buckinghamshire	120.0	Brighton and Hove	4.1	Brighton and Hove	49.2
England Average	78.2		144.4		6.2		63.8

[a] 2011-2013; [b] 2009-2011

Table 3.8: Bottom five English local authorities for key health indicators[75]

CVD deaths (<75 years per 100,000)[a]		Cancer deaths (<75 years per 100,000)[a]		Diabetes % (> 17 years)[a]		% Obese or overweight (> 16 years)[b]	
Manchester	137.0	Manchester	198.9	Leicester	8.7	Doncaster	74.4
Blackpool	125.2	Liverpool	195.2	Walsall	8.6	County Durham	72.5
Tameside	121.2	Middlesbrough	194.4	Harrow	8.5	Milton Keynes	72.5
Hackney	116.3	Kingston upon Hull	192.2	Sandwell	8.3	Blackpool	72.1
Salford	115.9	South Tyneside	192.0	Slough	8.2	Northumberland	71.9
England Average	78.2		144.4		6.2		63.8

[a] 2011-2013; [b] 2009-2011

Disturbingly, the North–South health divide is growing – since 1965, the Northern health penalty (excess mortality compared to the South) averaged at around 14%, or 1.5 million excess premature deaths.[76] Between 1965 and 1995, there was no health gap between younger Northerners (aged 20–34) and their Southern counterparts. However, now mortality is 20% higher among young people living in the North.[77] The health divide is now highest among those aged 0–9 and 40–74 and lower for those aged 10–39 and over 75. Overall, the North has 20% more premature deaths (deaths before aged 75) than the South, a consistent and increasing pattern between 1965 and 2008.[78] This is particularly the case for the most deprived areas. Figure 3.12 shows how the health of deprived areas (defined as the 20% most deprived of the English local authorities) in the North has become worse than the health of equally deprived areas in the South. It shows how, since 2001, life expectancy in deprived Southern areas has improved more quickly than in deprived Northern areas. On average, people living in the most

Figure 3.10: Percentage of the adult population that is obese or overweight, by English local authority[79]

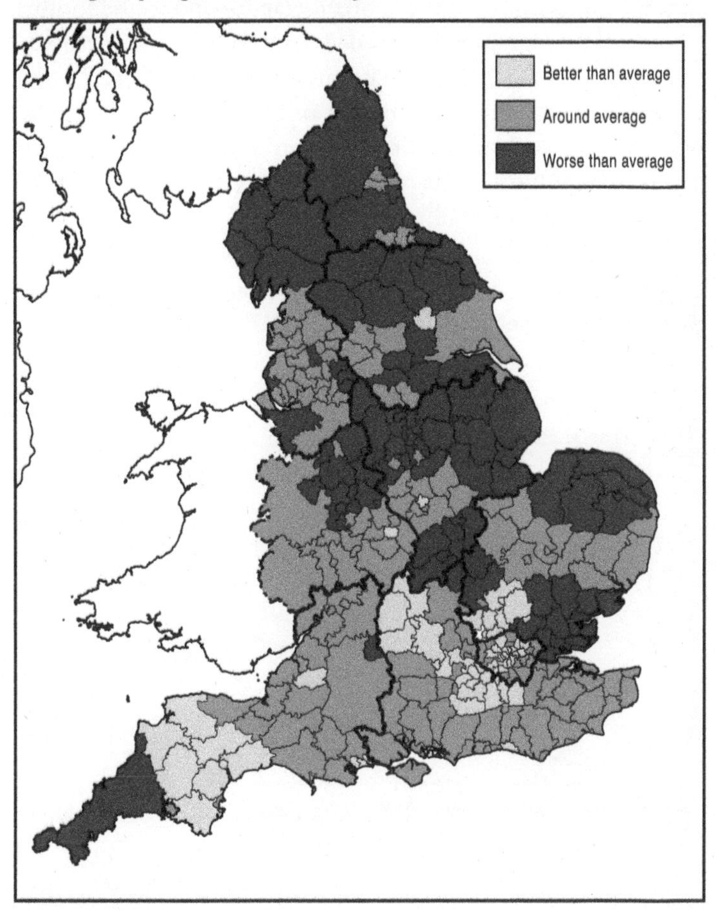

Figure 3.11: *Daily Mirror* headline, 27 October 2014

Which region is Britain's FATTEST? (Clue: two-thirds of northerners are now obese)

deprived local authorities in the South have a life expectancy of around six months longer than those in the North: the North is falling behind.

Another way to think about differences in health in England is to return once more to the sports metaphor and to use football teams as the geographical reference point. Bill Shankly (manager of Liverpool FC, 1959–74) famously commented that "Some people believe football is a matter of life and death, I am very disappointed with that attitude. I can assure you it is much, much more important than that." So what if football really was a matter of life and death?

Figure 3.12: Comparison of trends in life expectancy in deprived areas in the North and the South of England since 2001[80]

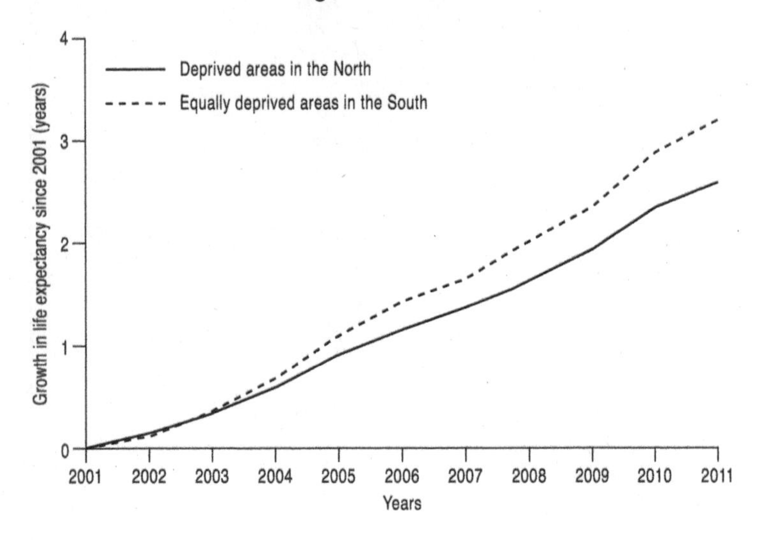

Table 3.9 shows a Public Health League (PHL) that ranks the 2014–15 Premier League football clubs from best to worst, using health indicators:

P (played)	Percentage of smokers
W (won)	Weight – percentage of obesity and overweight
D (drawn)	Deaths – all-cause mortality rates per 100,000 people
L (lost)	Life expectancy for males in years
F (for)	Female life expectancy in years
A (against)	Alcohol-related hospital admissions per 100,000 people
GD (goal difference)	Gap or difference in life expectancy for men between the most and least deprived areas of the local authority in years
Pts (points)	Points representing the sum of ranks for each health indicator

The final league points (Pts) represent the sum of ranks for each outcome. For example, Chelsea's Championship winning score of 114 points comes from ranking 18th for P, 19th for W, D, L, F and A and 1st for GD, where 19 is the best score and 1 the worst (ranks are 1-19 not 1-20, as Liverpool and Everton have the same data, as their grounds, Anfield and Goodison, are in the same local authority, only 1 mile apart). Premier League clubs are geo-referenced to the local authority with which they are most associated (for example, Manchester United data is for Trafford Council, Chelsea FC is represented by data from the Royal Borough of Kensington and Chelsea, Swansea is represented by data from the local health board although the Welsh average is used for the alcohol variable A).

Imagine the newspaper headlines if, on the final day of the 2014–15 season, three of the biggest English football clubs were relegated from the Premier League: Manchester City, Everton and Liverpool. Sounds unbelievable, but this is exactly what would happen if football were really a matter of 'life and death', as the PHL shows. Chelsea would still be the champions, but it would be Crystal Palace, Manchester United and Tottenham joining them in the top four.

Table 3.9: Public Health League, 2014–15[81]

		Public Health League								
		Team	P	W	D	L	F	A	GD	Pts
C	1	Chelsea	18	46	786	83	86	426	14	114
	2	Tottenham	19	59	904	80	85	653	7	114
	3	Crystal Palace	17	62	968	80	84	526	9	105
	4	Man Utd	20	60	920	80	84	560	9	103
	5	West Ham	19	57	1060	79	83	620	7	100
	6	QPR	21	50	936	79	84	631	9	97
	7	Arsenal	22	54	1025	78	83	849	5	89
	8	Aston Villa	19	64	1062	78	82	691	8	80
	9	Southampton	22	65	1053	78	83	726	8	73
	10	Leicester	24	57	1078	77	82	573	8	72
	11	Swansea	24	56	1065	78	82	562	12	66
	12	Burnley	20	65	1297	78	82	698	10	57
	13	West Brom	23	66	1112	77	81	791	8	52
	14	Newcastle	24	60	1110	78	82	828	12	47
	15	Stoke	19	67	1198	77	81	996	10	38
	16	Sunderland	23	69	1203	77	81	1071	10	33
	17	Hull	29	60	1210	77	81	837	12	31
R	18	Man City	24	63	1280	76	80	852	9	30
R	19	Everton	23	67	1206	76	81	810	10	29
R	20	Liverpool	23	67	1206	76	81	810	10	29

In terms of local derbies (nearest neighbour rivalries), if health outcomes are used then, for example, the Merseyside derby between Liverpool and Everton would be a draw (on all outcomes), Manchester United, who play in red, would win the Manchester derby against Manchester City, who play in blue (for example, death rates on the red side of the city are lower),

Tottenham would win the North London derby with Arsenal (for example, female life expectancy is higher in the Tottenham locale), while Newcastle would win the North East derby with Sunderland (for example, alcohol-related hospital admissions are lower in Newcastle).

Apart from throwing up some unusual league places – at least in football terms – the PHL also further demonstrates the extent of the North–South divide in health in England: the top half of the table is dominated by Southern clubs, and the relegated trio are all from the North West. The contrast between champions Chelsea and relegated Manchester City in terms of life expectancy is immense, at 7 years for men and 6 years for women.

The PHL also demonstrates the local health inequalities that exist within our towns and cities with, for example, Manchester United who qualify for the Champions League (with data from Trafford Council) faring much better than their 'noisy neighbours' – relegated Manchester City (with data from Manchester City Council). Life expectancy for men and women on the red side of Greater Manchester is four years higher than for those on the blue side, only a couple of miles down the road. Further, even within local authorities there are high inequalities in life chances with, for example, a 14-year gap in male life expectancy between the most and least deprived areas of Chelsea. These local health inequalities are the subject of the next section.

All cities have a North

These regional differences in health are replicated at a smaller geographical scale, with local health divisions within major towns and cities of wealthy countries as stark today as they were in Victorian times: all cities have a north. Indeed, many of the places that were poor and unhealthy in the past are poor and unhealthy today.[82] This section examines these localised health inequalities in the UK, North America and Europe in general terms before looking in more detail at particular examples of health divides in Liverpool, Manchester, Newcastle and Stockton-on-Tees in England, as well as local urban health divides in Washington DC in the US and Paris (France). These cities were also examples in Chapter 2 that discussed health in the 19th century.

Table 3.10 ranks the top five and bottom five local authorities in England in terms of the gaps in life expectancy for men and women between neighbourhoods across each local authority (LSOAs, see Chapter 1). The highest divide in life expectancy within one local authority in years is in Stockton-on-Tees in the North East at over 17 for men and 11.5 for women, the lowest divide for men is 2.4 years in Barking and Dagenham in London and for women it is in Islington in London where the difference is less than one year. The gaps are significantly larger for men than for women. All but one (Bedford) of the five local authorities with the highest health inequalities for women are in the North, although for men there is no clear North–South divide in this table, with areas like Kensington and Chelsea in London exhibiting very high health gaps. However, for both men and women, all of the five with the smallest gaps in life expectancy are in the South.

Figure 3.13 maps local authority life expectancy gaps across all of England. It also shows a clear spatial patterning with the authorities with the highest health gaps falling largely within the North. However, deprivation is not exclusively Northern

Table 3.10: Top and bottom five English local authorities ranked by inequalities in life expectancy across neighbourhoods[83]

	Top Five Local Authorities (smallest health divides)	Region[a]	Life Expectancy Gap in years 2012-2013[b]	Bottom Five Local Authorities (largest health divides)	Region[a]	Life Expectancy Gap in years 2012-2013[b]
	Barking and Dagenham	South (L)	2.4	Stockton-on-Tees	North (NE)	17.3
	Slough	South (SE)	4.5	Kensington and Chelsea	South (L)	14.3
Men	Brent	South (L)	4.7	Middlesbrough	North (NE)	14.2
	Kingston upon Thames	South (L)	4.8	North East Lincolnshire	South (EE)	12.7
	Greenwich	South (L)	4.8	Derby	South (EE)	12.4
	Islington	South (L)	0.6	Stockton-on-Tees	North (NE)	11.5
	Redbridge	South (L)	2.1	Bedford	South (EE)	11.1
Women	Telford and Wrekin	South (WM)	2.1	Sefton	North (NW)	10.4
	Bracknell Forest	South (SE)	2.4	Salford	North (NW)	10.3
	Oxfordshire	South (SE)	2.5	Newcastle upon Tyne	North (NE)	10.1

[a] EE = East of England; L = London; NE = North East; NW = North West; SE = South East; SW = South West; WM = West Midlands.
[b] Rounded to one decimal place

and all towns and cities across the UK have areas that are more deprived than others – leading to ubiquitous local health divides. By way of example, Table 3.11 shows how the key health outcomes vary across deprived to affluent areas of Scotland. This shows that people living in the most deprived neighbourhoods of Scotland have a death rate from coronary heart disease that is twice as high as those living in the most affluent areas (using the Scottish version of the IMD, as discussed in Chapter 1). It also shows that cancer deaths are 70% higher. There is a 10-year life expectancy gap between the most and least deprived areas and a

Figure 3.13: Map of English local authorities by the deprivation gap in average life expectancy[84]

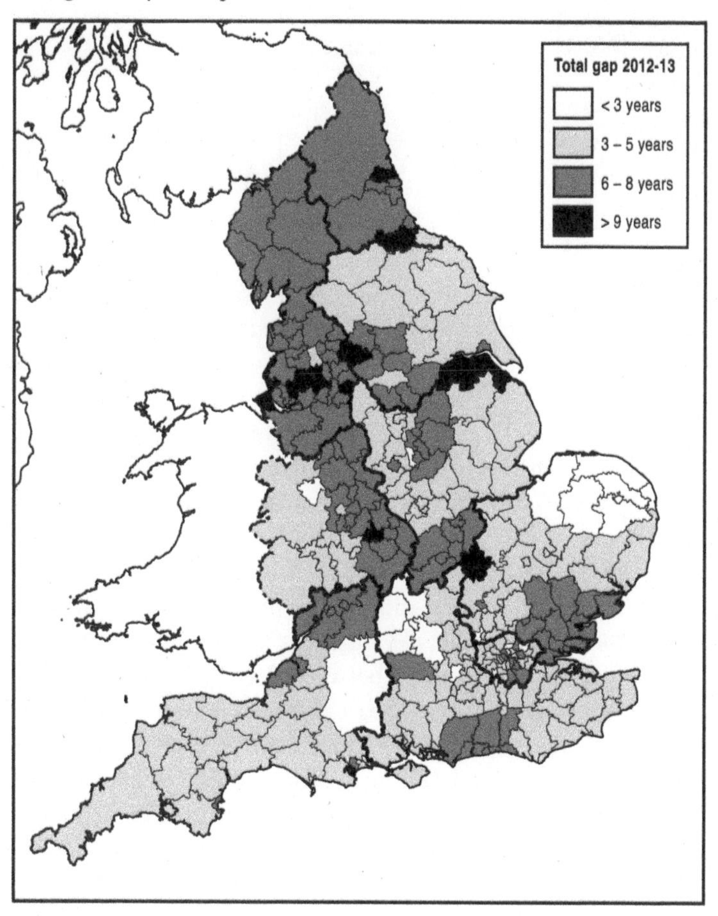

20-year gap in terms of healthy life expectancy – for both men and women. Obesity rates are 70% higher among women living in the most deprived areas compared to the least deprived areas and 20% higher for men – over a third of women in deprived areas are obese compared to less than a fifth in more affluent areas. A clear gradient is evident for each of the key health outcomes, with every step up the ladder of area level affluence accompanied by a decrease in mortality and morbidity. Diabetes is also twice as prevalent in the most deprived compared to the least deprived areas.[85]

Table 3.11: Key health outcomes by deprivation quintile, Scotland[86-89]

		CHD deaths per 100,000	Cancer deaths per 100,000	Life expectancy (years)		Healthy life expectancy (years)		Obesity % (BMI > 30)	
		All	All	Men	Women	Men	Women	Men	Women
Most deprived	Quintile 1	212	439	71.3	77.2	48.3	51.5	29	33
	Quintile 2	183	369	75.1	79.5	56.4	58.3	27	32
	Quintile 3	167	322	77.3	81.5	61.0	63.7	26	29
	Quintile 4	133	283	79.5	82.8	65.7	66.8	26	28
Least deprived	Quintile 5	110	257	81.7	84.0	69.1	71.9	24	19

The spatial gradient – whereby every step up the area-level deprivation ladder is associated with better health outcomes – is common to all high-income countries. For example, a study in Germany found an association between neighbourhood deprivation and the prevalence of diabetes and obesity – diabetes and obesity rates increased with increasing deprivation for both men and women.[90] The differences between the most and least deprived were substantial: the risk of diabetes among men in the most deprived neighbourhoods of Germany was 9% compared to 5% in the least deprived, and the risk of obesity among women was 22% compared to 17%. Similarly, in Sweden, research has found strong relationships between level of neighbourhood deprivation and coronary heart disease for both women and men, with the risk of developing coronary heart disease 87% higher for women and 42% higher for men in the most deprived neighbourhoods than in the most affluent neighbourhoods.[91] Likewise in the US, living in highly deprived neighbourhoods is associated with higher average BMI.[92] In Canada, neighbourhood deprivation has been found to be significantly associated with self-reported health status, with every increase in neighbourhood deprivation resulting in a 40% increased risk of reporting fair or poor health.[93] Likewise in France, living in a deprived neighbourhood increases the probability of reporting poor health.[94] In short, local health divides – between neighbourhoods of different levels of deprivation – are universal in wealthy countries.[95] This is explored further through examples of specific towns and cities in the UK and a variety of wealthy countries.

As was the case in the 19th century, there are local health divides present in the North West cities of Liverpool and Manchester. Like many Northern cities, Liverpool experienced significant economic decline over the 20th century. It was particularly affected by deindustrialisation and the closure of the docks in the 1980s (examined further in Chapters 4 and 5), and has areas of sustained and high deprivation, in close proximity to others of relatively high affluence. Today, as the PHL table showed (see Table 3.9), on average, the City of Liverpool continues to have some of the worst health outcomes in England. By way of example, Liverpool has above-average rates of CVD mortality before age 75 at 109 per 100,000 compared to an England average of 78 per 100,000. Likewise for cancer deaths for those under 75, Liverpool has rates of 195 per 100,000 compared to the England average of 144 per 100,000.[96] Further, within the Liverpool city region there are some stark local inequalities in health. These are shown in Figure 3.14, which uses the Mersey rail train line (local public transport system) to visualise spatial inequalities in life expectancy. Average life expectancy drops by 10 years in just a 20-minute rail journey between Formby (a commuter town to the north west of Liverpool, where less than 1 in 20 children live in poverty), where average life expectancy is 83, to Bootle (a small town to the west covering the former docks, where 1 in 5 children experience poverty), where average life expectancy is 73.

Like Liverpool, Manchester has experienced significant economic changes in the later part of the 20th century, and while it has some thriving new sectors (such as finance) resulting in areas of high affluence, it also has some of the highest pockets of unemployment and deprivation in England. This has led to

Figure 3.14: Life expectancy on the Mersey rail system[97]

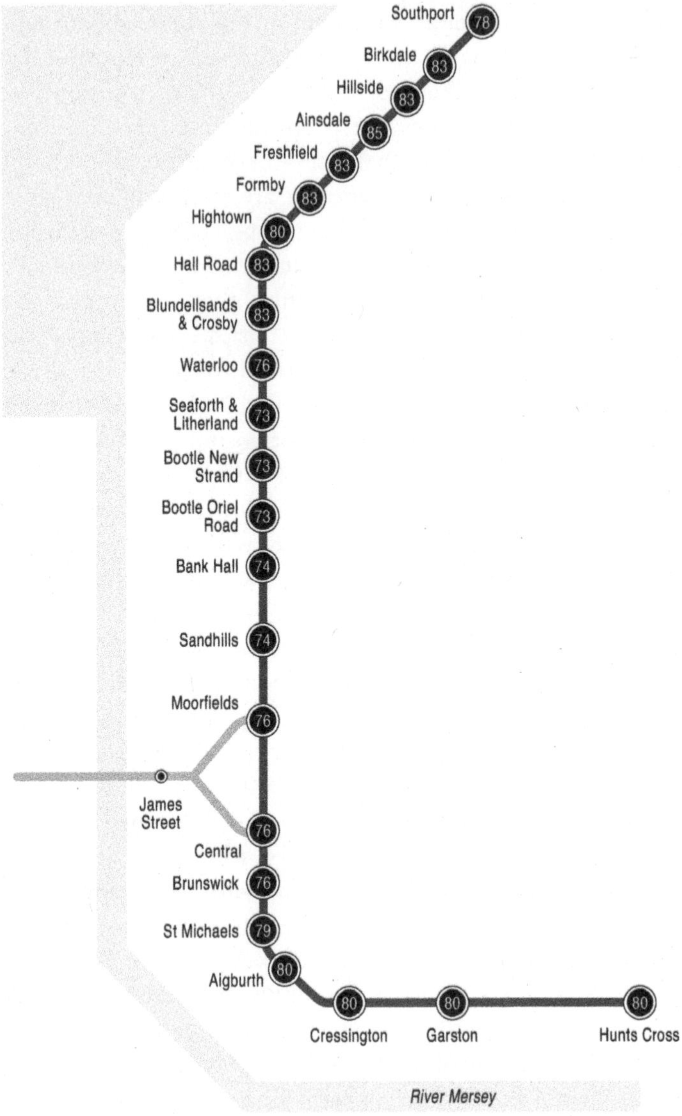

great contrasts across the city with, for example, the ward of Didsbury East in the south of the city being one of the least deprived wards in England (top 20% nationally in terms of its affluence), while the Harpurhey ward in the north of the city is the most deprived ward in Manchester and one of the top 10 most deprived wards in England. Table 3.12 shows how health contrasts between these areas:

Table 3.12: Health outcomes for the Didsbury East and Harpurhey wards of Manchester[98]

Health Indicator	Didsbury East (affluent)*	Harpurhey (deprived)*	Manchester (city average)*	England (national average)*
Bad / very bad health	5%	10%	7%	6%
Limiting long term illness	14%	23%	23%	18%
Obese 11 year olds	15%	25%	25%	19%
Obese adults	15%	26%	26%	24%
Male life expectancy	80 yrs	71 yrs	74 yrs	79 yrs
Female life expectancy	85 yrs	77 yrs	79 yrs	83 yrs
All cause mortality*	87	167	134	100
Cancer mortality**	96	152	127	100
Cardiovascular mortality**	83	152	131	100

* Rounded to nearest whole number

** Standardised Mortality Ratios (SMR) have the average for England as 100; an SMR above 100 is thereby worse than the national average; and an SMR below 100 is better than the national average.

The key health outcomes are worse on all counts in Harpurhey compared to Didsbury East; the latter is consistently better that the English or Manchester average, while the former is consistently worse. For example, bad and very bad self-reported health is twice as high in Harpurhey than Didsbury East (10% compared to 5%); one in four adults and children are obese in Harpurhey compared to only one in seven in Didsbury East; there is a nine-year gap in life expectancy for men and an eight-year gap for women; and mortality rates are significantly higher in Harpurhey than Didsbury East.

Local health inequalities are also evident today in the towns and cities of the North East of England. Newcastle suffered from declining employment since the 1980s and the loss of industrial jobs, particularly in terms of shipping (employment and health is examined further in Chapter 4). Health inequalities in Newcastle are visualised in Figure 3.15, which shows the differences in healthy life expectancy for people aged 55 across the metro system which links the two cities Newcastle and Gateshead. This shows that those aged 55 living near the South Gosforth metro stop (where less than 1 in 10 children experience poverty) can expect to live for a further 17 years in good health (disability and disease free) until they are almost 72 years old. In contrast, those in the nearby area of Byker (where over 2 in 5 children live in poverty) will on average only have an additional 9 years in good health (until they are aged 64). On average then, those over 55 living in Gosforth will have more than twice the number of healthy years ahead of them than those in Byker. These differences in health are on a journey that only takes 10 minutes: 'Rich and poor people live in very different epidemiological worlds, even within the same city.'[99]

Figure 3.15: Healthy life expectancy across the Newcastle metro[100]

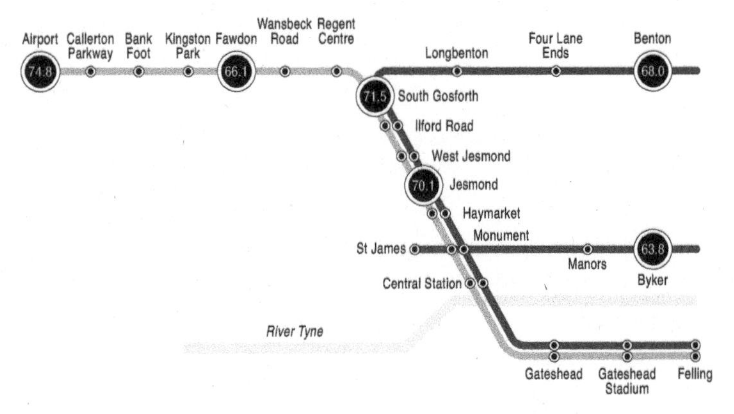

Stockton-on-Tees in the North East of England is a highly differentiated place as it has areas with above-average rates of poverty existing alongside areas that are very affluent: in the town centre ward, almost half of children live in poverty, while in the Hartburn ward only 2 miles away, less than 1 in 10 children live in poverty. This is also reflected in political terms with the borough returning one Conservative and one Labour MP in the 2015 general election. In terms of health inequalities, the gap in life expectancy for men is 17 years between the most (for example, Hartburn) and least affluent (for example, Town Centre) areas – the largest gap within a local authority in England. For women it is 12 years. However, life expectancy is only a headline indicator – it is important to look behind it and to explore what the other health issues are in this area.

Exploring the Stockton health gap in more detail is the subject of a Leverhulme Trust-funded research study by a Durham University team that I am leading.[101] This mixed methods study examines in detail the health of people living in the most and least deprived neighbourhoods (LSOAs, as defined in Chapter 1) of Stockton, areas which, as Figure 3.16 shows, are only a few miles apart.

Table 3.13 shows the underpinning health divides within this small town across a variety of indicators: people living in more deprived areas are more likely to have a health condition (33% higher), a mental health condition (20% higher), CVD (16% higher), a respiratory condition (50% higher), and almost twice as likely (90% more) to have multiple health conditions. In terms of health scores, rates of general wellbeing (EQ5D and EQ-VAS scales), physical health (SF8-PCS) and mental health (WEDMHS and SF-8MCS) are all between 8% and 16% higher in the most deprived areas. BMI is also slightly higher (27 compared to 26 on average). The causes of these health inequalities are multiple (the determinants of the Stockton health gap will be discussed further in the next chapter).

The health divides evident in UK towns and cities are also present internationally: urban health inequalities are universal. In Washington DC, the capital of the US, life expectancy increases about a year-and-a-half for each mile travelled along the metro system, from the deprived and predominantly black South Eastern areas of the city to the affluent white suburbs of Maryland, a gap of 20 years overall.[102] Inequalities in health in Paris in the 19th century were discussed in the previous chapter. Today, differences in life expectancy across the arrondissements of the Ile de Paris (central Paris) stand at five years between people living in the more affluent western arrondissements and those in the less affluent eastern ones. The 1st arrondissement (the location of the Louvre Museum) has an average life expectancy

Figure 3.16: Map of Stockton-on-Tees Study neighbourhoods

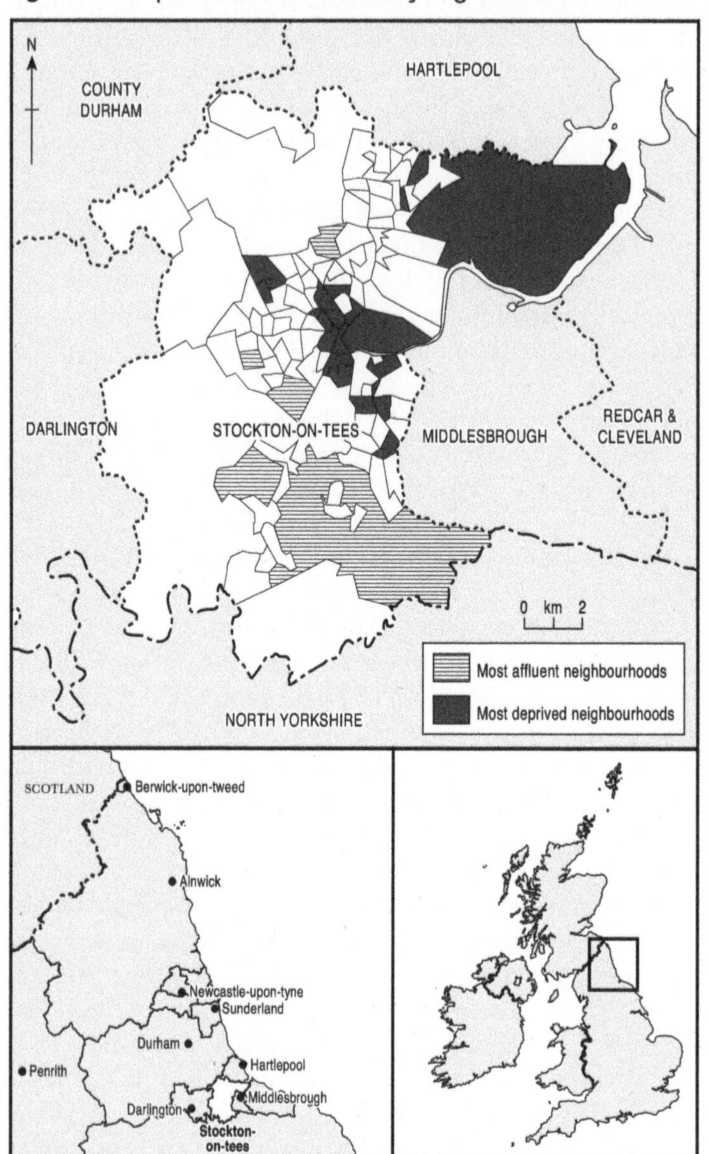

Table 3.13: Health inequalities in Stockton-on-Tees[103]

	Most deprived areas*	Most affluent areas*	Health Gap*
Health Condition			
Any health condition	60%	45%	+33%
Mental health	12%	10%	+20%
Cardiovascular	21%	18%	+16%
Respiratory	12%	8%	+50%
3 or more conditions	19%	10%	+90%
Health Scores			
EQ5D[a]	75	87	+15%
EQ-VAS[b]	64	74	+16%
WEDMHS[c]	50	55	+10%
SF8-MCS[d]	50	54	+8%
SF8-PCS[e]	46	50	+8%
BMI[f]	27	26	+6%

* Rounded to nearest whole number
[a] EQ5D is the European Quality of Life Scale which is a validated and well used measure of health and wellbeing. Higher scores = better health.
[b] EQ-VAS is a visual scale of 1-100 for general health. Higher scores = better health state.
[c] WEDMHS is the Warwick-Edinburgh Mental health Scale. Higher scores = worse health.
[d] SF88-MCS is the short form mental health scale. Higher scores = better health.
[e] SF-8 PCS is the physical component scale. Higher scores = better health.
[f] Body Mass Index

for men and women of 85 (2007 data). In contrast, people living in the 18th arrondissement (where the famous Moulin Rouge is based) have an average life expectancy of 80.

Health where you live

So this chapter has demonstrated how health varies internationally, nationally, regionally and locally, with a breadth of data and a variety of examples. The latter has shown that people living in very close proximity to one another effectively inhabit very different 'epidemiological life worlds',[104] with very different chances of having a healthy and long life. We will explore why this is the case in Chapters 4 and 5. But for now, it is worth thinking more about what health is like where you live. To support this book, there is an interactive explorer of how health and the determinants of health (see Chapter 4) vary across the local authorities of England. Using the explorer, anyone living in England can see what their local area is like by inputting their postcode. The explorer is free to use and is available at www.healthdivides.org.uk. It has details of health as well as education, unemployment rates and so on for each local authority (the latter are examined further in Chapter 4).[105] Using the 'health divides' explorer, I can compare the place where I grew up (Lincoln) with the places where I went to University (Birmingham), as well as where I have worked in the past (Liverpool and Sheffield) with where I now live (Durham). The explorer enables me to build up an area-level health profile – or biography – of the places connected to me. Check out the explorer – what is health like where you live? What it is like where your friends or family live? We use the 'health divides' explorer again in the next chapter, when we start to look at how *place* influences *health* and *why* it is that *where you live can kill you*.

CHAPTER 4

Placing life and death

The relationship between health and place is traditionally explained by geographers in terms of both compositional (*who lives here*) and contextual (*what is this place like*) factors. The compositional explanation asserts that the health of a given area, such as a town, region or country, is a result of the characteristics of the people who live there (individual-level demographic, behavioural and socioeconomic factors), whereas the contextual explanation argues that area-level health is also in part determined by the nature of the place itself in terms of its economic, social and physical environment. These two approaches are not mutually exclusive, and indeed places are about both people and the wider environment. The complexity of how place shapes health is explored further in this chapter through a series of examples. These approaches are then applied to the case study health divides of the US health disadvantage, the 'Scottish health effect', the North–South divide and local health inequalities via a case study of Stockton-on-Tees in the North East of England. The chapter concludes that health divides are a matter of both *poor people* and *poor places*, with economic factors being the key at this scale of analysis.

Who lives here?

The compositional view argues that 'who lives here' – the demographic (age, sex and ethnicity), health behaviour (smoking, alcohol, physical activity, diet, drugs) and socioeconomic (income, education, occupation) profile of the people within a community determines its health outcomes: that *poor people* result in *poor places*.

Demographic and health behaviours

Generally speaking, health deteriorates with age. For example, in the 2011 Census, those aged 45 to 64 were almost twice as likely (42%) to report a long-standing illness than those aged 16 to 44 (22%).[1] Most analysis of health data takes into account age differences between populations to account for these important effects on health – so-called age-standardisation. In wealthy countries, women live longer than men – for example, life expectancy for women in the UK is four years higher than for men (English men, 78.7 years, women, 82.7 years; Scottish men, 76.2 years, women, 80.6 years; Welsh men, 77.8 years, women, 82.0 years; Northern Irish men, 77.7 years, women, 81.8 years). Similarly, on average, American women live five years longer than American men (81 compared to 76 years). However, women (particularly older women) also generally experience worse health: *women get sick, men die.*[2] For example, in the UK limiting long-term conditions are higher among older women than among older men. Women also have higher rates of mental ill health (particularly in terms of depression and anxiety) across all age groups, although suicide rates are higher among men.[3]

Health differences between men and women are partly explained in biological terms, that is, sex-based, and partly in social terms, that is, gender-based. Sex refers to the biological differences between men and women, while gender is the social construction of sex-related roles and relationships – how men and women are expected to act within particular societies.[4] Research on differences in health between men and women focuses on the interaction of these two different elements although the social tends to be privileged. For example, men's poorer longevity is ascribed by some to men's higher rates of risky health behaviours such as alcohol consumption and drug abuse, or the fact that men are less likely than women to access healthcare services. These are linked to gendered assumptions of what it means to be a 'man' within dominant forms of masculinity. Social factors are also important as women have less access to higher paid jobs and therefore less access to health-promoting resources. Employment is often gendered, with men and women therefore experiencing different working conditions. Women also continue to bear the brunt of the unpaid domestic labour and caring responsibilities. And institutional or structural sexism is also important – for example, studies have shown that in countries where men and women are more equal, the health of both men and women tends to be better.[5]

Health also varies by ethnicity/race.[6] In the UK, for example, all-cause mortality rates are more than 25% higher among men and women of West/South/East African descent, even after adjusting for other factors.[7] In the US, African Americans have a life expectancy four years lower than that of White Americans,[8] while indigenous populations in the US, Canada, New Zealand or Australia experience life expectancies of 7–12 years less than their non-indigenous counterparts.[9] Historically, these ethnic/racial differences in health were explained through biological and genetic differences. More recently, however, the social aspects of the relationship have been more privileged by researchers. One such explanation is the cultural one that focuses on differences in diet, alcohol and other health-related behaviours between ethnic groups. Others link ethnicity to social-economic status – highlighting the differences in terms of income, housing conditions and so forth by ethnic group. Indeed in the US 'race' is quite often used as a proxy for social economic status.[10] Racial discrimination is another explanation put forward by researchers – how people from minority ethnic groups experience discrimination in terms of education, employment, housing and other opportunities, which has a negative impact on their health over the life course. Areas with a higher proportion of older people, with more men, or minority ethnic groups, would, on average – and all other things being equal – have worse health.

Smoking, alcohol, lack of physical activity, diet and drugs – the five so-called 'lifestyle factors' or 'risky' health behaviours – all influence health significantly. Smoking remains the most important preventable cause of mortality in the wealthy world, and is causally linked to most major diseases such as cancer and CVD.[11] Likewise, excessive alcohol consumption is related to some cancers as well as other key risks such as high blood pressure. Alcohol-related deaths and diseases are on the increase. Poor diet and low exercise rates can lead to obesity, which, as discussed in the previous chapter, is a major risk factor for poorer health and longevity. Drug abuse is an increasingly important determinant of death among the young.[12] People who do not smoke, have only moderate alcohol intake, consume a high amount of fruit and vegetable and engage regularly in physical activity will on average have a 14-year higher life expectancy than individuals achieving no healthy behaviours.[13] So, on average, areas with higher rates of these unhealthy behaviours among their populations would have worse health than others, all things being equal. However, things are seldom equal, and the following sections examine why some areas are more likely to have higher proportions of people engaging in unhealthy behaviours.

Socioeconomic status

As noted in Chapter 1, the socioeconomic status of people living in an area is also of huge health significance. Socioeconomic status – or social class in 'old money' – is a term that refers to occupational class, income or educational level.[14] People with higher occupational status (for example, professionals such as teachers or lawyers) have better health outcomes than non-professional workers (for example, manual workers). By way of example, English data shows that IMR was 16% higher in children of manual workers compared to professional and managerial workers.[15] People with a higher income or a degree have better health outcomes on average than those with a low income or no qualifications. The poorer someone is, the less likely they are to live in good quality housing, have time and money for leisure activities, feel secure at home or work, have good quality work or a job at all, or afford to eat healthy food – the social determinants of health (as discussed further in the following section).

In terms of the leading causes of death that were examined in Chapter 3, mortality and morbidity from CVD and cancer are unevenly distributed across society, with a disproportionate burden in low-income groups. Cancer mortality rates are two-fold greater in unskilled workers compared with professionals.[16] Although survival rates are improving in relation to some types of cancers, the deprivation gap between those living in deprived and affluent areas is continuing to widen.[17] Data from the British Heart Foundation indicate that there are 2.7 times more CVD deaths among men in the 20% most deprived neighbourhoods compared with the 20% most affluent.[18] Men in the most deprived neighbourhoods also have a 50% greater risk of mortality from stroke than those in the least deprived.[19] Similarly, socioeconomic status was shown to be related to lung cancer incidence, with people with low levels of education having a higher incidence of cancer.[20]

Obesity also disproportionately occurs in certain population groups. In wealthy countries, obesity is associated with social and economic deprivation across all age ranges, and research suggests that this gradient is embedded with little evidence of change over time.[21] The social gradient in obesity is more clearly demonstrated in women (and girls) than among men (and boys). It is estimated that in the UK some 10% of obesity in men and up to 33% in women is attributable to socioeconomic inequalities.[22] Further, it is known that minority ethnic groups in the UK and individuals with a mental health problem or physical disability are disproportionately affected by obesity.[23]

Mental health is intimately connected with social and spatial inequality. Consistent associations have been found between mental ill health and various markers of social and economic adversity, for example, low education, low income, low socioeconomic status, unemployment and poorer material circumstances.[24] The social gradient is particularly pronounced for severe mental illness. For example, in the case of psychotic disorders, the prevalence among the lowest quintile of household income is nine times higher than in the highest.[25] This is not just a result of downward social mobility (as it is harder to find and maintain employment when suffering from severe mental illness). The social gradient is also evident for common mental health problems, with a two-fold variation between the highest and lowest quintiles.[26] In general, socioeconomic status is also associated with suicide mortality and self-harm.[27]

These socioeconomic health divides are demonstrated in Table 4.1, which shows the percentage point gap in limiting long-term illness between the highest income tertile (the richest third in terms of income) and the lowest tertile (the poorest third) for men and women in 23 European countries. By way of example, in the UK, the rate of long-term illnesses is more than 20 percentage points higher among the lowest income men and over 17 percentage points higher among the lowest income women compared to those men and women in the top third of the income distribution.

However, these socioeconomic inequalities in health are not restricted to differences between the most privileged groups and the most disadvantaged; health inequalities exist across the entire social gradient, which runs from the top to the bottom of society, and 'even comfortably off people somewhere in the middle tend to have poorer health than those above them'.[28] Most major diseases, including cancer, heart disease, stroke, diabetes and obesity, as well as health behaviours, follow this social gradient. By way of example, in England, obesity rates are 27% and 34% among men and women routine and manual workers compared to 21% and 14% among men and women professional and managerial workers.[29] However, incidence rates of breast, skin and prostate cancer increase with socioeconomic status, although mortality rates from these cancers are still higher in deprived groups.[30]

Social determinants of health

Individual socioeconomic position leads to differential exposure to the social determinants of health. These are the conditions in which people work and live – what have been referred to as the 'causes of the causes'.[31] As noted in Chapter 1, there are clinical 'causes' of disease, proximal causes (health behaviours) and then underpinning them are social causes (and ultimately political ones; see Chapter 5). For example, one of the underpinning clinical 'causes' of stroke is hypertension (high blood pressure), the 'proximal cause' of the high blood pressure could be poor diet, smoking, alcohol consumption and so on, while the social causes of these proximal and clinical causes could be workplace

Table 4.1: Inequalities in prevalence rates of limiting long-term illness for the lowest income tertile compared to the highest income tertile, men and women in 22 European countries[32]

	Percentage point gap in limiting long term illness between highest and lowest income tertiles	
Country	**Men**	**Women**
Austria	10.8	4.2
Belgium	7.4	8.3
Czech Republic	4.0	7.7
Denmark	15.1	20.0
Estonia	22.8	12.4
Finland	14.8	15.4
France	11.7	10.3
Germany	11.5	12.1
Greece	8.9	12.0
Hungary	23.5	13.4
Ireland	8.0	10.8
Luxembourg	11.9	8.0
Netherlands	12.9	6.0
Norway	10.9	13.9
Poland	17.0	10.6
Portugal	14.6	7.1
Slovakia	16.2	9.6
Slovenia	18.8	19.1
Spain	13.3	6.8
Sweden	11.6	13.1
Switzerland	9.5	6.1
United Kingdom	20.8	17.5

stress or a low income and the subsequent inability to afford a healthy diet. The main social determinants of health are widely considered to be: (1) working conditions; (2) unemployment and worklessness; (3) access to essential goods and services (specifically water, sanitation and food); (4) access to healthcare; and (5) housing.[33]

The work environment has long been acknowledged as an important determinant of health and health inequalities. Historically, physical working conditions, such as exposure to dangerous substances (for example, lead, asbestos, mercury), as well as physical load or ergonomic problems, were a major cause of ill health in the working-age population.[34] However, despite a decline in wealthy countries in the number of jobs in manufacturing and heavy industry since the 1970s, adverse physical working conditions are still experienced by a significant proportion of the working-age population. For example, across Europe, 15% of workers are still regularly exposed to hazardous chemicals at work, 20% are exposed to vibrations and 33% are regularly exposed to noise, heavy loads or repetitive work.[35]

Hazardous chemicals include aluminum, cadmium, lead, mercury and benzene as well as toxic gases such as carbon monoxide and hydrogen cyanide.[36] These are associated with increased risk of respiratory diseases, certain cancers and hypertension (high blood pressure). Vibrations, most commonly experienced by those working in construction, road repair or mining, machinery operators or drivers, are associated with vibration syndrome and vibration-induced white finger, and musculoskeletal disease (particularly of the hand, arm or lower back).[37] Noise exposure is associated with acoustic shock injuries, tinnitus, hypertension, stress and fatigue, while heavy loads and repetitive work are associated with musculoskeletal disease, stress and anxiety.[38]

The health problems associated with the physical work environment are more prevalent among manual than non-manual workers. European data shows that the lowest occupational groups have 50% higher exposure to the majority of physical hazards compared to the top occupational groups. By way of example, a US study of hospital workers found an occupational gradient in the risk of lower back problems, which was largely explained by differences in the physical nature of work undertaken by different occupational grades.[39] Similarly, a Finnish study of municipal employees found that physical workload explained up to 95% of inequalities by occupational class in physical functioning.[40] The physical work environment remains an important contributory factor behind the social gradient in health.[41]

In addition to physical working hazards, research has shown that people in lower grade occupations also experience higher exposure to adverse psychosocial working conditions. The 'psychosocial work environment' is a collective way of referring to psychological and social influences on health such as time pressure, monotonous work, social reciprocity, job control and autonomy, fairness, work demands, job security, as well as social contact between co-workers and supervisors.[42] Low control over your work (for example, little choice over what tasks you do or when you do them) coupled with high job demands (such as frequency of tasks, high pressure environments and short deadlines) combine to produce chronic stress – this is called the 'demand-control' model of work stress.[43] This type of work is associated with an increased risk of stress-related morbidity including coronary heart disease,[44] adverse health behaviours (for example, consumption of unhealthy foods, physical inactivity, heavy drinking and smoking),[45] obesity,[46] musculoskeletal conditions[47] and mental health problems.[48]

There are considerable occupational inequalities in the distribution of adverse psychosocial working conditions, with jobs at the lower end of the occupational scale more likely to entail a higher exposure to adverse conditions than those towards the higher end.[49] European data shows that job demands are 50% higher and control at work 50% lower among the lowest occupational groups compared to the highest.[50] By way of example of how this contributes to the association between socioeconomic status and health, a study of the social gradient in coronary heart disease among British civil servants found that it was 50% higher in the lowest grade employees. Adjustment for differences in adverse psychosocial work environment factors halved this inequality between occupational grades among women, while adjustment for health behaviours only reduced the inequality by a quarter.[51]

Studies have consistently shown that unemployment increases the chances of poor health.[52] Research into the economic recessions of the 1980s and 1990s have shown that unemployment is associated with an increased likelihood of mortality,[53] poor mental health and suicide,[54] self-reported health and limiting long-term illness[55] and risky health behaviours.[56] The negative health experiences of unemployment are not just limited to the unemployed, but also extend to their families and the wider community.[57] Links between unemployment and poorer health have conventionally been explained through two interrelated concepts: the psychosocial effects of unemployment (for example, stigma, isolation and loss of self-worth) and the material consequences of unemployment (for example, wage loss, poverty and resulting changes in access to essential goods and services).[58]

Lower socioeconomic groups are disproportionately at risk of unemployment, and it is a key contemporary determinant of the social gradient in health. Unemployment is concentrated in lower socioeconomic groups.[59] For example, in London, over 90% of men and 80% of women with a university degree are employed compared to just 70% of men and 50% of women with no qualifications.[60] For both men and women, not being in paid employment accounts for up to 80% of the inequalities in the prevalence of self-rated poor health between the highest and lowest socioeconomic groups in England.[61] Ill health-related job loss also has a social gradient, with adverse employment consequences more likely for those in lower socioeconomic groups.[62]

The development of ill health can also result in long-term unemployment – so-called 'health-related worklessness'.[63] Across Europe, experiencing poor health is a significant risk factor for unemployment as people who develop chronic health problems while in employment are twice as likely to become workless as those who remain healthy.[64] Men and women in poor health are 60% and 40% less likely to enter paid employment than men in good health.[65] The employment rates of people with a limiting long-term illness or a disability are 50% lower than those without an illness or disability.[66] Studies have shown similar patterns in the US.[67] Health-related worklessness is also concentrated among less skilled workers, and there are significant educational inequalities in the employment rates of people with a limiting long-term illness or a disability. For example, in the UK men and women with a low education and a limiting long-term illness or a disability are almost 70% less likely than their highly educated healthy counterparts to be in employment.[68] These patterns are replicated in other wealthy countries to a greater or lesser extent.[69]

Access to clean water and hygienic sanitation systems are the most basic prerequisites for good public health. In the advanced capitalist democracies, access to water and sanitation were among the first major public health reforms of 19th-century Europe, although it was often only with the slum clearances and the advent of the post-war welfare state that access became universal. Agricultural policies affect the quality, quantity, price and availability of food, all of which are important for public health.[70] While overall increases in life expectancy may be partly attributed to better nutrition, increases in the prevalence of obesity in many countries point to the contribution food policies continue to make to malnutrition. Access to services is socially stratified, for example, access to food and a balanced diet is restricted by income (food poverty), as is access to energy (fuel poverty).

By way of example, food poverty is increasing in wealthy countries like the UK – best represented by the emergence of food banks and food redistribution programmes. The Trussell Trust, a Christian social action charity, is the largest food bank franchise within the UK. It operates a voucher system for those seeking emergency food provisions. Food bank clients bring their 'red' voucher to a food bank centre where it can be redeemed for three days of emergency food, up to three times within one period of crisis.[71] The Trussell Trust reported that almost 1 million people accessed food banks between the financial year 2013–14, a three-fold rise compared to the previous year 2012–13.[72] People who use food banks are generally those on the lowest incomes, for example, those on low wages, welfare benefits or with no source income at all (as a result of sanctions applied to benefits whereby they are removed for periods of weeks or months, leaving the recipient with no source of income with which to buy food). Recent research conducted in the town of Stockton-on-Tees in the North East of England suggests that such food insecurity has an impact on the health of the poorest.[73]

The poorest socioeconomic groups also disproportionately experience fuel poverty. A household is defined as being in fuel poverty if it needs to spend more than 10% of its income on fuel to maintain a satisfactory heating regime, which means 21°C for the main living area, and 18°C for other occupied rooms. In 2011, the number of fuel-poor households in England was estimated at around 2.39 million, representing approximately 11% of all English households.[74] The poorest tenth of households spent more than a fifth of their budget on fuel, and the number of UK children living in fuel poverty stands at over 1.5 million.[75] Fuel poverty is associated with health conditions such as respiratory problems and also with 'excess winter death' due to cold, particularly among elderly women.[76]

As noted in Chapter 2, housing has long been recognised as an important material determinant of health. Health concerns underpinned the slum clearances of the 1930s and the early post-war welfare state in the UK. Damp housing can lead to breathing diseases such as asthma, infested housing leads to the rapid spread of infectious diseases, and overcrowding can result in higher infection rates and is associated with an increased prevalence of household accidents. Expensive housing (for example, as a result of high rents) can also have a negative effect on health as expenditure in other areas (such as diet) is reduced.[77] Housing costs may also have an impact on health as the burden of debt involved in home ownership or high rents may lead to anxiety and worry.[78] Other internal housing conditions also have the potential to influence health.[79] In particular, poisoning may be caused by carbon monoxide from faulty gas fires, and injuries may be caused by accidents in poorly designed/maintained or overcrowded properties – particularly among children and the elderly. Lack of smoke alarms, fire extinguishers and sprinklers may exacerbate the risk of injury from fire.[80] Housing tenure may have psychosocial impacts on health – owning one's one home may confer greater feelings of security or prestige than social or private renting, and is often used as an indicator of greater long-term command over resources.[81] Again, exposure to poor housing, or unaffordable housing, is more of a risk for lower socioeconomic groups than higher ones – indeed, living in socially rented homes is often used as a way of classifying socioeconomic status.

Access to healthcare is a key determinant of health, particularly in terms of the treatment of pre-existing conditions. In most wealthy countries, some kind of access to healthcare is universal. However, there are variations in terms of how healthcare is funded (for example, social insurance, private insurance or general taxation), the role and level of co-payments for treatment and the extent of provision – what has been collectively termed 'healthcare decommodification'.[82] Inequalities in health outcomes may be influenced by inequalities in healthcare utilisation of prevention (reception and efficacy of health education and promotion messages, preventive attitude of GPs), diagnosis (delay or inaccuracy of diagnosis, missed recognition or denial of symptoms and need, ability to 'jump the queue') and treatment (cultural sensitivity of pattern of care, failure to empower patients/families, access to appropriate care, lack of comprehensive social and health care networks).[83] Some factors in healthcare may affect utilisation: accessibility (due to geographic, legal, informative barriers), affordability (due to the service and purchasing power of the individual) and quality and acceptability (due to professional training and practice, patient–professional interaction, compliance, continuity and appropriateness in supply organisation).[84] Research over several decades has shown that people in lower socioeconomic groups are less likely to access and use healthcare services than those in higher socioeconomic groups with the same health need.[85]

Explaining socioeconomic inequalities in health

Building on the importance of the social determinants of health are several different explanatory theories for why health inequalities exist between different socioeconomic groups in wealthy countries: materialist, behavioural-cultural, psychosocial and life course.[86]

- *Materialist:* This argues that it is income levels and what a decent or high income enables compared to a lower one such as access to health-benefiting goods and services (for example, healthcare access, schools, transport, social care) and limiting exposure to particular material risk factors (for example, poor housing, inadequate diet, physical hazards at work, environmental exposures).

- *Behavioural-cultural:* This theory of socioeconomic health inequalities asserts that the causal mechanisms are higher rates of health-damaging behaviours in lower socioeconomic groups. A more cultural explanation suggests that such differences in health behaviour are a consequence of disadvantage, and that unhealthy behaviour may be more culturally acceptable among lower socioeconomic groups.
- *Psychosocial:* This focuses on the adverse biological consequences of psychological and social domination and subordination, superiority and inferiority. The socioeconomic gradient in health is therefore explained by the unequal social distribution of psychosocial risk factors such as control at work and in the community or social support.
- *Life course:* This approach combines aspects of the other explanations, thereby allowing different causal mechanisms and processes to explain the social gradient in different diseases. It also highlights the role of the accumulation of disadvantage over the 'life course' – combining the amount of time different people have spent in more/less disadvantaged circumstances. Health inequality between social groups is therefore a result of inequalities in the accumulation of social, psychological and biological advantages and disadvantages over time.

A study using data from Norway compared the relative contribution of these material, psychosocial and behavioural explanations (alongside biomedical factors) of socioeconomic (educational and income) inequalities in mortality. It concluded that material factors were the most important in explaining income inequalities in mortality, while psychosocial and behavioural factors were the most important in explaining educational inequalities.[87] People exposed to one sort of factor (for example, material) may also be exposed to another (for example, psychosocial), and have interacting influences on their health. So these explanations of health inequalities are overlapping rather than competing.

Indeed, people of higher socioeconomic status (be it higher education levels, higher income or higher occupational class) have access to better resources, money, knowledge, prestige, power and beneficial social networks, while those of lower socioeconomic status (lower income, education or occupational class) have less access. People of higher socioeconomic status also have access to better contexts (as described in the next section) in terms of workplaces and neighbourhoods.[88] The health advantage of having a higher socioeconomic status is robust to varying degrees over time and place such that, while the clinical and proximal causes of socioeconomic inequalities in health have changed, the gradient still exists. For example, in the 19th century, as noted in Chapter 2, the leading causes of death were fevers and consumption, while in the 20th and early 21st centuries (as seen in Chapter 3), the main causes of death are cancers and CVD. Socioeconomic inequalities existed in the 19th century as they do today – despite the diversity of the actual causes of death. This is because high socioeconomic status in the 19th century enabled people to have better sanitation or to live away from polluting factories, for example, while in the 20th and 21st century, it enables better health behaviours or access to healthier work environments. People of high socioeconomic status use their resources to adapt to the disease threat of the day, and gain a health advantage over those of lower socioeconomic status who do not have the resources to adapt. This has led to socioeconomic status being called a 'fundamental cause' of ill health that persists despite competing causes of death.[89]

Intersectionality is another way of looking at multiple influences on health. It focuses on how socioeconomic status, ethnicity and gender are experienced not separately but in combination, and that we all have different aspects of social identity that coexist with one another. Intersectionality therefore looks at the *axes of inequality*, particularly socioeconomic status, gender and ethnicity together.[90] It also considers gender and ethnicity as social factors rather than simply demographic ones (as has traditionally been the case in compositional approaches to health and place), viewing them as socially structured, constructed and experienced. So, for example, health differences between men and women arise not just because of biological differences, but also as a result of the social construction of sex-related roles and relationships (gender). Likewise, ethnic inequalities in health can arise through racism, with minority ethnic groups more likely to experience discrimination personally, institutionally (systematic exclusion and disadvantage) and economically.[91]

Health is therefore affected by each of these axes of inequality. For example, as a professor I am in the most educated group in terms of my socioeconomic status; in terms of ethnicity, I am white; and in terms of gender I am a woman. So these factors all have influences on my health, and they influence together and at the same time. Intersectionality therefore draws recognition to the fact that any individual has 'such multiple aspects of identity with relevance for their relationships with others and with the structures and systems of power – and, therefore, for their health'.[92] Intersectionality looks at the whole individual and how they experience the various aspects of their social identity within particular contexts, and with specific health effects. Context – in its more geographical sense – is the subject of the next section.

What is this place like?

So, while the compositional view argues that it is 'who lives here' that matters for area health – and that essentially 'poor people make poor health' – the contextual approach instead highlights the fact that 'what is this place like' also matters for health: that health differs by place because it is also determined by the economic, social and physical environment of a *place*,; that 'poor places lead to poor health'. Place mediates the way in which individuals experience social, economic and physical processes on their health: places can be salutogenic (health-promoting) or pathogenic (health-damaging) environments – place acts as a health ecosystem. These place-based effects can also be seen as the *collective* effects of the social determinants of health. Indeed, it is a way of looking at population health as more than just the aggregate or average health of the health of individuals – it provides one of the collective dimensions of public health (public health is more than the aggregate of individual health). There are three contextual aspects to place that have traditionally been considered as important to health: economic, social and physical.

Economic environment

The effects of individual socioeconomic position on health status were examined in the compositional section earlier. Area-level economics instead looks at the health effects of the local economic environment, independent of individual socioeconomic position. Area-economic factors that influence health are often summarised as 'economic deprivation'. They include area poverty rates, unemployment rates, wages and types of work and employment in the area. They form a key part of the IMD (as described in Chapter 1) that is used to define the relative deprivation of neighbourhoods in the UK. The mechanisms whereby the economic profile of a local area has an impact on health are multiple. For example, it affects the nature of work that an individual can access in that place (regardless of their own socioeconomic position). It also has an impact on the services available in a local area, as more affluent areas will attract different services (such as food available locally or physical activity opportunities) from more deprived areas, as businesses adapt to the dominant demands (see the 'Social environment' section).

Area-level economic factors such as poverty are a key predictor of health including CVD, all-cause mortality, limiting long-term illness and health-related behaviours.[93, 94] For example, a Scottish study found that both individual socioeconomic indicators and area-level economic factors contributed to increased mortality risk.[95] This is demonstrated further in the examples below of neighbourhood deprivation and health behaviours in the East of England and on CVD in the US. Moreover, changes in local economic factors can have important effects on health, as an example of deindustrialisation and health demonstrates.

A number of studies have found an independent effect on health – across all socioeconomic groups – of living in an economically deprived area. For example, the East of England study (based on health surveys of adults aged over 16 in Cambridgeshire) found that individual socioeconomic status and area-level economic deprivation were both independently associated with adverse health behaviours.[96] As neighbourhood deprivation increased, residents were more likely to smoke and less likely to consume fruit and vegetables (even after adjusting for individual socioeconomic factors – employment and occupational social class). Similar relationships were shown for a composite healthy lifestyle score, which ranged from 0–4 whereby not smoking, moderate alcohol consumption (1–14 units/week for women and 1–21 units/week for men), high or moderate levels of physical activity, and eating five or more portions of fruit or vegetables on at least five days/week, each scored 1 point. Across all six of the individual occupational class categories used in the analysis, those living in deprived areas scored lower than their comparators in more affluent neighbourhoods. This is demonstrated in Figure 4.1.

Similar findings were reported for coronary heart disease in a study of middle-aged adults (aged 45–64) in four US states: North Carolina, Mississippi, Minneapolis and Maryland. Over the nine-year study period, people living in economically disadvantaged neighbourhoods in these localities had a 50-60% higher risk of

Figure 4.1: Mean healthy lifestyle score across quintiles of neighbourhood deprivation and six categories of occupational social class[97]

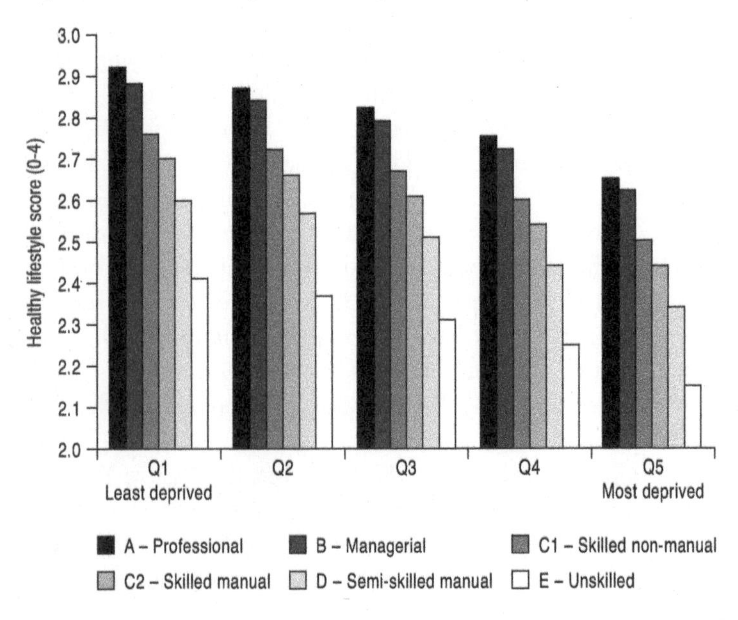

disease than those living in advantaged neighbourhoods, even after taking into account individual-level socioeconomic status (income, education and occupation) and health behaviours.[98] The pathways underpinning such relationships between area-level economic deprivation and health are not straightforward. They relate to both the social and physical aspects of place, as discussed in subsequent sections.

There is a widespread literature that considers the health effects of the shift from industrial to post-industrial production, and how this has been associated not only with economic but also environmental and social decline since the 1970s.[99] Such deindustrialisation (or devastation, as some have argued, given the scale and rapid pace of change – explored further in Chapter 5) has had significant implications for long-term job prospects, job security, migration patterns, housing quality and many other social determinants of health and health inequalities. For example, it is asserted that spatial inequalities in the current rates of unemployment levels in the UK reflect 'the loss of jobs in manufacturing and mining, which has not only been large overall, but has also clearly been concentrated in the cities and coalfields'.[100] The main areas affected in the UK were in the North East and North West of England, the South of Wales and the West of Scotland. These communities lost their main sources of employment, such as the coal, steel and shipping industries, in the rapid restructuring of the 1980s and 1990s, when manufacturing jobs were lost at a rate of up to 1,000 per week in industrial centres.[101] This rapid loss of employment is demonstrated for 10 regions of Europe in Table 4.2, where lost employment amounts to up to 63% of industrial jobs since the 1970s. There has not been enough in the way of new local employment to replace these large industries, and the service sector jobs that have emerged do not match the skills of the existing workforce. Deindustrialisation has meant that some communities have been left behind, with collective feelings of loss experienced by those still living there.[102] Deindustrialisation led to more than just the loss of employment; it also led to the fracturing of working-class cultures and communities.[103]

Chapter 3 demonstrated that the deindustrialised regions of the UK and Europe have higher rates of mortality and morbidity.

Table 4.2: Overview of employment changes in 10 post-industrial regions of Europe[104]

Post-industrial region	Country	Historical Industries	Industrial Job Loss (%) 1970s to 2005
West Central Scotland	United Kingdom	Shipbuilding and support industries (iron, coal, engineering)	-62%
Northern Ireland	United Kingdom	Shipbuilding, textiles, manufacturing	-20%
Merseyside	United Kingdom	Shipping, docks, manufacturing (e.g. cement), engineering	-63%
Swansea and South Wales	United Kingdom	Coal	-51%
Nord-Pas-de-Calais	France	Coal, textiles, steel	-43%
Wallonia	Belgium	Mining, metal working, textiles	-39%
The Ruhr	Germany	Coal, iron, steel	-54%
Saxony[a]	Germany	Steel, construction, engineering, textiles	-47%
Northern Moravia[b]	Czech Republic	Coal, steel	-19%
Silesia[c]	Poland	Coal, steel, automobiles, zinc	-55%

[a]1991-2005; [b]1993-2005; [c]1980-2005

Indeed, a study of such areas in England (characterised by having persistently low or deteriorating employment rates relative to the national average) found that they had higher rates of mortality and morbidity, even after adjusting for migration and the socioeconomic individual characteristics of residents.[105] Deindustrialisation has therefore been proposed as a mechanism to explain health divides such as that between the North and South of England or between the East and West of Scotland.[106]

The latter is examined in more detail in the case study of the 'Scottish health effect' later in this chapter.

Social environment

Places also have social aspects that have an impact on health. Opportunity structures are the socially constructed and patterned features of the area that may promote health through the possibilities they provide.[107] These include the services provided, publicly or privately, to support people in their daily lives such as childcare or transport, food availability or access to a GP or hospital, as well as the availability of health-promoting environments at home (for example, good housing quality, access and affordability), work (good quality work) and education (such as high quality schools).

Local environments can shape our access to healthy – and unhealthy – goods and services, thus enhancing or reducing our opportunities to engage in healthy or unhealthy behaviours such as smoking, alcohol consumption, fruit and vegetable consumption or physical activity. One example is the 'obesogenic environment'. The local food environment (such as the availability of healthy and unhealthy foods in the neighbourhood) as well as opportunities for physical activity (are there parks or gyms? Is the outside space safe and walkable?) are both central components of the obesogenic environment. Research has shown that in some low-income areas 'food deserts' exist where there is a paucity of supermarkets and shops selling affordable fresh food on the one hand, alongside an abundance of convenience stores and fast food outlets selling energy-dense junk food and ready meals on the other.[108, 109] Low-income neighbourhoods – particularly urban ones – may also inhibit opportunities for physical activity. Associations have been found between neighbourhood availability of fast food and obesity rates in a number of wealthy countries including the UK, the US and New Zealand,[110, 111] although evidence for the existence of food deserts is much stronger for North America than elsewhere. Similarly, associations between the local availability of alcohol or tobacco have been associated with health outcomes. For example, in Scotland studies have found that areas with a higher density of alcohol-selling outlets have higher alcohol-related hospitalisation rates and alcohol-related mortality, and that residents of areas with a higher number of tobacco-selling outlets are more likely to smoke.[112,113]

Similarly, access to healthcare varies by place. From the 1970s until the early 2000s, an 'inverse care law' was seen to exist in the UK whereby 'the availability of good medical care tends to vary inversely with the need for it in the population served'.[114] However, there was substantial investment in improving access to primary care services in deprived areas during the UK Labour governments of 1997–2010 (new facilities were built, there was an increase in medical school places and more efforts were put into recruiting GPs [primary care physicians] to work in areas of high deprivation). Studies have subsequently found that geographical access to GP services in more deprived areas of England tends to be as good, if not better, than more affluent areas. The most recent analysis suggests that 85% of the population in England live within a 20-minute (1 mile) walk of a GP – 98% in the most deprived areas.[115] Similarly, 90% of the population can access a community pharmacy within a 20-minute walk and, in the areas of highest deprivation, almost 100% of households can – the so-called *positive pharmacy care law*.[116] However, GP and community pharmacy access varies considerably between urban and rural areas, with only 36% of people living in the most deprived rural areas having access to a GP within a 20-minute walk and 42% to a community pharmacy.[117]

A second social aspect of place is collective social functioning. Collective social functioning and practices that are beneficial to health include high levels of social cohesion and social capital within the community (explored further below). More negative collective effects can also come from the reputation of an area (for example, stigmatised places can result in feelings of alienation and worthlessness) or the history of an area (for example, if there has been a history of racial oppression). In contrast, place attachment (an emotional bond that individuals or groups have with specific places) can have a protective health effect.[118] Local attitudes, say, around smoking, can also influence health and health behaviours either negatively or positively.[119]

Social capital – 'the features of social organisation such as trust, norms, and networks that can improve the efficiency of society by facilitating coordinated actions'[120] – is analogous to notions of physical and human capital: social networks matter. The key features of social capital at a neighbourhood level are collective reciprocity, trust, civic identity, civic engagement and the feelings of belonging created by community networks. Social capital consists of various aspects: bonding, bridging and vertical. 'Bonding' social capital refers to relationships between individuals in the same social group or community, that is, cooperation for mutual benefit or what is otherwise known as 'community spirit'.[121] Cross-cutting ties between heterogeneous groups of people are assumed to create so called 'bridging' social capital. 'Vertical' or 'linking' social capital is a hierarchical dimension whereby processes create bonds within a place across the socioeconomic hierarchy.[122] Welfare systems are an example of vertical social capital as they can be integrating in that everybody contributes to and benefits from them.

Social capital has been credited with having positive effects on a diverse range of political, social and economic factors affecting people's lives. It has been put forward as a mechanism through which place mediates the relationship between individual socioeconomic status and health outcomes.[123] Some studies have found that areas with higher levels of social capital have better health, such as lower mortality rates, self-rated health, mental health and health behaviours.[124] Indeed, some economically deprived areas exhibit better health than expected (referred to as area-health resilience), and this has partly been explained by higher levels of social capital and community control in these communities.[125] The processes involved include enhancing self-efficacy and self-esteem or the reduction of anxiety and fear as a result of improved levels of trust in society.[126] However, the relationship between social capital within an area/community and health is not uncontested, as other studies have suggested that close involvement in a community that has a prevalence of high-risk behaviour may result in poorer health outcomes due to a process of 'contagion',[127] and that not all types of social capital have positive influences on health.[128]

It is well established that how residents feel about their area is associated with health outcomes. The individual notion of stigma[129] – 'the situation of the individual who is disqualified from full social acceptance' – has been extended to examine how certain places become marginalised by obtaining a 'spoiled identity' and subsequently become stigmatised and discredited. This can be as a result of environment factors such as air pollution or 'dirt' as well as from social stigma, such as being labelled the 'obesity capital' of Britain, as happened with Copeland in West Cumbria (North West England), or economic stigma such as low property prices.[130] Residents of stigmatised places can also be discredited by association with these place characteristics. For example, a study of (post)industrial Middlesbrough in the North East of England found that 'even the birds cough round here'.[131] Local people had absorbed the perceptions of their local area as polluted and dirty. Indeed, inhabitants of Teesside are nicknamed 'Smoggies', associating the smog with which the area was historically associated with the individual residents. Other notable cases of such place-based stigma are Love Canal in New York, the location of a toxic waste dump. Research has shown that such place-based stigma can result in psychosocial stress and associated ill health alongside feelings of shame, on top of the physical health effects of air pollution such as respiratory disease.[132]

Physical environment

The physical environment is widely recognised as an important determinant of health and health inequalities.[133] There is a sizeable literature on the positive health effects of access to green space,[134] as well as the negative health effects of waste facilities,[135] brownfield or contaminated land,[136] and air pollution.[137] One (in)famous example of the latter is the so-called 'Cancer Alley', the 87-mile stretch in the US state of Mississippi between Baton Rouge and New Orleans, the home of the largest petrochemicals site in the US.[138] Awareness of how such factors differ by place has led to the development of the concept of 'environmental deprivation'.[139]

Environmental deprivation is the extent of exposure to key characteristics of the physical environment that are either health-promoting or health-damaging.[140] By way of illustration, researchers from the Centre for Research on Environment, Society and Health at the Universities of Glasgow and Edinburgh[141] developed a UK index of health-related multiple environmental deprivation (MED-Ix), a composite index that contained small area (ward level; see Box 1.1 in Chapter 1) measures of air pollution, climate temperature, solar UV radiation, proximity to industry and access to green space.[142] In a study testing the index, they found an area-level association between environmental deprivation and all-cause mortality: mortality was lowest in areas with the least environmental deprivation and highest in the most environmentally deprived.[143] Similarly, mortality was higher than average in four types of environment (industrial; fair weather conurbations; cold, cloudy conurbations; and isolated, cold and green areas), and lower than average in three (London and London-esque; mediocre green sprawl; and sunny, clean and green).[144]

The health geography literature has established the role of natural or green spaces as 'therapeutic' or health-promoting landscapes. So, for example, studies have found that walking in natural, rather than urban, settings reduces stress levels,[145] and people residing in 'green areas' report less poor health than those with 'less green' surroundings.[146] Research also indicates that green space can have an impact on health by attention restoration, stress reduction and/or the evocation of positive emotions.[147] Biophilia also underpins green space research. Biophilia theory argues that 'our response to nature today is influenced by universal, inherited human characteristics, which would have conveyed primeval evolutionary advantages for the human species'.[148] Subsequently, humans have preferences for natural settings, which offer resources for life and protection.[149] Natural settings (including green space, but also 'blue space' – rivers, lakes and the coast) are also theorised to have an impact on health as they constitute 'therapeutic landscapes'. A therapeutic landscape is defined as 'a place that is conducive to physical, mental, spiritual, emotional and social healing.'[150] However, a more straightforward explanation for the association of green space and better health outcomes is that green spaces may encourage exercise (for example, walking or jogging in a green park).[151]

Another example of how the physical environment of areas varies is in respect to brownfield land. Land is a finite resource, and redevelopment of previously used sites is common in wealthy countries. The term 'brownfield' land is often applied to such previously used sites. It is estimated that there are some 62,000 hectares of brownfield land in England.[152] Brownfield land has long been recognised as a potential health hazard from a toxicological perspective, as there is a large degree of overlap with contaminated land.[153] Contaminants include potentially toxic elements (such as lead or arsenic), inorganic chemicals (for example, asbestos), organic compounds (for example, petroleum hydrocarbons) and in some cases, radiation. The health effects of these contaminants vary, but as an example, chronic lead exposure includes neurological disturbances, anaemia, anorexia, fatigue, depression, vomiting, hypertension, gastrointestinal conditions, and in some cases, renal failure.[154] However, aside from the direct toxicological effects of contamination, it has also been suggested that low-quality, previously developed, open spaces (brownfield land that may or may not be contaminated), particularly in low-income urban areas, could have wider negative impacts on the general health of communities potentially operating through psychosocial mechanisms, as outlined above in respect to green spaces.[155, 156]

The health effects of brownfield land at an area level were examined by Litt and colleagues[157] in a district of Baltimore, US. They found that among those aged over 45, mortality rates from cancer, lung cancer and respiratory diseases (causes of death that are plausibly linked to the toxicological effects of brownfield land) were 27%, 33% and 39% higher respectively in areas with larger amounts of brownfield land. Similarly, an English study of differences in exposure to brownfield land found that areas with larger amounts of brownfield land have 15% higher rates of poor health and limiting long-term illness compared to areas with little to no brownfield land, after controlling for other area-level factors such as economic deprivation.[158] This is demonstrated in Figure 4.2, which shows brownfield land density by region (percentage of brownfield) alongside standardised rates of 'not good health' (NGH SMR), limiting long-term illness (LLTI SMR) and mortality (DEATHS SMR). The North West, North East and London have higher rates of brownfield land *and* higher rates of poor health.[159] Areas with higher amounts of brownfield land are also those that experienced deindustrialisation; indeed, brownfield land can be seen as an environmental legacy of previous industrial activity.

Figure 4.2: Prevalence of brownfield land (%), standardised mortality rates (deaths SMR) and standardised morbidity rates for limiting long-term illness (LLTI) and not good health (NGH) by English region[160]

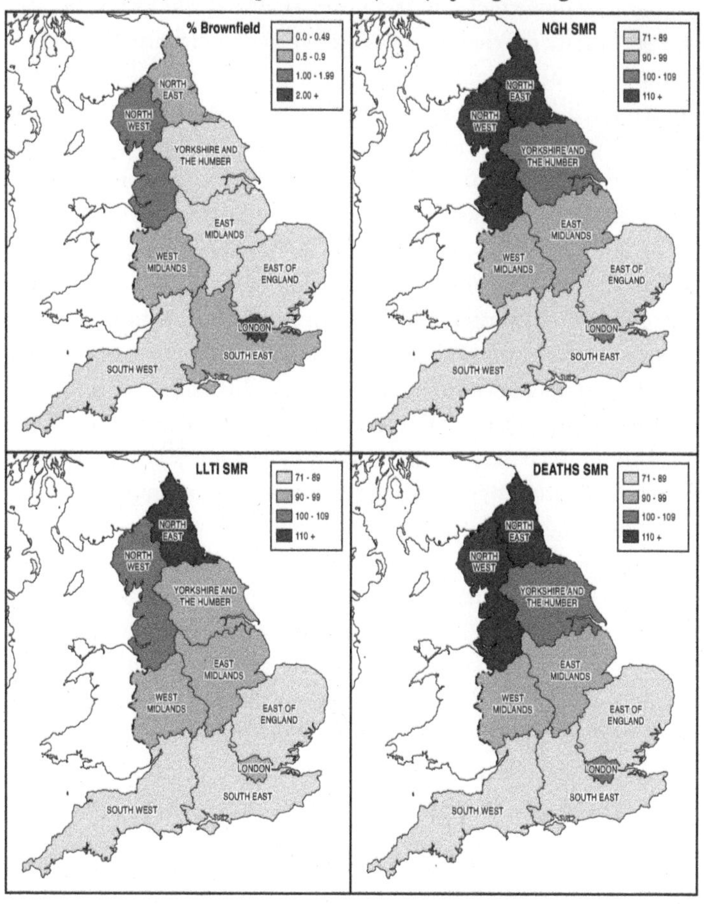

Poor people *and* poor places

The contextual and compositional explanations for how place relates to health are not mutually exclusive, and to separate them is an over-simplification and ignores the interactions between these two levels.[161] The characteristics of individuals are influenced by the characteristics of the area, for example, individual employment status can be determined by local school quality and the availability of jobs in the local labour market. Health is influenced by the interaction of *both* individual (compositional) and collective (contextual) factors.[162] For example, children might not play outside due to having no garden (a *compositional* resource), because there are no public parks or transport to get to them (a *contextual* resource), or because it might not be seen as appropriate for them to do so (*contextual* social functioning).[163]

Further, the characteristics of places and people are highly interrelated as, for example, 'the lives of children growing up in a particular neighbourhood may be shaped by the social and material aspects of the neighbourhood: but the social interactions and behaviour of these children, and how as adults they might operate in the same neighbourhood, also shapes the local social and physical environment and helps create context for their neighbours'.[164] Similarly, areas with more successful economies (for example, more high-paid jobs) will have lower proportions of lower socioeconomic status residents. This 'collective resources' approach suggests that all residents, and particularly those of low income, enjoy better health when they live in areas characterised by more/better social and economic collective resources. This may be especially important for those on low incomes as they are usually more reliant on local services. Conversely, the health of poorer people may suffer more in (deprived) areas where collective resources and social structures are limited, a concept known as 'deprivation amplification': that the health effects of individual deprivation, such as lower socioeconomic status, can therefore be *amplified* by area deprivation.[165] For example, in England, the health of low-income women is worse in areas of high deprivation than in more affluent areas. Equally, the social gradient in health is starker and steeper in the North than the South,[166] suggesting a potential *amplification* effect within the

North. The health of socioeconomic groups also varies by country – with, for example, the health of the unemployed worse in countries like England and Ireland than in other European countries.[167]

Composition and context should not therefore be seen as separate or competing explanations, but as entwined.[168] Both contribute to the complex relationship between health and place, an ecosystem made up of people, systems and structures: physical, social, economic and political (Chapter 5 examines the latter). As Professor Steven Cummins of the London School of Hygiene and Tropical Medicine and colleagues have argued, 'there is a mutually reinforcing and reciprocal relationship between people and place'.[169] The four case study health divides examined in this book are now used to illustrate this further by looking at the compositional and contextual determinants of the US health disadvantage, the 'Scottish health effect', the North–South health divide and local health inequalities in Stockton-on-Tees, the English town with the greatest health divide.

Stars and *stripes*

As previously shown in Chapter 2, the US has a significant health disadvantage relative to other wealthy countries, especially in terms of key outcomes such as IMR, CVD and obesity. The latter threatens to continue the disadvantage long into the future unless something changes. The US health disadvantage became particularly prominent from around 1980. A National Academies report examined the US health disadvantage – setting out the extent of the issue, examining the potential causes as well as exploring what can be done about it.[170, 171] In terms of understanding why the US does so badly, they examined both compositional factors – differences between the US and other countries in terms of individual health behaviours and in terms of poverty rates and other indicators of socioeconomic status – as well as the wider contextual influences including the role of the social and physical environment. This section summarise the results of their investigation.

So, from a comparative perspective, do Americans engage more in 'risky' health behaviours than people in other countries? In terms of tobacco, the report found that in the 1950s the US had the highest rates of smoking among high-income countries. Today, however, it is one of the lowest – around 16% of US adults smoke compared to 22% of UK adults.[172] Indeed, of comparable countries, only Sweden has lower smoking rates. There is some evidence that around 20% of the US health disadvantage in terms of life expectancy and mortality of the over-50s is attributable to these historical differences in smoking rates,[173] although smoking does not explain differences in health at younger ages.[174] There are significant differences in diet between the US and other countries. For example, average calorie intake per US adult is 3,770 per day (when a healthy intake is around 2,000 for women and 2,500 for men) – the highest in the world. In contrast, Swedish adults consume an average of 3,130 kcals per day – 17% less than the US average.[175] A higher amount of calories in the US diet also come from fats and sugars. It is estimated that the US obesity epidemic (examined in Chapter 3) accounts for 40–70% of the differences in life expectancy among Americans aged over 50.[176] The results of studies that examine cross-national differences in physical activity rates vary, with some suggesting that the US population has about average rates of activity, while others suggest it is lower. The National Academies report therefore concluded that there was insufficient evidence to determine the contribution of physical activity to the US health disadvantage.[177] In terms of alcohol, the research is conflicting as while there is tentative evidence that heavy drinking and binge drinking might be higher among young Americans, the overall prevalence of alcohol consumption among Americans is lower than for Europe.[178]

The National Academies report also explored the role of differences in socioeconomic factors, specifically poverty rates and educational outcomes among the US population compared to other high-income countries. In terms of poverty, the report found that the US has relatively high rates of poverty, with over 17% of US citizens experiencing 'relative poverty' (defined as having less than 50% of the average [median] national income) compared to 11% in the UK and around 7% in Denmark.[179] The US also has the highest rates of child poverty among wealthy countries – in excess of 20% of US children live in poverty (disproportionately concentrated among African American children). Poverty rates in the US – as with other wealthy countries – have increased since the 1980s. Given the long-established links between poverty and poor health, the report authors concluded that 'poverty and child poverty are especially plausible explanations for the pervasive US health disadvantage across multiple causes of illness, unhealthy behaviours, and mortality'.[180]

Alongside the health disadvantage, the US also has an educational disadvantage with a 'mixed but overall mediocre – and in some cases very low – comparative standing',[181] with lower levels of skills and attainment among younger people, which could be contributing to some of the adverse health trends among young Americans such as accidents and violence, drug use, dietary intake and sexually transmitted diseases.[182] The US also has the highest rates of incarceration in prisons of comparable countries.[183] The US population differs compositionally from other wealthy countries in terms of its ethnic make-up – with higher rates of immigration than other countries, especially European ones. However, there is evidence that 'first generation' immigrants are healthier than the native population that they join. So the US health disadvantage is not explained by immigration. However, the high levels of current and historical racial inequalities in the US might also be a factor – African Americans live four years less on average than white Americans, compounding the higher levels of socioeconomic inequalities.[184]

The National Academies report also examined differences between the US and other wealthy countries in terms of contextual factors. In regard to aspects of the social environment, such as social cohesion, there is limited cross-national evidence, and what exists is rather mixed in terms of the relative standing of the US. However, in terms of voting participation rates or levels of trust, an Organisation for Economic Co-operation and Development (OECD) report found that the US ranks among the lowest of wealthy nations.[185] In terms of the physical environment, again, the National Academies report found that cross-national research is sparse, but it did note that there is growing evidence that the built environment, particularly in US cities, is less conducive to physical activity than similar urban environments in other countries – US-built environments are 'less walkable'. Also, the report found evidence of food deserts in the US, particularly concentrated in poorer communities. Car ownership is much higher in the US – 800 motor vehicles per 1,000 people compared to just over 500 in the UK or Sweden.[186] This adds up to an 'obesogenic' urban environment in the US. However, the US is around average for wealthy countries in terms of environmental factors such as air pollution, albeit with large socioeconomic inequalities in exposure with higher rates of harmful toxins experienced in poorer neighbourhoods.[187]

So, to summarise, compositional behavioural factors might be contributing to the excess mortality and lower life expectancy among older Americans, and diet differences might be contributing to differences between Americans and people in other wealthy countries in terms of obesity and diabetes, but such differences in health behaviours do not fully explain the US health disadvantage. Why are Americans more likely to consume more unhealthy food? There are also differences between the US and other wealthy countries in terms of the socioeconomic status of the population – particularly in terms of poverty – that could be contributing to the health disadvantage. But why does the US have worse poverty rates than other wealthy countries? Why has it increased since the 1980s? It is, after all, the richest country in the world. There is also evidence of a more 'obesogenic' urban environment in the US. But what is creating – or allowing – this environment in the US? An analysis of compositional and contextual factors can only take us so far along the chain of causality. To understand more fully why some countries are more or less healthy than others, we need to go further 'upstream' in our analysis and examine the political economy of health – how political choices and policy decisions create, sustain or reduce health divides. This is the subject of Chapter 5, where we will return to the example of the US health disadvantage.

Men behaving badly?

In Chapters 2 and 3, the relative health disadvantage experienced by Scotland in comparison to the other countries of the UK – and especially in comparison to England – was set out in both a historical (Chapter 2) and a contemporary context (Chapter 3). It was in 1950 that Scottish health deviated from the rest of Western Europe, and 1980 when the deviation became more marked.[188] The immediate clinical causes of the 'Scottish effect' post-1950 were differences in CVD, stroke, respiratory disease and cancer. However, since 1980 there have been differences in alcohol and drug-related deaths, suicide, violent deaths and road traffic accidents.[189] The 'Scottish effect' has therefore been linked, to an extent, to higher rates of unhealthy behaviours (proximal causes), particularly the higher rates of alcohol consumption and smoking in Scotland and the infamously less healthy diet, which includes unofficial national dishes of deep-fried chocolate bars.[190] There are also other compositional differences in the Scottish population that might be important such as higher rates of LBW babies and higher rates of teenage conceptions.[191]

Looking further upstream to the social determinants, the 'Scottish effect' has also been linked to the 'Scottish anomaly' in terms of workplace health and safety, whereby Scotland has higher levels of workplace deaths and accidents, as against the UK average.[192] Using comparisons across the UK and with other industrial areas in Europe, however, research has shown that the 'Scottish effect' (and associated proximal cause of health behaviours) is not due to different levels of poverty, and nor is it an issue of any outward migration of healthier Scots.[193] A prominent view until recently has been that the country as a whole, and the West of Scotland in particular, suffered from especially rapid and extensive deindustrialisation during the 1980s, and that this had an adverse impact on health through increasing unemployment, poverty and alienation, and resulted in the increase (or continuation of) negative health behaviours.[194] This deindustrialisation hypothesis, however, was tested in a comparative study of 20 post-industrial regions across Europe, which found that, despite being more affluent than the other deindustrialisation areas, Scotland fared *worst* since the 1980s in terms of health outcomes.[195] So if it is not poverty or deindustrialisation, what explains the persistence of the 'Scottish effect'? Why are the Scots more likely to 'behave badly' in terms of health behaviours? Why is suicide and violent death higher? And what explains the increasing prominence since the 1980s?

The compositional and contextual factors examined in this chapter are not able to fully explain the 'Scottish effect' – there is a need to look even further upstream to the political determinants. The latter is the subject of the next chapter, and the 'Scottish health effect' will be revisited there.

The North or Northerners?

Chapter 3 outlined the stark differences between the North and the South of England in terms of a range of health conditions and in terms of life expectancy: Northerners, on average, live two years less than Southerners. This section examines how compositional and contextual factors contribute to the Northern health penalty: to what extent is the 'Northern health effect' a result of differences in the social and behavioural characteristics of Northerners (compositional)? And to what extent is it a result of the wider economic, social and physical environment of the North (contextual)?

In terms of compositional factors, the North has a higher proportion of people in lower occupational groups than the South. For example, in the North East, 20% of the population are in the lowest occupational groups compared to 14% in London. 17% of people in the North East, 15% in the North West and 14% in Yorkshire and Humber are in receipt of welfare benefits compared to just 9% in the South East.[196] Poverty rates are also higher in the Northern regions: 22% in the North East, 23% in the North West and 24% in Yorkshire and Humber, compared to 17% in the South East. Rates of debt are also higher in the North – people living in the North East have the most debt, owing 34p for every pound in gross income in contrast to 17p and 12p respectively for the South East and South West.[197] Likewise, health behaviours are worse in the North – 20% of people in the North West smoke compared to 17% in the South East. Physical inactivity rates are also higher – for example, in the North East 32% of people do no exercise compared to 25% in the South East.[198] So certainly there would be an expectation – based on the links between socioeconomic status, behaviours and health outcomes – that these compositional factors will be contributing to the health divide. Indeed, statistical analysis has suggested that around four-fifths of the mortality gap between the North and South is explained by these compositional factors.[199]

However, the North also differs from the South in terms of the wider economic, social and environmental context. In terms of economic factors, unemployment is highest in the North East (12%) and lowest in the South East (6%).[200] Average weekly wages (gross, or before tax) are also lower: £477 in the North East, £484 in the North West, and £479 in the Yorkshire and Humber region – much lower than in the South East, where wages average £567 per week.[201] There are also differences between North and South in terms of opportunity structures, with poorer transport links across the North – 84% of national transport investment was spent in London and the South East.[202] Access to healthcare services such as pharmacies or GPs, however, is fairly equitable between the North and South.[203] In terms of collective social functioning, it could be argued that the 'grim up North' reputation might result in negative feelings of alienation, lack of collective control and worthlessness. However, place attachment levels in the North and the sense of a Northern identity could be protective, and the North on the whole has more stable communities than the South. The physical environment of the North also has some disadvantages with post-industrial legacies of higher rates of brownfield land (for example, 27% of wards in the North West are exposed to brownfield land compared to 10% in the South West) and other aspects of environmental deprivation.[204] Statistical modelling suggests that around a fifth of the North–South mortality gap can be explained by these contextual factors.[205]

So the 'Northern health effect' can be accounted for in terms of both compositional and contextual factors, with the former accounting for the majority of the gap. However, compositional factors are strongly influenced by contextual ones – it is hard to have a job, for example, when there are few in the local area. Further, as with the US and Scottish examples, compositional and contextual factors can only go so far in explaining the North–South divide – why has nothing been done to reduce it? Why does it persist? Why has it been allowed to increase? This requires a more fundamental determinants analysis – that politics determines the size and scale of health divides. The North–South case will be examined again in the next chapter when it will be contrasted – unfavourably – with the gap between the East and West of Germany, a gap that was closed in a generation.

A tale of two towns

In Chapter 2 we examined gaps in health in a number of towns and cities in the UK and across the world. Here we use Stockton-on-Tees again, as the place in England with the largest health gaps between its most and least deprived areas, as an example through which to explore the compositional and contextual determinants of these local health divides. It should also be noted that Stockton, too, experienced significant deindustrialisation in the 1980s, and lost a high proportion of its manufacturing, engineering and shipping jobs. Indeed, Mrs Thatcher made her famous 'walk in the wilderness' survey of the effects of her deindustrialisation policies here in 1987.

Again, using data from the Stockton-on-Tees Health Study (see www.durham.ac.uk/health.inequalities), Table 4.3 shows the results of statistical modelling that examines how much of the health gap in Stockton is explained by compositional and contextual factors. The compositional factors used relate to the main theories of health inequalities between socioeconomic groups: material (income, unemployment etc), psychosocial (loneliness, isolation etc), and behavioural (smoking, drinking, diet, exercise), while the contextual data relates largely to the physical environment (noise, pollution, dirt, crime, safety, housing quality). Three different measures of health are used: general wellbeing (EQ5D and EQ-VAS scales) and physical health (SF8-PCS).

As with the North–South divide, most media reports about differences in health between rich and poor areas focus on differences in health behaviours: poorer areas have worse health because the people living there do not take as much care of themselves, they smoke more, they drink more, they eat fast food and they don't exercise. However, as Table 4.3 shows, while differences in smoking, alcohol consumption, diet and exercise account for between 2% and 7% of the gap

Table 4.3: Explaining the health gap in Stockton-on-Tees, England[206]

% Gap explained	Health Measure		
	Measure 1 (SF8PCS)	Measure 2 (EQ5D)	Measure 3 (EQVAS)
Behavioural	2.3%	7.3%	5.3%
Psychosocial	21.9%	26.1%	18.6%
Material	22.8%	14.0%	23.2%
Environment	7.9%	10.9%	2.7%
Clustered	18.3%	30.0%	24.6%
Total Explained	73.2%	88.3%	74.4%
Unexplained	26.8%	11.7%	25.6%

(depending on the measure), material and psychosocial factors explain more – between 14% and 23%, and 19% and 22%, respectively, or between 33% and 45% when taken together; physical environment factors account for a further 3% to 11%. Of course, the different causes of health gaps often cluster together – people who experience poor material factors often also experience poor psychosocial factors and poorer environments, and are more likely to engage in less healthy behaviours. This clustering is also shown in Table 4.3, and it accounts for between 18% and 30% of the gap. As often with statistical models there is a certain proportion of the gap that remains unexplained. So, when thinking about local health divides, both contextual and compositional factors matter – the latter the most, particularly psychosocial and material factors. But why do some people and places suffer from material deprivation in a rich country like England? This is examined further in the next chapter, which focuses on the politics of health.

Home town health

This chapter has examined how place matters for health – both in terms of *who lives there* and *what the place is like*. This has shown the multiple different influences on health, and how health divides emerge. We explore more on why health divides are *allowed* to exist and how they could be different in Chapters 5 to 7, but for now, let's return to the interactive 'health divides' explorer we first used at the end of Chapter 3 (see www.healthdivides.org.uk). We can use it to think about what it is like where you live, and how this might have an impact on the health of your home town.

As we saw in Chapter 3, this explorer links health data in England to local authorities. It also has data on education, unemployment, smoking rates and so on for each local authority. Using the explorer, I can revisit my personal 'places of interest': where I grew up (Lincoln), where I went to university (Birmingham and Manchester), where I have worked in the past (Liverpool and Sheffield) as well as where I now live (Durham), as well as the places that are important in my family history – where my parents grew up (Kent and Newcastle), or where my brother now lives (Nottingham). Adding the new place data on the determinants of health enables me to see why there are such differences in health between my places of interest, linking to the compositional and contextual factors discussed earlier in this chapter. Check out the explorer – what is it like where you live? What it is like where your friends or family live? Does health vary alongside the determinants of health? The explorer helps to illustrate some of the contextual and compositional factors that influence health and place where you live.

This chapter has shown the importance of individual and environmental factors – particularly economic ones – in explaining the relationship between health and place, and offers some insight into the existent of health divides. However, the examination of compositional and contextual factors only goes so far – it looks at the influence of very local and proximate factors, and does not look upstream at the determinants of these factors themselves. To do this, we need to scale up our thinking to *fundamentally* explain why health divides exist: *what determines the contextual and compositional influences on health?* Traditional health geography analysis is unable to fully answer this question as it is fundamentally a political one and as such, it requires an engagement with the political determinants of health: place matters for health, but politics matters for places. In the next chapter we explore what *really* explains why it is that *where you live can kill you.*

CHAPTER 5

It's the (political) economy

> Medicine is a social science, and politics nothing but medicine at a larger scale.
>
> Rudolf Virchow, 1821–1902

The previous chapter examined the role of compositional and contextual factors in health divides. However, by only focusing on these individual characteristics or localised neighbourhood effects, geographical analysis misses the bigger picture, as these compositional and contextual determinants of health are themselves shaped by wider political and economic factors, and therefore the relationship between health and place (and the health divides that exist between places) are *politically* determined:[1] place matters for health, but politics matters for place. Indeed, as Professor Tom Slater of the University of Edinburgh has argued, we need to think not just about how 'where you live affects your life chances', but also how 'your life chances affect where you live': 'if where any given individual lives affects their life chances as deeply as neighbourhood effects proponents believe, it seems crucial to understand why that individual is living there in the first place'.[2]

Ultimately, people live where they can afford to live. Private housing markets produce social sorting, and the emergence of spatial concentrations of poverty and poor neighbourhood infrastructures due to lack of investment. Understanding how place relates to health therefore requires insights from the political economy to think about the more fundamental causes of health divides: *the politics of health*. This 'scaling up' of our understanding of the relationship between health and place is sometimes referred to as the 'political economy' or 'political geography' explanation.[3, 4] The title of this chapter reflects the primacy of these causes. In 1992, 'It's the economy, stupid!' was used by Bill Clinton in his successful US presidential campaign against George Bush Senior. The comment reflected the recession that the US was experiencing at the time, but it is used here as it also encapsulates what is the most fundamentally important driver of health divides. The political addition reflects the fact that the economy we have is the result of political choices we make – as Clinton was, in fact, suggesting. This chapter examines how politics is the fundamental determinant of health divides, outlining key insights from political economy research, and using them to analyse the case studies of the US health disadvantage, the 'Scottish health effect', the North–South health divide in England and local health inequalities. It shows how political ideas and ideologies influence health, place and inequalities, concluding that, above all, geographical health divides are a matter of political and economic choices rather than individual characteristics or local conditions.

Political causes

The 'political economy' approach to explaining health divides focuses on the 'social, political and economic structures and relations' that may be, and often are, outside the control of the individuals or the local areas they affect.[5] Individual and collective social and economic factors such as housing, income and employment – indeed, many of the issues that dominate political life – are key determinants of health and wellbeing.[6] Why some places and people are consistently privileged while others are consistently marginalised is ultimately a political choice, and political choices can thereby be seen as the 'causes of the causes of the causes'.

To return to our examples of the causes of stroke or heart disease from earlier chapters, the immediate clinical 'cause' could be hypertension (high blood pressure). The 'proximal cause' of the hypertension itself could be lifestyle factors such as poor diet, of which the 'social cause' is having a low income or living in a low-income neighbourhood, the causes of which are political – low incomes and low-income neighbourhoods exist because the political and economic system *allows* them to exist. Wages could be regulated so that they are higher (an example being the living wage), or laws could make it easier to organise collectively in trade unions to bargain for better wages, or food prices could be controlled or subsidised (for example, in the US it is meat and corn oil that receive government subsidies, not fruit and vegetables, and likewise in the EU, farmers are encouraged to produce dairy), and neighbourhood food provision does not have to be left to the vagaries of the market (which leads to clustering of poor food availability in poor neighbourhoods). As noted in Chapter 1 (see Figure 1.13), another way to think about this is to imagine a river – downstream are the individual clinical and proximal compositional factors, mid-stream are the contextual factors and upstream are the macro-economic and political factors. The latter are largely controlled by national governments, although increasingly influenced by international and global levels of governance such as those of the EU or IMF.[7] If something polluting is put in the river upstream, it will contaminate all the water in the river – mid-stream and downstream. In terms of health, our political choices result in particular economic and social policies being pursued, and these can be either salutogenic or pathogenic to the people and areas they affect as they have an impact on all the other 'downstream' determinants of health.

In this sense, patterns of health and disease are produced by the structures, values and priorities of political and economic systems.[8] Area-level health – be it local, regional or national – is determined (at least in part) by the wider political, social and economic system and the actions of the state (government) and international-level actors (supranational government bodies such as the EU, inter-state trade agreements such as the proposed TTIP between the US and the EU, as well as the actions of large corporations): politics can make us sick – or healthy.[9] Politics and the balance of power between key political groups – notably labour and capital – determine the role of the state and other agencies in relation to health, and whether there are collective interventions to improve health and reduce health inequalities, and also whether these interventions are individually, environmentally or structurally focused. In this way, politics (broadly understood) is the *fundamental* determinant of our health divides because it shapes the wider social, economic and physical environment and the social and spatial distribution of salutogenic and pathogenic factors, both collectively and individually.[10]

Politics, power and the state

This section outlines the key concepts of politics, power and the state. 'Politics' is derived from 'polis', the Greek for city-state, and in broad terms, politics is about community organisation, how people choose to live together, and collective decision-making about resources, or, 'who gets what, when, how'.[11] There are different definitions of politics (see Box 5.1), but to a greater or lesser extent, politics is about power.[12] At the general level, power is about the ability to achieve a desired outcome (power to do something), but more narrowly it is used to mean power over something or someone and to make, or influence, decisions[13] (see Box 5.1). The state is one of the key instruments of power in any territory. The 'state' is an 'essentially contested concept'[14] with various definitions, the most widely used of which is the narrow theory of the state as simply the institutions of central and local government, the police, the army and the civil service. Government relates to a set of institutions that together make (legislative), implement (executive) and interpret (judicial system) policies and laws.[15] In wealthy democracies (such as in the US, the UK or other Western European countries), the state is often presented as neutral and independent – above party political disputes or the conflicts of economic interests. Political power is dispersed among a wide variety of social groups that compete with one another for dominance and control of the independent institutions of the state. The state can also be seen as the embodiment of the collective will.

An alternative perspective, however, has been put forward by political economists, which broadens the parameters of the state to include many aspects of civil society including schools, the healthcare system, the professions (such as medicine) and the media.[18] In this sense, it is harder to exert democratic control over the state, and it is not neutral but dominated by vested interests, particularly those of big business. Disputes about the role of the state underpin many discussions about healthcare (for example, how much should be publicly provided by the state), and health status (for example, the extent to which individuals are responsible for their own health compared to collective [state] responsibility for providing the conditions in which all can achieve the best possible health). This is examined further in the next section.

Box 5.1: Politics and power[16]

There are four aspects of politics:

- *Politics as government:* traditionally politics has been associated with the art of government and the activities of the state, and its academic study focuses on the personnel and machinery of government, excluding the many arenas in which political activities take place in civil society.
- *Politics as public life:* politics is primarily concerned with the conduct and management of community affairs through the institutions of the state (for example, the courts, the police, the NHS), excluding the political activity of families, personal relationships and so on.
- *Politics as conflict resolution:* politics is concerned with the expression and resolution of conflicts through compromise, conciliation, negotiation and other strategies. Politics is thus seen as a process privileging debate and discussion.
- *Politics as power:* politics is the process through which the production, distribution and use of scarce resources is determined in all areas of social existence, including personal relationships. Politics is thus a term that can be used to describe any 'power-structured relationship or arrangement whereby one group of persons is controlled by another'.[17]

At the general level, power is about the ability to achieve a desired outcome – power to do something – but more narrowly, it is used to mean power over something or someone and to make decisions. Influence is the external ability to have some effect on the content of these decisions. There are three forms of political power:

- *The power of A to influence the behaviour of B.* This exercise of power is observable and is tied to public conflicts over interests (such as access to resources – education, decent housing, healthcare etc). It is performed in the public arena as part of decision-making processes.
- *The power of A to define the political agenda*, thus preventing B from voicing their interests in public (policy) decision-making processes. Potential issues and conflicts are kept off the agenda to the advantage of A and to the detriment of B. The use of this type of power can be obvious or concealed. An example is political lobbying by corporations or other third sector agencies.
- *The power of A to define the values and beliefs that B ought to hold* (for example, what counts as fair/who gets what). B's perceptions and preferences are moulded by A in such a way that B accepts that these are the norm. This dimension of power is played out, for example, in processes of socialisation, ideological hegemony, the control of information and the control of the mass media.

Power therefore not only exists when it is attributable to a specific agent (intentionalist), but also when it is a feature of systems (structuralist), such as economic systems.

Politics of health

'Health, like almost all other aspects of human life, is political in numerous ways.'[19] There are three key aspects to the political nature of public health: how it is distributed and determined; the role of the state in improving the public's health; and the fact that a right to health is a fundamental human right. Ultimately, health is political because it is a resource over which *power* is exercised. The health of populations and places is not only under the control of individual citizens or local communities, but it is also subject to the wider political relations of the state, the economy and society. Further, changing society is only achievable through politics and political struggle.

As demonstrated in Chapter 4, there is a large evidence base showing that 'the most powerful determinants of health in modern populations are to be found in social, economic, and cultural circumstances'.[20] As this book has shown, however, there are large health divides between areas. That these inequalities exist is a matter of political choice, and how these health inequalities are approached by society is also highly political and ideological: are health inequalities to be accepted as the 'natural' and inevitable results of differences in respect of compositional factors (e.g. lifestyle factors) or the 'silent hand of the market' determining your socioeconomic status, where you live or what your area is like? Or are they a moral, social and economic abhorrence that needs to be tackled by a modern state and a humane society?[21] Underpinning these different approaches to health and health inequalities are not only divergent views of what is scientifically or economically possible, but also differing political and ideological opinions about what is desirable. Some people and places – such as Scotland, the North or deprived areas – are economically, politically and socially marginalised by those in power, and their health suffers as a result. Further, factors such as housing, income, employment – indeed, many of the issues that dominate political life – are all important determinants of health and wellbeing. As seen in previous chapters, these determinants (or resources for health) are unequally distributed between people and places.

Health is political because any purposeful activity to enhance population health needs 'the organised efforts of society'[22] or the engagement of 'the social machinery',[23] and both of these require political involvement and political actions. Population health can only be improved through the organised activities of communities and societies. In most countries, the organisation of society is the role of the state and its agencies. The state is the focus of politics. Furthermore, it is not only who has the power to organise society in the interests of health promotion, but also whether and how that organisational power is processed and operated that makes it political.[24]

Finally, health is political because it is a human right:[25] 'Everyone has the right to a standard of living adequate for the health and wellbeing of himself [sic] and of his family, including food, clothing, housing and medical care and necessary social services, and the right to security in the event of unemployment, sickness, disability, widowhood, old age or other lack of livelihood in circumstances beyond his control.'[26] While the right to health includes the right to healthcare – a scarce commodity that is the subject of much political debate – it goes beyond healthcare to encompass the underlying determinants of health, such as safe drinking water, adequate sanitation and access to health-related information and a standard of living adequate for health and wellbeing.

In democratic systems, human rights are embedded within citizenship. Citizenship is 'a status bestowed on those who are full members of a community. All who possess the status are equal with respect to the rights and duties with which the status is endowed.'[27] Human rights are therefore in principle universal and independent from the market (socioeconomic status) position of the individual.[28] While the majority of high-income democratic states (except the US) have ratified the UN's International Covenant on Economic, Social and Cultural Rights (ICESCR), the extent to which health is a right of citizenship is a continued and constant source of political struggle. The post-war welfare states of Western Europe to a large degree ensured that certain health services and a certain standard of living, via welfare provision, became a right of citizenship. However, Professor Ted Schrecker of Durham University has argued, the human rights ethos 'stands in dramatic contrast to much contemporary economic policy wisdom', where the majority of states pursue economic liberalisation (neoliberalism, discussed later in this chapter), entailing the dismantling of the state provision of resources provided on the basis of citizenship, and replacing them with market-based provision that varies by how much you can pay.[29] The gap between the right to health of citizens and the reality on the ground is evident in that, for example, 33 million US residents currently lack access to healthcare, and the right to a standard of living adequate for health and wellbeing is not possessed by the 1 million children living in absolute poverty in the UK.[30]

Political ideologies and health[31]

This section focuses on the key political ideologies of wealthy democracies and how they have informed approaches to health and health inequalities: conservatism (associated with the Conservative Party in the UK, the Republican Party in the US or the Christian Democratic Parties of Western Europe), liberalism (associated with the Liberal Democrats in the UK, the Democrats in the US and in its neoliberal form, with parties of both left and right) and socialism and social democracy (associated with the Labour Parties of the UK, Australia or New Zealand, and the Social Democratic Parties of Western Europe).

Ideology is a system of interrelated ideas and concepts that reflect and promote the political, economic and cultural values and interests of a particular societal group.[32] Ideologies, like societal groups, are therefore often conflicting, and the dominance of one particular ideology within a society to a large extent reflects the power of the group it represents. Ideology can be used to manipulate the interests of the many in favour of the power and privileges of the few.[33] So, for example, liberal democratic ideology, with its emphasis on the individual, the market and the neutral state, can be seen as a reflection of the power of business interests within capitalist society.[34] A hegemonic – universally prevailing or dominant – ideology is usually one that has successfully incorporated and cemented a number of different elements from other competing ideologies, and thereby fuses the interests of diverse societal groups and classes.[35] There is emerging evidence that ideologies, via the different economic and social systems they produce, can play a key role in determining differences in health between places (as will be examined in the first case study presented later in this chapter).

Conservatism

The literal interpretation of conservatism is to 'conserve', to maintain what has been tried and tested, rather than to seek radical change. Part of maintaining the traditional order of things includes a belief that human talent varies naturally, and consequently, that attempts to 'level' things out (equality of any kind) are artificial and destined to fail. The existence of a social hierarchy is not only viewed as inevitable but also desirable, as it is thought to promote innovation and success, and allows the majority to benefit from the leadership of particularly talented individuals. Rich people tend to be thought of as creators of prosperity rather than plunderers of the poor (a view that contrasts with socialist and communist ideas about wealth). Hence, conservatism differs from many other political ideologies in its vindication of inequality.[36] Conservative preferences for maintaining tradition are associated with preserving the dominance of particular groups (for example, the wealthy) or of a religion (for example, Christianity) or culture (for example, 'Britishness'). These preferences are also associated with a morality emphasising the importance of self-discipline, decency, the 'nuclear family unit' and a respect for the rule of law.

As well as a tendency towards tradition, other features of conservatism include a view of society as a collection of self-interested individuals, a belief that underlies Margaret Thatcher's infamous claim that 'there's no such thing as society'. Of particular importance to health, Conservatives tend to see the role of the state as minimal, with a preference for limited (if any) welfare provision. While some Conservatives favour a society in which the privileged classes provide basic welfare (for example, housing) to the 'deserving poor' on a charitable basis, there is agreement that too much provision by the state removes incentives from the poor to improve or help themselves, creating a dependency culture and a permanent underclass of what Thatcher called 'moral cripples'. The only exception to Conservative preferences for minimal government intervention in society tends to be around law and order, where significant state intervention is often viewed as essential to maintain the smooth running of society.

Under Conservative thinking, health is an individual good. Its unequal distribution across populations and places as well as the influence of unequal social and spatial exposure to the wider determinants of health is both natural and acceptable: health divides are not a political or collective concern.

Liberalism (and neoliberalism)

At its heart, liberalism is essentially an economic approach but, like all economic doctrines, it has far-reaching political and social repercussions. With its focus on freedom and choice, liberalism emphasises the importance of individual over collective rights.

So liberalism promotes the equality of individual political and religious rights (so-called 'socially liberal'). In economic terms, individuals are also given primacy over collective entities (for example, social classes or communities). Liberalism believes in a small state and a lack of state interference in the market and in the lives of individuals.

Classical liberals believe that a free market guarantees social justice, allowing all those with talent and a willingness to work to succeed. This genre of liberalism was popular in the 18th and 19th centuries, when its proponents advocated minimal state intervention in the economy and the importance of the 'invisible hand of the market' and free trade. Popular discontent with the social consequences of this approach (for example, the Great Depression of the 1930s) put pressure on Liberal Parties to adapt. Out of this situation, 'modern liberalism' emerged, which conceded that state intervention to reduce the excesses of market economics and mitigate its negative effects was desirable in order to provide 'equality of opportunity'. In post-war Europe, alongside the elections of Social Democratic Parties, this helped with the creation of the welfare state and the implementation of a more interventionist approach by the state to the economy (known as Keynesianism).

The 'crisis of the welfare state' in the late 1970s led to the re-emergence of more classical liberal ideas, especially in relation to economics. This form of liberal thinking, which resurrected market economics, is known as 'neoliberalism' ('neo' meaning 'new'). Some strands of modern conservatism, such as the 'New Right' movement of the 1980s (strongly associated with Thatcherism in the UK and Reaganism in the US), while employing a traditionally conservative moral rhetoric, also encapsulated a drive towards the free market and competitive individualism, taking inspiration from liberal thinking – 'neoliberalism'.[37] Geopolitically, neoliberalism is associated most with the US, but economic globalisation means it has increasingly become hegemonic (that is, globally dominant) to the extent that some commentators argue there is now no alternative.[38] Indeed, neoliberal approaches even infiltrated European Social Democratic Parties in the 1990s (for example, Blair's New Labour in the UK).

The individualistic nature of liberal ideology means that, as with conservatism, health is an individual matter, and health divides are essentially compositional in nature. However, there is acknowledgement that they are not natural or inevitable, but the result of 'risky individual health behaviours'. This shifts responsibility for health improvement away from governments and onto individuals, thereby allowing the kind of minimal state intervention advocated by liberalism. (Neoliberalism and health is examined further later in this chapter.)

Socialism and social democracy

Socialism is the broadest of political ideologies as it contains a variety of perspectives, from revolutionary communists to reformist social democrats. The meaning of socialism is therefore not fixed and it differs by time and place. Originally socialism was associated with the Marxist/communist tradition, and used to describe the desire for economic equality (common ownership of the productive wealth and a classless society) in contrast to the purely political or religious equality (for example, the right to vote and be represented) advocated by liberals.[39] The Social Democratic Parties (SDP) of Western Europe were originally based within this Marxist tradition, but by the early 20th century a split occurred: the Communist Parties continued to advocate revolution and the overhaul of the capitalist system as the only way of achieving economic equality, while the SDP supported the reform of capitalism and proposed a parliamentary road to socialism. The British Labour Party was always of the latter type.

In the immediate post-war period, social democrats used increased state intervention (such as the public ownership of key parts of the economy, the redistribution of income and the establishment of the welfare state) to mitigate the effects of capitalism and thereby increase economic equality[40] – part of a consensus with more social liberalism. However, there is little agreement among social democrats about how much state intervention is required in the economy or how much economic equality is desirable. The most recent evolution of social democracy in the 1990s – the 'Third Way' (associated particularly with Blairism in the UK)[41] – saw the abandonment of previous commitments to public ownership and a dilution in views of the extent to which the state needs to intervene to ensure equality.[42] Indeed, Social Democratic parties started to embrace the individualism and market fundamentalism of liberals and conservatives. This, alongside the collapse of the communist Eastern bloc, has led to claims that socialism has died in the face of the resurgence of neoliberalism.

In terms of health, the socialist tradition embraces social rights (including the right to health and a decent standard of living) and, historically at least, privileges collective rights over individual ones. This is demonstrated through such things as increasing access to healthcare (for example, the British Labour Party set up the NHS), and a concern for creating the collective economic and social conditions in which all can obtain the best possible health state. Health divides are therefore a concern for government and for collective political action.

Political health divides

To date, the *political geography* approach, which takes the theories and concepts outlined above and uses them to analyse the fundamental political causes of health divides, has largely focused on the analysis of differences between wealthy countries. Research here has indicated that political choices are important in terms of explaining these international differences.[43, 44] For example, it has shown that long-term rule by more left-wing, redistributive, Social Democratic parties results in better national health outcomes such as IMR, life expectancy or LBW babies (birth weight of an infant of less than 2.5kg) than rule by more right-wing, neoliberal governments.[45, 46] This is examined in more detail in the international health divides case study in this section. However, the *political geography of health* approach can, and should, also be applied to aid understanding of other health divides including local and regional ones. Examples of the effects of politics (power, ideologies and the exercise of state power) on the other key health divides of this book – between the countries of the UK, the regions of England and local ones within towns and cities – are also examined in this section with regards to neoliberalism and the politics of the 'Scottish health effect', lessons from German reunification for the English health divide and the effects of austerity and welfare reform on regional and local inequalities in health in the UK.

Rules of the game

Chapter 3 set out differences in health between wealthy countries, particularly noting the US health disadvantage. These differences in health among the richest nations are not explained by medicine or genetics. As discussed in Chapter 4, conventionally, these differences have therefore been assumed to be as a result of compositional explanations in terms of variations in health behaviours between the populations of countries or, more recently, in terms of contextual factors such as levels of social cohesion or the physical environment.[47] In Chapter 4 we examined these explanations for the US health disadvantage. This examination started to unpack why the US does worse than other wealthy countries – but it also created new questions. It showed that diet and poverty could contribute to the divide between the US and other wealthy countries, but, as this section will show, the reasons why the US has higher rates of poverty and why Americans consume more unhealthy food are ultimately political ones. There are, indeed, significant political and institutional arrangements that differentiate the US from other rich democracies.[48]

While all these countries are in economic terms capitalist, and in political terms liberal democracies, they still differ in important ways in terms of how they implement, manage and structure their societies, which in turn lead to subtle but important differences in the social determinants of health. Key among these are (1) social welfare benefits in the areas of health, pensions and unemployment insurance; (2) income inequality; (3) collective bargaining and political incorporation; and (4) public health regulation.[49] All of these are important for health – and the US does comparatively badly on these *and* badly on health. Could there be a connection? Politically designed institutions set the wider 'rules of the game', shaping the environment within which the other contextual and compositional determinants of health play out.[50] So let's now examine whether the 'rules of the game' vary in the US compared to other wealthy countries.

These 'rules of the game' can best be captured through the concept of welfare state regimes.[51] The 'welfare state' is a contested term within social and political analysis.[52] Conventionally, it has been used as a means of referring to the provision of key welfare services in terms of the state provision of education, healthcare, housing, poor relief and social insurance (cash benefits for the unemployed, the sick or the old, for example), and other social services as well as the regulation of key areas.[53] More broadly, the welfare state can be considered as a particular form of capitalist state, or a specific type of society and economy, which emerged in advanced market democracies in Western countries during the early post-war period.[54] It therefore encompasses the full political 'rules of the game' – the setting in which other processes take place, including the social and proximal determinants of health.

For most of the 19th century, there was minimal state provision of welfare beyond very basic 'poor relief' – the provision of basic food rations and shelter (often provided via institutions such as the English workhouse system). Beyond these provisions welfare came via family members or charity (particularly the Church). This began to change in the early 20th century with the introduction of rudimentary and highly selective (non-workers that included most women were typically excluded from such schemes) state-organised welfare systems that provided basic pensions, unemployment and sickness benefits funded via social insurance payments (for example, the National Insurance Act 1911 in the UK or the Bismarckian welfare reforms of 1880s Germany).

It was not until after the Second World War (1945) that a fuller welfare state – what is often referred to as the 'Keynesian welfare state' – was established in most wealthy countries. To a greater or lesser extent, this 'golden age' of welfare state capitalism was characterised by centralism, universalism and Keynesian economics (active macroeconomic management by the state, such as interventionist fiscal policy, a large public sector and a mixed economy), full (male) employment and high public expenditure, and the promotion of mass consumption via a redistributive tax and welfare system. There was also a mainstream political consensus in favour of the welfare state and the redistribution it encompassed. In the 'golden age' of welfare state expansion (from the 1940s to 1960s), Western countries experienced significant improvements to public housing, healthcare and the other main social determinants of health including workers enjoying the highest share of national income ever.[55] 'Golden age' welfare states varied considerably, however, in the services they provided and the generosity and coverage of social insurance and welfare benefits.

In this period, welfare state capitalism could be divided into broadly three different types, or regimes:[56] Liberal, Bismarckian and Social Democratic (see Table 5.1). These are described below, although there were, of course, significant differences even within these regimes as, for example, in the case of the Liberal regime where New Zealand and the UK provided nationalised health services while the US relied largely on a private insurance system (discussed later). There are also debates among academics about the number of different regimes and which countries should be in which group.[57]

Broadly speaking then, in the welfare states of the Liberal regime (the Anglo-American countries of Australia, Canada, Ireland, New Zealand, the UK and the US), state provision of welfare was fairly minimal, social insurance benefits were modest and often attracted strict entitlement criteria, recipients were often subject to means testing and receipt was stigmatised.

Table 5.1: Welfare state regimes[58]

Liberal	Bismarckian	Social Democatic
Australia	Austria	Denmark
Canada	Belgium	Finland
Ireland	France	Iceland
New Zealand	Germany	Sweden
United Kingdom	Italy	Norway
United States	Japan	
	Switzerland	
	Netherlands	

In this model, even in the post-war period, the dominance of the market was encouraged by guaranteeing only a minimum level of support, and by subsidising private welfare schemes. In the Liberal welfare state regime a stark division existed between those, largely the poor, who relied on state aid, and those who were able to afford private provision.

The Bismarckian welfare state regime (Austria, Belgium, France, Germany, Italy, Japan, Switzerland and the Netherlands) was characterised by its 'status differentiating' welfare programmes in which benefits were often earnings-related, administered through the employer, and geared towards maintaining existing social hierarchies. The role of the family was also emphasised, and the redistributive impact of this regime was minimised. However, the market was marginalised more than in the Liberal regime.

The Social Democratic regime type (Denmark, Finland, Iceland, Sweden and Norway) was characterised by universalism, comparatively generous social transfers, a commitment to full employment and income protection, and a strongly interventionist state, both in terms of the economy and regulation (for example, a strong public health policy). The state was actively used to promote social equality through a redistributive social security system. Unlike the other welfare state regimes, the Social Democratic regime type promoted an equality of the highest standards, not an equality of minimal needs.

The 'golden age' of the welfare state effectively ended with the economic crisis of the 1970s (with high inflation, slow economic growth and the end of full employment), during which there was a general loss of confidence in the ability of welfare state capitalism to adequately maintain profitability and to safeguard the capitalist economic system. This was the emergence of neoliberal economics, initially in the Anglo-American countries, but then spreading across continental Europe (neoliberalism is discussed further in the next case study). The political consensus of the early post-war years broke down as governments started to dismantle and restructure the welfare state, under the justification of neoliberal ideology. Reforms (which largely occurred in the 1980s and 1990s) were characterised by the privatisation and marketisation of welfare services; entitlement restrictions and increased qualifying conditions for benefits, and a shift towards targeting and means testing; cuts or limited increases to the actual cash values of benefits; modified funding arrangements (with a shift away from business taxation); and an increased emphasis on an active rather than a passive welfare system.[59]

This neoliberal restructuring of the welfare state has been analysed by some commentators as a shift from Keynesian welfare state capitalism, which could afford and required a high level of public welfare expenditure, to a system of 'workfare state capitalism', in which high welfare expenditure is considered to be incompatible with a profitable economy. Workfare state capitalism is characterised by decentralisation and welfare pluralism (with a strong role for the private sector), the promotion of labour market flexibility, supply-side economics, the subordination of social policy to the demands of the market, and a desire to minimise social expenditure. Like welfare states, there are variants on the workfare model reflecting the historical constraints presented by the policy hangover of existing welfare state regime structures and politics, variations in public opinion between countries and differences by regime in policy responses to common challenges.[60] The neoliberal workfare state emphasises the privatisation of state enterprise and welfare services and the deregulation of the private sector.[61] The neo-Bismarckian workfare state is characterised by an economic policy increasingly geared to the microeconomic level and a smaller role for the state as key welfare services, such as health or pensions, become increasingly self-regulated and welfare becomes more pluralistic and privatised.[62] The neo-social democratic response relies on a state-guided approach to economic reorganisation. Flexibility is provided through an active labour market policy, which emphasises training, skills and mobility while retaining a generous out-of-work benefit system. Welfare provision is also more mixed, but the new providers are more likely to be from the charitable and voluntary sectors than private capital.

The welfare state is thereby understood as more than a set of transfers and services; it consists of systems and processes, which themselves shape society and structure socioeconomic and demographic stratifications – the 'rules of the game'.[63] The welfare state is therefore potentially an important macro-level political and economic contextual determinant of health that also mediates the extent, and impact, of socioeconomic inequalities in exposure to the social determinants on health.

Research has demonstrated that countries with more generous welfare and healthcare benefits have lower IMR, lower overall mortality rates, less mortality at younger ages and, albeit to a lesser extent, increased life expectancy at birth.[64, 65] Indeed, a study found that the type of welfare state accounted for 20% of the difference in IMR between wealthy countries and 10% of differences in LBW babies.[66] Key welfare state policies – support for dual earners (where both men and women are encouraged to work) and generous basic pensions – decreased IMR and old age excess mortality respectively.[67] Social welfare benefits in the areas of unemployment insurance, pensions and health care are considerably lower in the US than in other wealthy countries.

For example, a comparative analysis of benefit generosity across three primary policy domains (unemployment insurance, sickness benefits and pensions) in 18 wealthy countries since 1970 found that the US has consistently been very ungenerous with a very low level of benefits in the early 1970s; it increased moderately until the late 1970s, then declined after the 1980s; and the US now provides the lowest level of welfare generosity.[68] More social democratic countries – such as Norway and Sweden – have the highest levels of generosity. In this study, benefit generosity was measured as the percentage of the average employee wage that is replaced by benefits; how long those benefits can be received; restrictions on benefit eligibility, such as waiting periods, retirement ages and work requirements; and the population coverage rate (the percentage of the workforce that is entitled to the benefits).

An example of how getting access to welfare benefits is harder in the US is provided by the treatment of mothers with young children. Historically since the 1960s, women with young children were entitled to welfare benefits (albeit of a fairly low, around federal poverty line, level). However, since 'reforms' implemented by President Clinton, a Democrat, in 1996, low-income women no longer had a guarantee of state-provided minimum income support unless they enrolled on workfare programmes ('workfare' requires benefit recipients to basically 'work for their benefits').[69]

The US spends the most on healthcare – in absolute terms, per head of population and as a proportion of national income. Around 18% of US GDP is spent on healthcare compared to around 6% in the UK.[70] However, a large proportion of this is wasted on funding and regulating a healthcare market, rather than going on patient care. Unlike other wealthy countries that operate a social insurance system (whereby the government, employers and employees co-fund healthcare via regular set contributions, for example, France and Germany) or a national health system (where healthcare is funded by the government based on general taxation, for example, the UK, Sweden or New Zealand), the US system is effectively a private market. Individuals are expected to buy insurance policies themselves to cover their health risk, and employed people might get coverage from their employers. There are some government-funded schemes for the very poor (Medicaid) and for the elderly (Medicare), but these are not as generous as schemes in other countries.

Although the (in)famous 'Obamacare' Patient Protection and Affordable Care Act reforms of 2010 did a lot to increase coverage rates, around 10% or 33 million Americans remain without health insurance of any kind, and therefore only have access to emergency care, not prevention or primary or secondary care.[71] Millions of others remain 'under-insured', whereby their healthcare policies do not cover the full range of health services or their health needs. They also face considerable out-of-pocket payments or co-payments for services.[72] This all means that healthcare access in the US is the most 'commodified' (market dependent) of wealthy nations – access is highly dependent on market position, so that richer people and places have better access than the poor and more deprived areas.[73] It is an extreme example of the 'inverse care law'. Access to healthcare plays an important role in certain health outcomes, particularly those amenable to medical intervention.

The National Academies report, mentioned previously in Chapter 3, also examined the role of income inequality in the US health disadvantage.[74] Income redistribution – to reduce the wage inequality that arises in market economies – is one of the key policy mechanisms available to governments. This is usually done by taxing higher earners and corporations, and redistributing this to others, via welfare benefits (as mentioned above) or via public services such as healthcare or education, for example. In *The Spirit Level*, Richard Wilkinson and Kate Pickett[75] found that the level of income inequality in a country (and in the US states) is associated with health outcomes. They found that countries and states with higher levels of income inequality between the top and bottom 20% of the income scale had worse health outcomes – higher IMR, lower life expectancy, higher rates of obesity, excess risk of premature mortality, homicide rates and higher levels of mental ill health. The relationship between income inequality and poorer health outcomes is also found at a smaller geographical scale in the towns and cities of the US: *more unequal places (almost always) do worse.* Of the wealthy countries, the US is the most unequal. On the widely used 'Gini coefficient' measure of income inequality (on a scale of 0–1, whereby 0 is complete income equality within a population, and 1 is complete inequality), the US scores 0.38, while more social democratic countries like Norway score 0.25.[76]

Collective bargaining and political incorporation have also been associated with health outcomes. Trade unions exist to protect and promote the rights and wages of workers. In countries such as the UK and the US, they developed in the late 19th century in response to the appalling and dangerous working conditions and low wages that industrial workers experienced. Countries with higher rates of trade union membership have more extensive welfare systems, higher levels of income redistribution, and, correspondingly, lower rates of income inequality. All of these, as mentioned above, are associated with better health outcomes.

In the 'golden age' of the post-war welfare state (1945–75), trade unions were also incorporated to varying degrees into policy-making (so-called 'corporatism', an approach to governance most favoured by Social Democratic governments). This declined with the rise of neoliberalism (discussed further in the next case study). Countries with greater levels of trade union density also have better health and safety regulations. Again, the US has historically had the lowest rate of trade union membership among wealthy countries, restricting the representation of working-class interests in policy and politics.

For example, in 2010 only 12% of the US workforce were members of a trade union. In contrast, the rates were 26% in the UK and 68% in Sweden.[77]

Further, research has shown that the political incorporation of minority groups is robustly associated with better health among those groups, suggesting a direct connection between political empowerment and health.[78] The US was a historical laggard in terms of the incorporation of minority groups, with equal civil rights for African Americans only achieved in the 1960s. An example of the effects of such political incorporation on health comes from a Harvard University study of the Democrats' 1964 Civil Rights Act abolition of the 'Jim Crow laws' in the Southern states of the US such as Mississippi. These effectively allowed racial discrimination and segregation, and were similar to the apartheid regime in South Africa. The study found that from 1960 to 1964, the African American infant death rate was 20% higher in the Jim Crow states than in the non-Jim Crow ones, whereas after abolition (and the increased political emancipation of African Americans in these states), the gap disappeared.[79]

A further example of how political institutions shape the wider 'rules of the game' is via regulation, particularly in areas relevant to public health. Preventative health policy such as increasing the price of (or restricting access to) cigarettes and alcohol reduces consumption of these harmful products. Regulating saturated fat levels in food can reduce CVD; reducing air pollution levels lowers risks for respiratory disease and CVD; and workplace health and safety regulations reduce workplace accidents and illnesses.[80]

The role of regulation in the US health disadvantage can be explored through the example of the obesity epidemic. Why does the US have the highest rates of obesity? Why do Americans consume more fast food and saturated fats than the citizens of other wealthy countries? Less regulation of products and of their advertising is part of the answer: *fat is a political issue*.[81] An analysis of 25 high-income countries between 1999 and 2008 found that the increased deregulation of fast food was associated with an increase in consumption – which, in turn, increased mean BMI.[82] During the 10 years studied, the average number of fast food transactions per year across the 25 countries increased by a fifth, from 27 per person in 1999 to 33 in 2008. Average BMI increased from 25.8 to 26.4kg/m^2. The more deregulated countries – such as the US – had faster increases in both fast food consumption and BMI. Social democratic governments favour public health regulation more than conservative or liberal governments as they are more prepared to intervene to reduce market-generated inequalities. Indeed, research suggests that among European countries, preventative health policies (especially in terms of alcohol and tobacco control) are better in those countries with longer periods of social democratic rule.[83]

So this case study has set out how politics and political institutions – 'the rules of the game' – may be the fundamental determinants of the US health disadvantage. It can also be argued that the escalation of the US health disadvantage since the 1980s is related to the rise of neoliberal politics – and this is the topic of our next case study.

Shock doctrine[84]

Since the 1980s, the social and spatial determinants of health have become much more stratified, with the poorest areas and poorest people faring worse in relative terms than they have at any point since the Second World War. In a previous book (written with Professor Ted Schrecker of Durham University) I have argued that this increase in health inequalities has been the result of the dominance of neoliberalism in economic and social policy. We called contemporary health inequalities a 'neoliberal epidemic'.[85] This section provides a brief summary of some of the key aspects of neoliberalism and health before examining the effects of neoliberalism on one of our key health divides, the 'Scottish health effect'.

The 'golden age' of the welfare state effectively ended with the economic crisis of the 1970s (when rising oil prices combined with high inflation and high unemployment) and the simultaneous rise of neoliberalism or 'market fundamentalism' as the dominant political and economic ideology. The fundamental presuppositions of neoliberalism are as follows: (1) markets are the normal, natural and preferable way of organising human interaction; (2) the primary function of the state is to ensure the efficient functioning of markets; and (3) institutions or policies that lead to outcomes different from those that would be expected from a market require justification.[86] The core tenets of neoliberalism remained on the margins of mainstream politics in the wealthy world until the 1970s.[87] At that point the economic uncertainties of 'stagflation' – the simultaneous occurrence of high inflation and high unemployment – created a newly receptive climate among both elites and, in many countries, electorates.

Various narratives of the advance of neoliberalism can be found in the literature. One regards neoliberal policies as pragmatic responses to a changing global economic environment that was largely outside the control of individual national governments. Under these new conditions, neoliberal policies were the only ones that 'worked'.[88] Another views neoliberalism as a political project aimed at the restoration of the class power of business (capital) that had been eroded by the rise of the welfare state and associated redistributive policies.[89] It is clear, however, that neoliberalism is best understood as having multiple dimensions, including concrete policy programmes and innovations (for example, scaling back the welfare state), more general reorganisation of state institutions (for example, privatisation and contracting out), and an implicit ideology that gives primacy to the individual as opposed to the collective, exemplified by Thatcher's (in)famous comment that 'there is no such thing as society, only individuals and their families'.[90]

The election of the Conservative government of Margaret Thatcher in the UK in 1979 (and of Republican US President Ronald Reagan in 1980 or Helmut Kohl in West Germany in 1982) represented key turning points. The political consensus of the 'golden age' began to break down as governments started to dismantle and restructure the welfare state. The 'reforms' were characterised by the privatisation and marketisation of welfare services; entitlement restrictions and increased qualifying conditions for welfare benefits, and a shift towards targeting and means testing; cuts or limited increases to the actual cash values of benefits; modified funding arrangements (with a shift away from business taxation and towards consumption taxes); an increased emphasis on an active rather than a passive welfare system; deregulation of the economy with the promotion of labour market flexibility, supply-side economics and a desire to minimise public social expenditure; and the subordination of social policy to the demands of the market.[91]

The advance of neoliberalism in the UK is shown in Figure 5.1. This uses data from the Economic Freedom of the World Index, produced by Canada's neoliberal Fraser Institute.[92] The Index measures the size of government (expenditures, taxes etc), the legal structure and security of property rights, access to finance, freedom to trade internationally and the regulation of credit, labour and business. It produces a scale of 1–10, with higher scores representing higher levels of 'economic freedom' as defined by neoliberals – meaning fewer rights for workers, lower taxes on businesses, easier (although not necessarily less costly) access to credit and less state regulation (that is, freedom for business/capital, but not necessarily for people/workers). So Figure 5.1 shows how neoliberal 'economic freedom' has increased since 1980 – it is much higher in 2010 than in 1980. This increase in 'economic freedom' (for capital/business) was achieved primarily by increasing economic insecurity, unemployment and income inequality, and decreasing the size of the social safety net for everyone else. These have had a particular impact on more deprived areas and certain parts of the UK and the US than others, with the former manufacturing heartlands in the North

Figure 5.1: The growth of neoliberalism in the UK, 1970–2010[93]

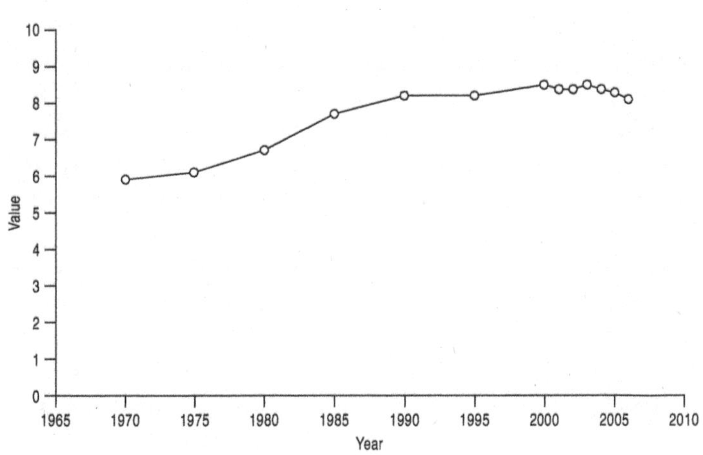

of England, the West of Scotland, South Wales and the 'rustbelt' in the northern US especially effected (as noted in Chapter 3).

During the neoliberal era, there has been a decline in the number of standard full-time, permanent jobs, and a sharp increase in flexible or precarious employment: more and more people are working on either temporary contracts or no contracts, with limited or no employment or welfare rights. This partly reflects a decline in manufacturing employment (deindustrialisation) in wealthy countries and the rise of the service sector. It also reflects the anti-trade union laws introduced since 1979 (the UK now has some of the most restrictive trade union rights of any wealthy democracy). In this new economy, skills, working hours, contracts, conditions, pay and location are all more flexible and precarious. The once standard full-time, permanent contract with benefits has been superseded by a number of atypical forms of employment that tend to be characterised by lower levels of security and poorer working conditions.[94] Rather than being a transitory stage in an individual's employment history, atypical forms of labour are becoming the norm for many workers in the labour force of high-income countries.[95] As an important ethnographic study of the Teesside area of North East England (where Stockton-on-Tees is located) found, 'Moving in and out of jobs, and above and below the poverty line, over a working life is ... now the normal experience for many working-class people.'[96] This 'low-pay, no-pay cycle' is an example of a broader international trend that has been described as the emergence of a new stratum of workers called 'the precariat'.[97] The expansion of the precariat is exemplified by what are called 'zero hours contracts', under which workers have no set hours of work and are not guaranteed even minimum hours from week to week. Such contracts also reduce entitlements to certain out-of-work benefits, and to pensions. In 2014, 1.4 million workers in the UK were on such contracts.[98]

Alongside the decline in manufacturing and the rise of economic insecurity, there has been an emergence of permanent or structural unemployment. Until the late 1970s, there was a government commitment to the pursuit of full employment (unemployment rates of <3% or employment rates of >80%). There were, of course, periods of unemployment during the early post-war years, but these were cyclical, following the boom and bust patterns of the economy (for example, the early 1960s in the UK): in periods of economic growth there were jobs for all, in periods of recession there was an increase in unemployment.

This was abandoned under the neoliberal monetarist pursuit of low inflation by the Thatcher (and Reagan in the US) and subsequent UK governments that accepted high unemployment and its social consequences as collateral damage. Indeed, Norman Lamont, Conservative UK Chancellor of the Exchequer, stated in 1991 that 'rising unemployment and the recession have been the price that we have had to pay to get inflation down. That price is well worth paying.'[99] This was echoed in 1998 by Eddie George, Governor of the Bank of England, who stated that 'northern unemployment is an acceptable price to pay for curbing southern inflation'.[100] At the same time, there was an expansion in terms of those (for example, women, lone parents, the sick) for whom work was expected or required as an alternative to falling behind economically.

Meanwhile, as part of the neoliberal project to shrink the state, neoliberalism reduced the support provided to people when out of work. For example, in the UK the percentage of an average production worker's wage that would be replaced by unemployment benefits (the unemployment replacement rate) for one earner supporting a partner and two children declined from 69% in 1971 to 36% in 1990, although increasing slightly under Labour governments post-1997 (examined further in the next chapter). For a single worker with no dependants, the decline was even more dramatic: from 54% in 1971 to 20% or less in every year post-1990s.[101] These figures apply only to those workers who are eligible for benefits; a further neoliberal 'reform' was restricting eligibility for any support at all, as noted in the previous case study of the US health disadvantage. The neoliberal policy turn has also seen the privatisation and marketisation of key public services such as housing and the NHS as well as infrastructure such as the railways. Since the 2007/08 financial crisis, the policy of austerity pursued by the UK government and the EU (for example, enforced on Greece) has led to further welfare state cutbacks, with (predictable) negative effects on our health divides (explored in the next case study).

Neoliberalism has also seen an increase in the concentration of wealth, with the share of UK wealth of the top 0.1% (one one-thousandth) of the population found to have increased from 7% in 1978 to 22% in 2012, comparable to the inequality of distribution before the Great Depression of the 1930s, and roughly equal to the net worth of the bottom 90% of the population, which had fallen from 35% in the mid-1980s to 23% today.[102] The growth in the income share of the top 1% that began around 1980 occurred contemporaneously with reductions in the marginal Income Tax rate for top earners – in the UK, from 83% in 1980 to 40% in 1988 under Thatcher's government. The top marginal rate was later raised to 50% under the 2005–10 Labour government, and then lowered again to 45% by the Conservative-led coalition (2010–15). Wealth inequality also widened considerably. This is shown in Figure 5.2 in terms of the percentage of wealth received by the richest 1% in the UK from the 1920s to the mid-2000s.[103] This fell until the 1980s, when it started to increase rapidly.

The effects of these neoliberal economic and social policies on health inequalities have been stark (or of 'epidemic' proportions, to use Schrecker and Bambra's term[104]), as it has meant that those at the bottom have fallen even further behind. It has also had an impact on health divides, and can therefore be seen as a political

Figure 5.2: Percentage share of wealth held by the richest 1% in the UK from the 1920s to the mid-2000s[105]

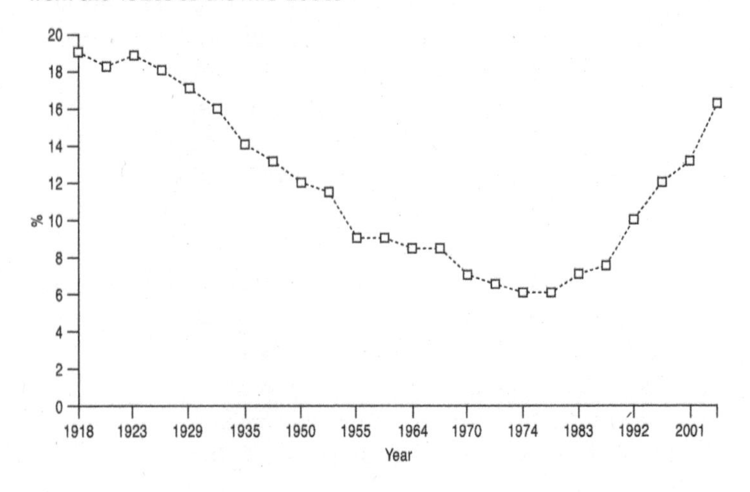

attack on public health.[106] The effects of neoliberalism on health have been extensively documented in terms of the rapid implementation of 'casino capitalism' in the former communist states of the USSR and Eastern Europe, whereby the collapse of the communist states in 1990 led to the rapid dismantling of their welfare and healthcare systems and policy of full employment. This led to unprecedented increases in poverty accompanied by deteriorations in health behaviours (with very high rates of alcohol-related mortality), and increased IMR and lowered life expectancy.[107] However, neoliberalism has also been linked to the post-1980 escalation of the 'Scottish health effect'.

Chapter 3 explored the 'Scottish health effect', whereby Scotland has worse health than the other countries of the UK. It examined some of the conventional explanations for it, drawing on compositional and contextual factors. However, some analysts have argued that while the 'Scottish health effect' is detectable since the 1950s, its rapid increase – and changing epidemiology from CVD, stroke, a respiratory condition and cancer to alcohol and drug-related deaths, suicide, violent deaths and road traffic accidents – since 1980 can be linked to the rapid implementation of neoliberalism in the UK in this period: a neoliberal 'shock doctrine' for Scotland.

In a powerful article, Scottish researchers Chik Collins and Gerry McCartney[108] argue that the neoliberalism implemented by the post-1979 UK Thatcher-led Conservative governments constitute a 'political attack' against the working class, and that Scotland (particularly Glasgow and the West of Scotland) became a particular target. While neoliberalism spread across wealthy countries in the 1980s, the UK was exposed in a way that other European nations were not, in a very rapid and intense manner that adversely affected health through unemployment, poverty, alienation and associated increases in 'risky' health behaviours. For example, deindustrialisation was implemented as a 'shock doctrine' with very rapid loss of employment within a few years in the UK, while in other Western European countries it was phased in more gradually, and often with more safety nets (such as employment services or inducements for new industry to come to the affected areas). In short, it was less ideologically driven elsewhere.[109] As described above, the political attack was not just in terms of the implementation of mass unemployment via deindustrialisation, but also via the assault on trade union and workers' rights, reductions in benefits, the intensification of poverty and wage compression, as well as vast reductions in the availability of social housing.

Collins and McCartney also argue that while the attack was on all of the UK working class, Scotland and the West of Scotland were more vulnerable to its health-damaging effects than other regions of the UK as a result of having higher rates of industrial and public sector employment (and trade union membership), higher levels of social housing occupation, higher rates of benefit receipt among the population, as well as heightened feelings of national (not just local) disempowerment and loss of control as a result of a democratic deficit, whereby the vote for the Conservative Party in Scotland was significantly below that of the rest of the UK.[110] The 'perfect storm' of all of these factors helps to explain why the 'Scottish health effect' became more pronounced since 1980, and why there was an epidemiological shift to causes of death most associated with poverty and despair. The neoliberal political attack on public health continues today, as is explored further in our final politics case study of austerity and regional and local health divides.

German lessons

As noted in Chapter 1, the scale of the North–South health divide in England is such that the life expectancy gap for women between the North East and North West of England and London in the South East is now greater than the gap between the former West Germany and post-communist East Germany in the mid-1990s.[111] After reunification in 1990, life expectancy for women in East Germany caught up with that of women in West Germany in little more than a decade, whereas the gap between the North East and North West of England and London has persisted for women. East German women now have a higher life expectancy than North Eastern English women. For men, the German life expectancy gap is now smaller than the English one (demonstrated in Figure 5.3). This section examines how the German health gap was closed and the lessons that can be learned from this for reducing the English divide.

Figure 5.3: Life expectancy trends for men and women in London, the North East and North West of England, and West and East Germany, 1980–2012[112]

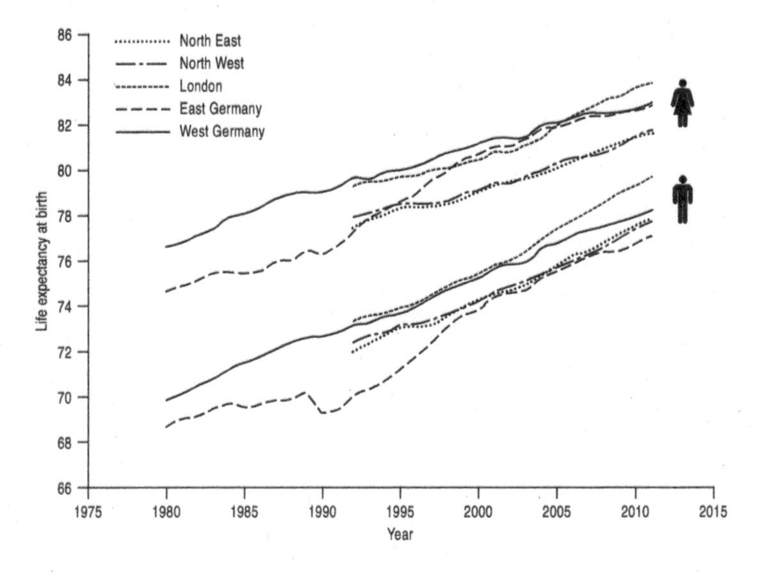

After the Second World War, Germany was split into two separate states: the German Democratic Republic (GDR/East Germany), a communist totalitarian state, part of the Warsaw pact or Soviet bloc, and the Federal Republic of Germany (FRG/West Germany), a liberal democratic state, a founder member of the EU and part of the North Atlantic Treaty Organisation (NATO). This also included – and was symbolised by – the division of Berlin into two halves, East and West, by the Berlin Wall. In 1989, tentative political reforms suddenly culminated in a peaceful 'velvet revolution' across the Eastern bloc countries. The East German state, arguably one of the most repressive and ideological of the Eastern bloc countries,[113] held out on political reforms but eventually succumbed to 'people power' when a hole in the 'Iron Curtain' around the Eastern Bloc was created between Hungary and Austria, and thousands of East Germans started to flee into West Germany via Hungary and Austria. The

Berlin Wall was then literally torn down in November 1989. This eventually led to the GDR's first free elections and to the creation of a unified Germany in 1990.

Between 1949 and 1990, East Germans inhabited a completely different world from West Germans (and the citizens of other wealthy democracies). The GDR was a totalitarian regime, dominated by a single political party, the Socialist Unity Party of Germany (SED), whose state communist ideology was vigorously enforced across all parts of society, with the economy, education, working life, domestic life, housing, healthcare and so on all within state control. Any deviance from party orthodoxy was suppressed including use of a repressive and violent secret state police (the infamous Stasi). Under this system, East Germany fell behind the West in terms of key indicators including economic development, healthcare provision and medical technology, living standards, environmental standards, and in terms of public health.

In terms of economic development, in 1990 the GDP of the GDR was $160 billion compared to $946 billion for the FDR – $10,000 per head in the GDR compared to $15,00 per head in the West, around 50% higher.[114] This had daily consequences as, for example, manufactured and luxury goods were in a short supply. For example, there were long waiting lists for cars, and a Czech Skoda car cost 25,000 East German Marks in 1988, equivalent to two years of average wages of 1,200 Marks per month.[115] Necessities were, however, very cheap in East Germany as, for example, rents were only about 6% of the average salary, although housing standards were also considerably less good (many East Germans lived in overcrowded houses, all allocated by the state).[116] Healthcare provision suffered in terms of having less well equipped hospitals, less well trained medical professionals and less spending per head on healthcare provision. In 1990 about a fifth of hospitals in East Germany were in a poor state of repair, a third of hospital beds were unusable, medical technology was 15 to 20 years behind the West, and only 2,000 different drugs were available in the East compared to 40,000 in West.[117] The physical environment also suffered as the regulation of, for example, air pollution, was less restrictive, and the lack of access to foreign energy imports entailed a dependency on highly polluting (dirty) 'brown coal'. Import restrictions also had an impact on the national diet, with very little access to fruit and vegetables such as bananas.[118]

The impacts of this GDR 'experiment' on public health are demonstrated in Figures 5.4 and 5.5, which show life expectancy trends between East and West from 1970 to 2010. There was a clear East–West life expectancy gap which peaked in 1990 at almost three years between women and three-and-a-half years between men. This gap has rapidly narrowed in the decades following reunification, particularly for women, so that by 1996, the East–West health divide for women was only around one year, and by 2010 it had dwindled to just a few months (West, 82.8 years; East, 82.6 years).[119] Among men, the gap decreased to just over one year by 2010 (West, 78.0 years, East, 76.6 years). Figure 5.6 shows health inequalities in the reunified City of Berlin today, some of the smallest local health divides in Europe. There is 'only' a three-year gap between the most and

Figure 5.4: Life expectancy trends in East and West Germany for women, 1960–2010[120]

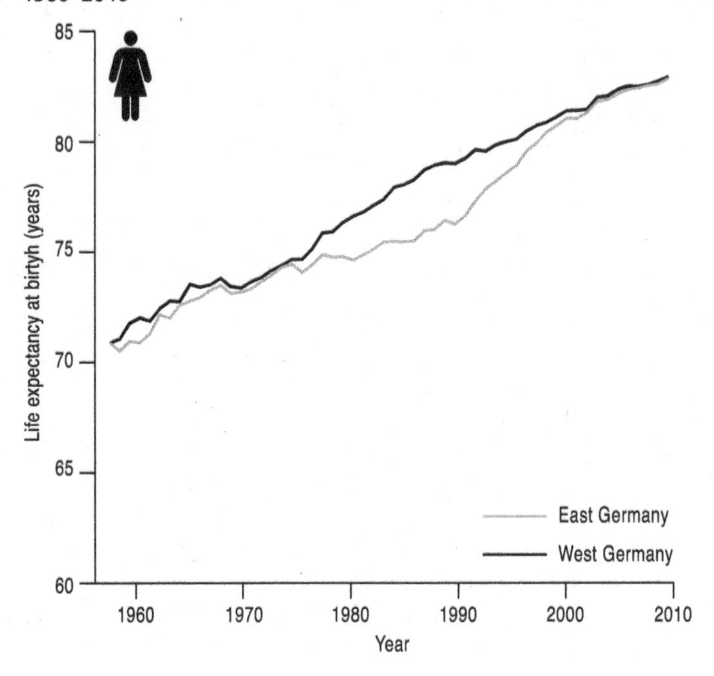

least affluent parts of Berlin (compared to 17 years in Stockton-on-Tees in England or 25 years in New Orleans in the US). Men in the Mitte district of the city centre will on average live to 76, and women to 81. In contrast, men in neighbouring Charlottenburg will live to 79.5 and women to 84.

So how did reunification lead to such rapid changes in the health of East Germans? There are two main factors: economic and medical.

First, the living standards of East Germans improved with the economic terms of the reunification, whereby the West German Deutsche Mark (a strong internationally traded currency) replaced the East German Mark (considered almost worthless outside of the Eastern bloc) as the official currency – a Mark for a Mark. This meant that salaries and savings were replaced equally, one to one, by the much higher value Deutsche Mark. Substantial investment was also made into the industries of Eastern Germany, and transfer payments were made by the

Figure 5.5: Life expectancy trends in East and West Germany for men, 1960–2010[121]

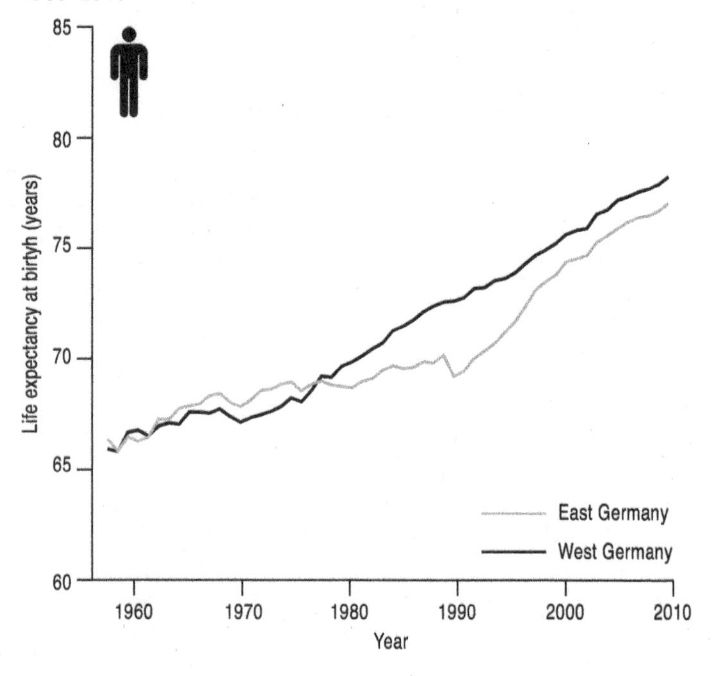

West German government to ensure the future funding of social welfare programmes in the East. This meant that between by as early as 1996, wages in the East rose very rapidly to around

Figure 5.6: Life expectancy by Berlin district[122]

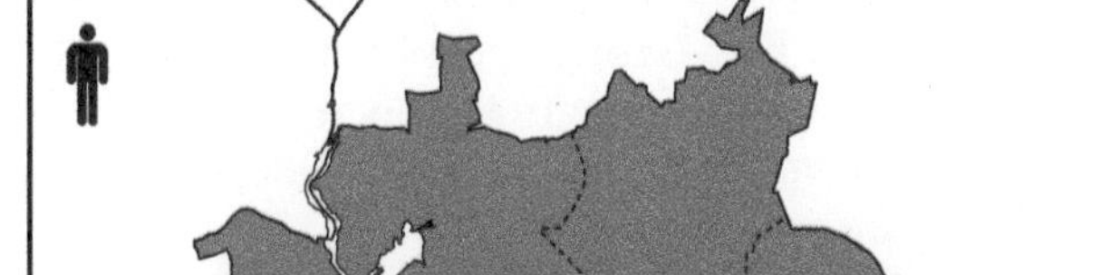

75% of Western levels, from being less than 40% in 1990.[123] This increase in incomes was also experienced by old-age pensioners. In 1985, retired households in the East had only 36% of the income of employed households while retirees in the West received 65%.[124] After reunification, the West German pension system was extended into the East, which resulted in huge increases in income for older East Germans: in 1990 the monthly pension of an East German pensioner was only 40% that of a Western pensioner, but by 1999 it increased to 87% of West German levels.[125] This meant that retired people were one of groups that benefited most from reunification – particularly East German women as they had, on average, considerably longer working biographies than their West German counterparts.[126] Research by the Max Planck Institute for Demographic Research in Rostock has shown that the rapid improvement in life expectancy in 1990s East Germany was largely a result of falling death rates among pensioners.[127]

Access to a variety of foods and consumer goods also increased as West German shops and companies set up in the East. It was not all Keynesianism for the 'Ossis' (Easterners), however, as unemployment (unheard of in the full employment socialist system) also increased as a result of the rapid privatisation and deindustrialisation of the Eastern economy. Unemployment remains nearly double that in West Germany today. These economic improvements were funded by a special Solidarity Surcharge, which was levied at a rate of up to 5.5% on income taxes owed (for example, a tax bill of €5,000 attracts a solidarity surcharge of €275).[128]

Second, immediately after reunification, considerable financial support was given to modernise the hospitals and healthcare equipment in the East, and the availability of nursing care, screening and pharmaceuticals also increased. This raised standards of healthcare in the East so that they were comparable to those of the West within just a few years.[129] This had notable impacts on, for example, improvements in neonatal mortality in East.[130] Falling death rates from conditions amenable to primary prevention (for example, cancer screening) or medical treatment accounted for 14% (men) and 27% (women) of the overall increase in life expectancy to age 75 in East Germany in the 1990s, while falling death rates from those conditions amenable to secondary prevention (public health policy measures) accounted for between 10% (women) and 22% (men).[131] Decreases in CVD (amenable to primary and secondary prevention, medical treatment and rising living standards such as better diet) amounted to a further 10% (women) to 17% (men).[132]

Both the economic reforms and the increased investment in healthcare were the result of the deep and sustained political decision to reunify Germany as fully as possible, so that 'what belongs together will grow together'. Meanwhile, in England, the economic development and living standards of the North compared to the South have declined since the 1990s. There has been little by way of public investment in the North to rectify these differences despite the rhetoric of the 'Northern Powerhouse' being used by the Conservative government since 2015. The North continues to lose out to the South in regards to things such as spending on transport infrastructure, 84% of which was spent in London and the South East.[133] More widely, capital infrastructure spend in 2013 amounted to £223 per head in the North East compared to £5,426 per head in London.[134] Indeed, the North East of England is now one of the poorest regions in Europe. While the German East–West health gap has almost disappeared, the English North–South health divide has, unsurprisingly, continued, with the life expectancy gap today standing at around two years for both men (North, 78 years; South, 79.8 years) and women (North, 81.9 years; South, 83.6 years).[135]

Germany's lessons for the English divide are therefore two-fold: first, even large health divides can be significantly reduced and within a short time period; and second, the tools to do this are largely economic but, crucially, within the control of politics and politicians. Ultimately, the German experience shows that if there is a sufficient political desire to reduce health divides, it can be done: where there is a will, there is a way.

All in it together?[136]

The financial crisis of 2007/08 was a result of a downturn in the US housing market, which led to a massive collapse in financial markets across the world. Banks increasingly required state bailouts (for example, in the UK the retail bank Northern Rock was nationalised, while in the US, Lehmann Brothers investment bank filed for bankruptcy and the mortgage companies Freddie Mac and Fannie Mae were given major government bailouts). Stock markets posted massive falls that continued as the effects in the 'real' economy began to be felt, with unemployment rates of over 10% in the US and the Eurozone. In 2009, the IMF announced that the global economy was experiencing its worst period for 60 years.[137] The global economic recession continued throughout 2009 and 2010, and while many wealthy governments injected liquidity into their economies (so-called 'quantitative easing'), it was also accompanied in many European countries (including the UK, but most notably in Greece and Spain) by escalating public expenditure cuts: austerity. Austerity – reducing budget deficits in economic downturns by decreasing public expenditure and/or increasing taxes – has exacerbated the recession in some European countries, most notably in the periphery Eurozone countries of Greece, Spain, Italy and Portugal. Even at the time of writing (2015), youth unemployment in these countries remained at over 50% in Greece and Spain and over 35% in Italy and Portugal. In Greece, general unemployment levels amounted to 25% of those aged 16–65 in 2015, while poverty rates had doubled since the financial crisis of 2007 to 40%, and government debt stood at 177% of GDP in 2015.

The UK, while not as affected as the Eurozone by the financial crisis and subsequent recession, still embarked on a programme of austerity. Here, no time was wasted in 'making the most of a crisis', with the 2010–15 coalition government (of Conservatives and Liberal Democrats) and then the Conservative majority government elected in 2015 enacting large-scale cuts to central and local government budgets, and increased NHS privatisation as well as steep reductions in welfare services and benefits. It is estimated that the UK welfare reforms enacted up until 2015 will take nearly £19 billion a year out of the economy. This is equivalent to around £470 a year for every adult of working age in the country (see Table 5.2 for details).

The biggest financial losses arise from reforms to incapacity-related benefits (£4.3 billion a year), changes to tax credits

Table 5.2: Austerity-driven welfare reform in the UK, 2010–15[138]

Date	Measure
January 2011	Child Trust Fund abolished
April 2011	Child benefit frozen until 2015
April 2012	A one year time limit to the receipt of contributory ESA for people in the Work Related Activity Group Tax credits withdrawn from 'middle income' families
May 2012	Lone Parent Obligations introduced
October 2012	Conditionality, sanctions and hardship payments introduced
January 2013	Child Benefit withdrawn from individuals earning more than £50,000
March 2013	Housing Benefit / Local Housing Allowance restricted to the Consumer Prices Index – as are other benefits
April 2013	Childcare costs covered by Working Tax Credit cut from 80% to 70% Council Tax Benefit – 10% reduction for welfare recipients in total payments to local authorities Up-rating of working-age benefits not related to disability restricted to 1% (inflation 3.5%) Household Benefit Cap (set at £26,000 maximum) Social Fund replaced by locally determined schemes for crisis loans and community care grants Under occupancy charge or 'Bedroom Tax' if claimant has one spare bedroom (14% reduction) or more (25% reduction) Restrictions in access to legal aid
April 2013-October 2017	Migration of all existing working-age Disability Living Allowance (DLA) claimants onto Personal Independence Payment (PIP)
June 2013	Replacement of DLA by PIP for all new claimants
October 2013	Universal Credit – new claims and changes
December 2013	PIP reassessment of DLA claims
April 2014	Universal Credit – transfer existing claims
February 2015	Roll out of Universal Credit
July 2015	Tax credits and family benefits under Universal Credit limited to the first two children only Working age benefits frozen for four years from 2016 Working element of Employment and Support Allowance (ESA) payments reduced to Job Seeker's Allowance (JSA) levels The benefit cap reduced to £20,000 Housing Benefit entitlement restricted for those aged between 18 and 21 Those earning more than £30,000 pay more if they rent social housing

(£3.6 billion a year) and the 1% up-rating of most working-age benefits (£3.4 billion a year).[139] The 2010–15 Housing Benefit reforms resulted in more modest losses – an estimated £490 million a year arising from the under-occupancy charge (most commonly referred to as the 'bedroom tax'), for example – but for the households affected, the sums are nevertheless still large (for example, £12 per week reductions per 'spare room' for those on benefits that are only around £65 per week). In this section, we examine the health effects of austerity and welfare reform through reference to local health divides in the UK.

Despite the claim by the UK Prime Minister David Cameron that 'we are all in it together', the financial impact of the welfare reforms varies greatly across the country. Professors Tina Beatty and Steven Fothergill of Sheffield Hallam University have shown that austerity will widen the gaps in prosperity between the best and worst local economies across England, increasing the socioeconomic divide between the most and least deprived areas of towns and cities and between richer and poorer parts of the country.[140] Britain's older industrial areas, a number of seaside towns and some London boroughs were hit hardest. Much of the South and East of England (outside London) escaped comparatively lightly. Blackpool, in the North West of England, was hit worst of all – an estimated loss of more than £900 a year for every adult of working age in the town. The three regions of Northern England alone can expect to lose around £5.2 billion a year in benefit income by 2017. More than two-thirds of the 50 local authority districts worst affected by the reforms are the Northern 'old industrial areas' – places such as Knowsley, Liverpool, Middlesbrough, Hartlepool, Stoke and Burnley. The higher reliance on benefits and tax credits in Northern, post-industrial parts of England means that the failure to up-rate with inflation and the reductions to tax credits have a greater impact here.[141] The unequal spatial distribution of welfare cuts is shown in Figure 5.7.

Local government spending (excluding the police, schools and Housing Benefit) fell by nearly 30% in real terms between 2008 and 2015 in England. In terms of the geographies of local authority budget cuts, a similar pattern to welfare reform emerges: as a general rule, the more deprived the local authority,

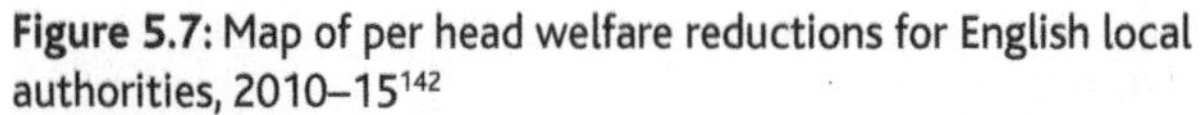

Figure 5.7: Map of per head welfare reductions for English local authorities, 2010–15[142]

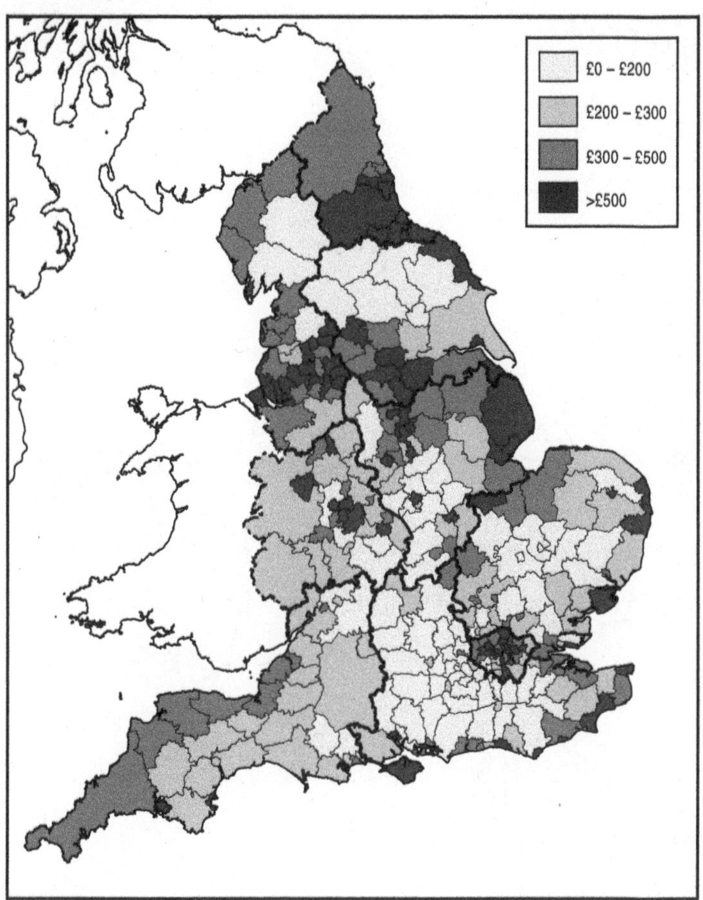

the greater the financial hit.[143, 144] At the extremes, the worst-hit local authority areas – mainly located in the North (for example, Middlesbrough) – lost around four times as much, per adult of working age, as the authorities least affected by the cuts – found exclusively in the South and East of England (for example, Hart in Hampshire). Here the cuts amounted to less than £50 per head in this period. In contrast, the loss per working-age adult in the worst-affected Northern districts was £470 a year. The geographical distribution of cuts to local authority budgets is shown in Figure 5.8.

Figure 5.8: Map of per head reductions in local authority budgets, England, 2010–15[145]

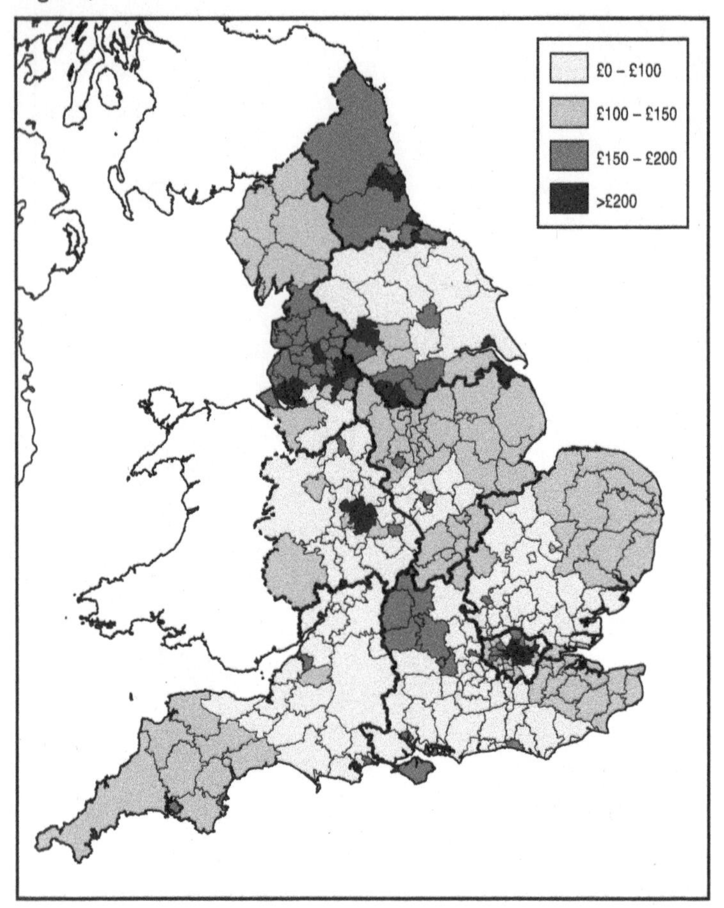

These 'upstream' politically driven changes of the UK government's austerity programme have already started to have an impact on the midstream and downstream determinants of health by unequally changing the social geographies of place and the social determinants of health.[146] For example, there have been spatially concentrated increases in poverty rates across the country – particularly in the North. In 2012, the regions with the lowest levels of poverty were the South East (17%) and East (18%). Rates were much higher in the Northern regions, with 22% in the North East, 23% in the North West and 24%

in Yorkshire and Humber. Child poverty rates follow similar geographies, with rates much higher in the Northern regions – 29% in the North East, 31% in the North West and 30% in Yorkshire and Humber, compared to 21% in the South East. In certain areas of the North, the child poverty figure is over 35% (for example, 38% in Manchester and 37% in Middlesbrough)[147] although this is also the case in London (36%).

Food poverty has also increased since the era of austerity, with almost 1 million people accessing emergency food banks in the financial year 2013/14. In 2013, 83% of Trussell Trust food banks reported that benefits sanctions – when payments are temporarily stopped – had resulted in more people being referred for emergency food, and 30% of visits were put down to a delay in welfare payments.[148] Alongside food poverty, many more are now also experiencing fuel poverty as energy costs rise.[149] The North East (21%) and North West (19%) have some of the highest levels of fuel poverty in England, while the South East (11%) has the lowest.[150]

So what will all this mean for regional and local health divides? There is an emerging literature that examines the repercussions of austerity for population health. In a wide-ranging and well-publicised analysis of the health effects of austerity, Stuckler and Basu[151] concluded that the overall effects of recessions on the health of different nations vary significantly by political and policy context, with those countries (such as Iceland or the US) that responded to the financial crisis of 2007/08 with an economic stimulus faring much better – particularly in terms of mental health and suicides – than those countries (for example, Spain, Greece or the UK) that *chose* to pursue a policy of austerity (public expenditure cuts to reduce government debt). It has also been shown that austerity will have a disproportionate impact on the health of vulnerable groups, especially those individuals and families, including children, on the lowest incomes or in receipt of welfare benefits.[152]

However, the effects on geographical health divides have been less explored. It is not yet possible to comprehensively assess the effects of the current austerity programme using contemporary data due to the long delays in collating and releasing health data,[153] as well as the lag period required to ascertain the effects on mortality. However, there are early indications that it is serving to increase existing divides such as that between the North and the South of England. For example, since 2007, suicide rates have increased across England, but at a greater rate in the North than the South: by 2012 they were 12.4 per 100,000 in the North West compared to 8.7 per 100,000 in London.[154] Similarly, antidepressant prescription rates have risen since 2007, again with the highest increases in the North: by 2012, antidepressant prescription rates were highest in Blackpool (331 per 1,000) and lowest in Brent (71 per 1,000).[155] Food bank use and malnutrition rates have also increased more in the North, with food banks in the South actually shipping food up to the North.[156] Recent data has also shown that there have been significant improvements in mortality rates among lower socioeconomic status women in the South (East, London and South East regions) but not in Northern regions, where they have actually increased since 2002/03.[157] Spatially concentrated increases in unemployment over recent years have also led to an increase in the North–South divide for both morbidity and mortality.[158]

We can also draw on previous studies of the health effects of austerity-style welfare reform policies (such as the welfare retrenchment of Reagan's US or Thatcher's Britain) and extrapolate from these. Previous research into austerity-style policies suggests that such geographically concentrated cuts to the social safety net will only serve to increase existing local divisions in health. Indeed, as Professor Jamie Pearce of the University of Edinburgh has argued,[159] these studies from the 1980s and 1990s 'are almost certain to understate the scale and multitude of the health consequences',[160] given the larger scale of the subsequent spending cuts this time around. Nonetheless, they provide the best available evidence at this stage of the effects on health inequalities of the 'austerity epidemic'.[161]

In terms of health inequalities between individuals of different socioeconomic status (compositional factors), for example, a US study found that while premature mortality (deaths under age 75) and IMR (deaths before age one) declined overall in all income quintiles from 1960 to 2002, inequalities by income and ethnicity decreased only between 1966 and 1980, and then increased between 1980 and 2002.[162] The reductions in inequalities (1966–80) occurred during a period of welfare expansion in the US (the 'War on Poverty') and the enactment of civil rights legislation that increased access to welfare state services. The increases in health inequalities occurred during the Reagan–Bush period of neoliberalism when public welfare services (including healthcare insurance coverage) were cut, funding of social assistance was reduced, the minimum wage was frozen and the tax base was shifted from the rich to the poor, leading to increased income polarisation.

These findings are mirrored in studies of welfare state reductions in New Zealand,[163-166] which found that while general mortality rates declined, socioeconomic inequalities among men, women and children in all-cause mortality increased in the 1980s and the 1990s, and then stabilised in the early 2000s. Likewise, spatial inequalities in health between local areas and regions increased. The increases in health inequality occurred during a period in which New Zealand underwent major structural reform (including a less redistributive tax system, targeted social benefits, the introduction of a regressive tax on consumption, the privatisation of major utilities and public housing, user charges for welfare services, and a more deregulated labour market). The stabilisation of inequalities in mortality in the late 1990s and early 2000s was during a period in which the economy improved, and there were some improvements in services (for example, better access to social housing, more generous social assistance and a decrease in healthcare costs).

Research into the health effects of Thatcherism (1979–90) has also concluded that the large-scale dismantling of the UK's social democratic institutions and the early pursuit of 'austerity-style' policies increased socioeconomic health inequalities. Thatcherism deregulated the labour and financial markets, privatised utilities and state enterprises, restricted social housing, curtailed trade union rights, marketised the public sector, significantly cut the social wage via welfare state retrenchment, accepted mass unemployment and implemented large tax cuts for the business sector and the most affluent.[167] In this period, while life expectancy increased and mortality rates decreased for all social groups, the increases were greater and more rapid among the highest social groups so that inequalities increased.

Area inequalities also increased in this period, with the North and Scotland falling behind the rest of the UK – as explored further in the next chapter.[168]

These historical increases in social and spatial health divides were not inevitable as in the UK, like the US and New Zealand, inequalities in mortality declined from the 1920s to the 1970s as income inequalities were reduced and the welfare state was expanded.[169, 170] Nonetheless, this all suggests that the health of the poorest people and places suffers the most in times of welfare retrenchment. As the North of England, Scotland and deprived areas of our towns and cities have higher rates of poverty, unemployment and welfare receipt, they will disproportionately suffer the social and health consequences of austerity. And this will only serve to increase local health divides.

This chapter and the case studies within it have demonstrated the importance of politics, ideologies, political institutions and policies as the fundamental determinants of health divides. The next chapter continues with this theme by examining how health inequalities policy in the UK has – or has not – addressed health divides since the 1980s.

CHAPTER 6

Too little, too late

Previous chapters have explored the relationship between health and place across different scales showing consistent evidence of spatial inequalities in health within local areas, between the regions and countries of the UK, as well as within and between countries internationally. They have shown that the causes of geographical inequalities in health are complicated and multifaceted, a combination of compositional (people), contextual (environment) and ultimately political and economic factors. This chapter examines how public policy has had an impact on health divides using a case study of the UK since the 1980s. It provides an overview of health inequalities policy since 1979, drawing on the key actions during this period. The successes and failures of UK policies in terms of reducing health inequalities are critically examined with reference to the wider context of the neoliberal political economy and the social and spatial determinants of health.

The UK is chosen as a case study because the Thatcher governments of 1979–90 played an important role in the promotion of the international neoliberal policy agenda, which remains influential today; because the Blair Labour governments from 1997 to 2010 implemented the most extensive health inequalities strategy in Europe;[1] and because the coalition and Conservative governments since 2010 implemented austerity. The chapter critically reflects on how policy has had an impact on health inequalities from 1980 to 2015, analysing some of the key developments in this period. It ends by reflecting on what *could* or *should* have been done, drawing on evidence from a series of government-commissioned reviews into tackling health inequalities.

Thatcherism and health inequalities, 1979–97[2]

The need to reduce health inequalities across the UK contributed to the decision to establish the National Health Service (NHS) in 1948. Yet, despite this universal, free at the point of use health service, by the 1970s it was becoming increasingly evident that free access to healthcare had not been enough to stem socioeconomic and spatial inequalities in health. In as far as a health inequalities policy existed at this time, it was within the NHS. So, in 1977, the Labour government (1974–79) faced fresh calls to do something about the issue. They responded by asking the Chief Scientist, Sir Douglas Black, to appoint a working group of experts to investigate the issue and to make policy recommendations for the government.[3] The resulting report, which is widely referred to as the Black Report,[4] argued that materialist explanations were likely to play the largest role in explaining health inequalities (see Chapter 4), and, therefore, that policy-makers ought to prioritise the reduction of differences in material and economic circumstances between socioeconomic groups and between deprived and affluent areas (see Table 6.1 for a summary of the report). The report was published in 1980 (on a Bank Holiday Monday in August to minimise publicity, and with only 260 copies produced), when the commissioning Labour government (left-wing, social democratic) had been replaced by the first Thatcher-led Conservative (right-wing, neoliberal) government (1979–83). The new government wholeheartedly rejected the report's recommendations (which included increasing welfare benefits and decreasing child poverty). In an infamous foreword to the report, Patrick Jenkins, the then Secretary of State for Social Services, claimed that the report was 'wildly unrealistic' and 'seriously flawed'. This set the tone for the next 20 years as, under the Conservative governments of 1979–97, health inequalities were not on the official policy agenda at all.[5] Even the term 'health inequalities' was discarded, and health differences between socioeconomic groups and places were instead referred to using the less emotive term, 'health variations', implying that health differences could be 'natural', individual and therefore not something for which politicians and policy-makers were responsible.

Table 6.1: Overview of the Black, Acheson and Marmot reports[6]

	Black Report	Acheson Report	Marmot Review
Background	The Black Report (1980) on health inequalities was commissioned by the outgoing Labour government in 1977 and brought health inequalities into the spotlight and represented the first example of a comprehensive strategy to draw attention to health inequalities over the life course. Health inequalities were not recognised as a problem by many at the time.	The Independent Inquiry into Inequalities in Health chaired by Sir Donald Acheson was commissioned by the newly-elected Labour government in 1997, which committed itself to implementing the evidence-based policy recommendations.	Following publication of the WHO report on the social determinants of health, Sir Michael Marmot was commissioned to consider the implications for health inequalities in England post-2010. As with the Acheson Inquiry, the Marmot Review was expected to make evidence-based recommendations.
Aims	1. To assemble available information about the differences in health status among the social classes and about factors which might contribute to these, including relevant data from other industrial countries; 2. To analyse this material in order to identify possible causal relationships, to examine the hypotheses that have been formulated and the testing of them, and to assess the implications for policy; and 3. To suggest what further research should be initiated.	1. To review the latest available information on inequalities of health, to summarise the evidence of inequalities of health and expectation of life in England and identify trends. 2. In the light of that evidence, to conduct – within the broad framework of the Government's overall financial strategy – an independent review to identify priority areas for future policy development, which scientific and expert evidence indicates are likely to offer opportunities for Government to develop beneficial, cost effective and affordable interventions to reduce health inequalities. 3. To report to the Secretary of State for Health. The report will be published and its conclusions, based on evidence, will contribute to the development of a new strategy for health.	1. Identify, for the health inequalities challenge facing England, the evidence most relevant to underpinning future policy and action 2. Show how this evidence could be translated into practice 3. Advise on possible objectives and measures, building on the experience of the current PSA target on infant mortality and life expectancy 4. Publish a report of the Review's work that will contribute to the development of a post-2010 health inequalities strategy.
Explanatory theory	Took a multi-causal approach to explaining health inequalities but suggested the role of behavioural and cultural determinants in producing inequalities in health were significantly outweighed by the role played by economic and social conditions.	Acheson (1998) also supported a multi-causal approach to explaining health inequalities, using a model composed of different layers including individual lifestyles and the socioeconomic environment. Similarly to Black, this approach emphasised the importance of material and structural conditions in shaping other key determinants, such as lifestyle-behaviours.	The distribution of health and wellbeing is once again understood to be caused by interplay of various determinants, with material circumstances playing an important role. However, psychosocial factors, such as social cohesion, and other social stresses are given more prominence in explaining the relationship between material inequalities and health inequalities.
Key recommendations	37 recommendations, prioritizing giving children a better start in life within a wider anti-poverty strategy	39 recommendations; key priorities similar to those of Black report, namely: 1. All policies likely to have an impact on health should be evaluated in terms of the impact on health inequalities. 2. High priority should be given to health of families with children. 3. Further steps should be taken to reduce income inequalities and improve living standards of poor households	6 policy objectives: 1. Give every child the best start in life 2. Enable all children, young people and adults to maximise their capabilities and have control over their lives 3. Create fair employment and good work for all 4. Ensure healthy standard of living for all 5. Create and develop healthy and sustainable places and communities 6. Strengthen the role and impact of ill health prevention

Understanding Thatcherism, Conservatism and New Right ideologies in this period helps explain why Thatcher's government made the decision to reject the recommendations put forward in the Black Report (1980). Margaret Thatcher (1925–2013) was UK Prime Minister from 1979–90. Her critique of UK social democracy during the 1970s and her adoption of key neoliberal strategies, such as financial deregulation, trade liberalisation and the privatisation of public goods and services, were popularly labelled 'Thatcherism'. Thatcherism was an ideological project that set out to radically re-cast the relationship between labour and capital and between the state, society and the individual.[7] Thatcherism and the New Right provided a narrative that explained the crisis of British capitalism in the 1970s as a crisis of the welfare state, high wages and low productivity, of the 'undemocratic' power of what in 1984 she called 'the enemy within', that is, the trade unions.[8] Thatcherism set out to systematically dismantle the structures of the post-war Keynesian consensus around the social wage, full employment, the corporatist state and the size and role of the public sector. This goal was pursued through the aggressive promotion of the free market alongside the 'hollowing out' of the state.[9]

Thatcher's political programme included: (1) deregulation of the labour and financial markets (including the 'big bang' deregulation of the City of London in 1986); (2) the privatisation and marketisation of the main utilities (water, gas and electricity) and state enterprises (for example, British Steel, British Rail and British Airways); (3) the promotion of home ownership (including the widespread sale of public housing stock under the 'Right to Buy' scheme); (4) the curtailing of workers' and trade union rights (for example, bans on the 'closed shop', obligatory membership ballots before any industrial action, restrictions on the right to picket including a ban on secondary picketing, and removal of trade union immunity from damages); (5) the promotion of free market ideology in all areas of public life (including healthcare and the civil service); (6) significant cuts to the social wage via welfare state retrenchment (for example, a 7% reduction in state expenditure on social assistance between 1979 and 1989; removal of 16- to 18-year-olds from entitlement; reductions in state pensions; abolition of the inflation link for welfare benefits); (7) an acceptance of mass unemployment as a price worth paying for the above policies; and (8) large tax cuts for the business sector and the most affluent (for example, during Thatcher's premiership, the rate of Income Tax for the top tax bracket was reduced from 83% to 40%).[10]

These changes all led to a fundamental rebalancing of British economic and social life that saw a reassertion of social class divisions. The growing economic equality experienced as a result of UK social reforms since 1945 was reversed, with income inequality increasing significantly (for example, the richest 0.01% had 28 times the mean national average income in 1978, but this increased under Thatcher's tenure to 70 times in 1990). Additionally, as a result of welfare state retrenchment, high unemployment and falling wages for many poorer workers (due to the decreased bargaining power of trade unions), there was a near doubling of poverty rates in the UK, from 6.7% in 1975 to 12.0% in 1985.[11] By the 1990s and 2000s, these new high levels of income inequalities and poverty became normalised. Social mobility gains were also stalled via changes to the education system as well as the 'lost generation' of young people who left school and went straight onto 'the dole' in the early 1980s. From 1980, the number of unemployment claimants rose from around 1 million to around 3 million in 1983, and a further peak was seen in the early 1990s. Meanwhile there was also a steady rise in the number of claimants of long-term sickness (disability) benefits. The rise in the number of disability benefit claimants has been attributed to a government desire to move people off the unemployment register and because of the lack of jobs in the economy.[12]

The new economy that emerged in the 1980s was seriously unbalanced. Manufacturing and extraction industries, public utilities and collective housing provision were displaced by finance and banking industries, privatised utilities and rampant property speculation. The 'big bang' of 1986 saw the deregulation of the City of London, and with that, the unleashing of hitherto unimaginable forms of financial speculation. The ostensible 'giving power back to the people' through privatisation led, in fact, to the radical de-democratisation of the power industry – now largely externally owned – and other utilities. And the ambition to create 'a nation of homeowners' produced a mushrooming of homelessness due to a chronic shortage of affordable social housing, creating the preconditions for the more recent emergence of a new breed of 'Buy to Let' landlords charging 'market rents'. It also underpinned a new culture of speculation and chronic indebtedness – on which a new breed of amoral 'entrepreneurs' in banking and finance would be able to prey. All of this generated sharply increased inequalities of income and wealth across Britain, and a dramatic increase in poverty. It also put in place most of the prerequisites for the great banking and finance crisis of 2008. In this way Thatcher's governments wilfully engineered an economic catastrophe across large parts of Britain, and began the dismantling of the welfare state and the privatisation of the NHS in England.[13]

The impact of these changes on other key social determinants of health was, in many cases, dramatic. Inequalities in educational outcomes and in access to healthcare, for example, both increased following policies implemented under Thatcher's leadership.[14] In housing, Thatcher's government quickly implemented a 'Right to Buy' initiative, which gave council tenants the right to purchase the homes they occupied, often at greatly discounted rates. This policy reflected the ideological belief in the superiority of the market and was popular among many of those it helped move into the housing market. However, it contributed to the growing wealth inequalities and, more broadly, the policies of Thatcherism sowed the seeds of the housing market crash in 1989, which left many homeowners trapped by 'negative equity'.[15] Meanwhile, as the better quality houses were sold off, local councils were left with responsibility for a far smaller and increasingly poor quality housing stock. All of this contributed to growing levels of homelessness.[16] Longer term, these significant changes in housing policy also resulted in the current housing crisis in the UK.

Although Thatcher backed off from any wholesale reform of the NHS, allegedly fearful of an adverse public reaction to such a move, her government did introduce a number of policy initiatives that set the NHS on a course from which it has not deviated since. That course might be characterised as a shift from a welfare state to a market state.[17] The most significant

NHS development that took place under her premiership was the introduction of a quasi-market in healthcare centred round competition and choice.[18] Among the most controversial changes Thatcher introduced was the policy of contracting out or outsourcing, introduced in 1983, whereby health authorities were required to set up competitive tendering arrangements for their cleaning, catering and laundry services. Additional non-clinical services were later added to the list. The main significance of this development was the establishment of the principle that the core responsibility of health authorities was no longer to directly provide non-clinical services, but merely to ensure that they were in place at the least cost. A key negative impact was a loss to the public sector ethos of the NHS in which, for example, cleaners were perceived as members of the ward team, whose friendly, reassuring presence made important contributions to the wellbeing of patients. This contribution disappeared once the tight schedules of competitive contract cleaning took over. Equally important was the perception that ward cleaning became substantially less thorough, leading over time to the current high prevalence of hospital-acquired infections.[19] The NHS and Community Care Act 1990 introduced market-style mechanisms into the NHS, notably the purchaser–provider separation and GP fundholding, whereby GPs were allocated budgets that they were free to spend as they saw fit, to meet their patients' needs. This marked a substantial break with the past, and opened up the NHS to market forces.

These significant and rapid social and economic changes had an impact on health divides in the UK. Mortality rates in the UK, and across Western and Central Europe, have been improving for around 150 years.[20] This long-run improvement continued throughout the period of the Thatcher government, with all-cause mortality rates declining at a similar rate to those in other countries and compared to the time periods before and after. However, underlying the overall improvement in mortality rates, some specific causes of mortality increased markedly, either during the period of the Thatcher government, or immediately afterwards. For example, alcohol-related mortality increased dramatically during the late 1980s and early 1990s in the UK in contrast to the improving trends in other parts of Europe.

Increases were also seen in drug-related mortality, suicide and violence at this time,[21] all of which are causes of death that are clearly socially produced rather than due to biological or physiological mechanisms. Further, within the UK, mortality rates improved much more slowly in Northern and inner-city areas than in the more affluent Southern England,[22] to the extent that in some local areas, mortality rates actually worsened.[23] Indeed, for young adults in Scotland there has been no improvement over the course of the last 30 years.[24] Figure 6.1 shows that the gap in mortality between the least and most

Figure 6.1: Trends in health inequalities in England and Wales, 1975–2003 (by occupational social class) and Scotland, 1981–2001 (by Carstairs area deprivation)[25]

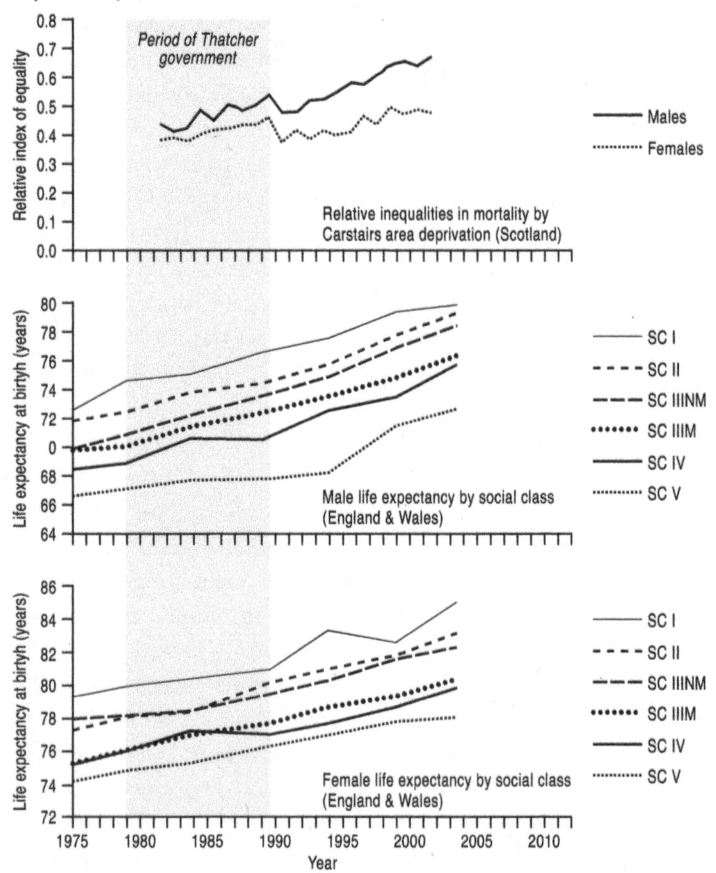

deprived postcode areas in Scotland increased rapidly between 1981 and 2001, to leave Scotland with the highest inequalities in Western and Central Europe.[26, 27] The rise in spatial inequalities in health during the 1980s was also reflected in a rapid rise in mortality inequalities by occupational social class in England and Wales. Life expectancy increased for all social class groups among males and females over time, but the increase was more rapid among higher social classes than in lower ones, such that the inequalities increased (see Figure 6.1). The rises in cause-specific mortalities such as alcohol- and drug-related deaths, suicide and violence, and the widening health inequalities occurred during the same time period in which unemployment, poverty and income inequality all rose.

New Labour and health inequalities, 1997–2010[28]

Labour was re-elected in 1997 with a landslide victory and a manifesto that had highlighted the need to tackle various social inequalities, promising to tackle the 'root causes' of ill health, such as poor housing and unemployment. The new government was keen to emphasise the previous Conservative government's failure to address health inequalities. The Labour government initially criticised the Conservatives for placing an 'excessive emphasis on lifestyle issues', casting the responsibility for ill health onto individuals rather than the economic and social structures of society and the places where people live.[29] In addition, and as promised in their manifesto, the Labour government commissioned a follow-up to the Black Report, announcing an independent inquiry into health inequalities.[30] The Acheson Inquiry, as it became known, was commissioned by Tessa Jowell, the first ever Public Health Minister. On publication in 1998, its recommendations were officially welcomed, used as the basis of a new health strategy, and the government stressed that they were already implementing many of them (see Table 6.1).

In broad terms, many of the resulting Acheson Report's[31] 39 recommendations reflected the conclusions of the earlier Black Report:[32] both highlighted the need to have a multifaceted approach to health inequalities, and both advocated a reduction in income inequalities, with a particular focus on child poverty.

The key difference was that the Acheson Report was released in a far more favourable political climate than its predecessor and might, therefore, have been expected to have more of a policy impact. However, Labour had also stipulated that the Inquiry's recommendations should recognise the government's fiscal commitments which, at that time, included a two-year agreement not to increase public spending. This restriction led to an under-representation of any attempt to tackle the fundamental economic and political determinants in the emerging policy initiatives that were linked to the report.[33]

A wealth of policy statements referring directly to the report were produced, indicating that policy decisions had, as promised, been directly informed – or at least influenced – by the recommendations of the report. Certainly in the period 1997–2003, health policy across the UK reflected some of the ideas set out in the Black and Acheson Reports, including a consistent rhetorical emphasis on the need to tackle the social and economic determinants of health inequalities as well as a commitment to employing cross-cutting government policies (that went beyond the Department of Health and the NHS) to tackle health inequality.[34] Most notably, by 2004, national targets to reduce health inequalities were also introduced with a focus on life expectancy and IMR.

These targets, however, reinforced the idea that policy-makers could tackle health inequalities through specialised health improvement measures, directing efforts to the least well-off individuals and areas such as the Spearhead local authorities that were the 70 most disadvantaged local authorities in England. They all received additional financial resources to improve area health, and area-based initiatives emerged. These tried to get different sectors – particularly the NHS, local authorities and the voluntary sector – to work in partnership together to improve the health outcomes of a specific deprived area. Examples from this period include Health Action Zones, Healthy Living Centres, Health Improvement Programmes and New Deal for Communities (summarised in Box 6.1). This target culture is perhaps one reason why, in the period 2004–07, public health policy moved away from the initial concern with social and economic determinants and instead focused increasingly on health services and lifestyle behaviours.[35] This shift was associated with a reduction in the level of responsibility that the central government appeared to be taking for health inequalities, as policy documents increasingly emphasised the importance of individual responsibility for health outcomes.[36] Targets to reduce health inequalities were abandoned across the UK in 2011.

Box 6.1: Description of area-based health initiatives, 1997–2010[37]

Health Action Zones (HAZs)

HAZs were area-based initiatives designed to tackle social exclusion and inequalities. Acknowledging the wider determinants of health, HAZs were intended to develop partnership working between the NHS, local government and other sectors with the aim of tackling ill health and persistent inequalities in the most disadvantaged communities across the UK. Initially 11 HAZs were launched in the first wave in April 1998, followed by a further 15 in April 1999. Collectively, HAZs were awarded £320 million over a three-year period. It was originally intended that the lifespan of HAZs would last between five and seven years, with successful services being mainstreamed thereafter. However, HAZs were effectively wound down by 2003. The projects facilitated by HAZs varied extensively, but included initiatives that aimed to address social and economic determinants (such as services providing advice on benefit support); promote healthy lifestyles (for example, breakfast clubs); empower individuals and communities (for example, a Gypsy and Traveller Project Advisory Group); and improve health and social care services (for example, the Integrated Substance Misuse Service).

Health Improvement Programmes (HImPs)

HImPs were action plans developed by NHS and local government bodies working together. They were introduced in 1999 and, despite being re-named Health Improvement and Modernisation Plans in 2001, they continue to form a key approach to public health in England. The plans set out how these organisations (with, where deemed appropriate, voluntary and private sector input) intend to improve the health of local populations and reduce health inequalities. The programmes offered a three-year plan for identifying local health needs and developing relevant strategies to improve health and healthcare services at a local level. HImPs were founded on the basis of multi-agency partnership working between local government and regional Strategic Health Authorities (SHAs).

New Deal for Communities (NDC)

As part of the Neighbourhood Renewal Strategy, NDC was developed to tackle health and social inequalities experienced by the 39 most deprived communities in the UK. In partnership with local communities, NDC sought to address embedded issues of deprivation and long-term poverty by improving outcomes in terms of housing, education, employment and health. Interventions mainly focused on promoting healthy lifestyles, enhancing service provision, developing the health workforce and working with young people.

Healthy Living Centres (HLCs)

HLCs were introduced in 1998 to tackle the broader determinants of health inequalities and to improve health and wellbeing at a local level. Funding was awarded for 352 community projects that varied in terms of focus, ranging from service-related issues to activities addressing unemployment, poverty and social exclusion. Example interventions included health-focused projects such as a physical activity outreach programme in rural localities, support programmes such as a Community Health Information Project that trained members of the local community to act as ambassadors for HLCs, and services such as 'Bumps to Babies', which provided midwifery and health visiting services for young families.

The effects on actually reducing health inequalities of these policies between 1997 and 2010, however, have only been partial, and even these small effects have been superseded by recent events such as austerity (as outlined in Chapter 5). Following the election of a Labour government on a mandate that included a commitment to reducing health inequalities and implementing evidence-based policy in 1997, the UK became the first European country in which policy-makers systematically and explicitly attempted to reduce inequalities in health.[38] A raft of policy measures designed to reduce health inequalities were introduced since 1997 (as previously described), and, although the UK's political system has become increasingly fragmented as a result of political devolution in Northern Ireland, Scotland and Wales, health inequalities have remained consistently high on policy agendas throughout the UK. However, despite having the most systematic policy around health inequalities in Europe, by the time Labour left office in 2010, mounting evidence indicated that local health inequalities in the UK and between the countries of the UK had not changed substantially, and in some cases had continued to get worse.

The key targets of the Labour government's strategy were to reduce the relative gap in life expectancy at birth between the most deprived local authorities (called Spearhead areas) and the English average by 10% by 2010, and to cut relative inequalities in IMR between manual socioeconomic groups and the English average by 10%, from 13% to 12%. The strategy failed to meet its own targets as the relative gap actually increased between 1995/97 and 2008 by 7% in terms of male life expectancy and by 14% in terms of female life expectancy.[39] However, the relative gap between manual socioeconomic groups and the England average for IMR actually fell between 1995/97 and 2007/09 from 13% to 12%, with a further fall to 10% in 2008/10 (see Table 6.2). The latter represents a reduction in relative inequalities of 25%. The absolute gap also decreased from 0.7 in 1997/99 to 0.5 in 2007/09 with a further fall to 0.4 in 2008/10, an overall reduction of 42%. This suggests that regarding its own – albeit very limited – terms, the English health inequalities strategy was partially successful.[40]

Another area of success of the strategy was around inequalities in 'mortality amendable to healthcare'. Amenable mortality is defined as mortality from causes for which there is evidence that they can be prevented given timely, appropriate access to high-quality care.[41] NHS funding was increased from 2001 when a 'health inequalities weighting' was added so that areas of higher deprivation received more funds per head to reflect their higher health needs. Analysis has shown that this policy – of increasing the proportion of resources allocated to deprived areas compared to more affluent areas – was associated with a reduction in absolute health inequalities from causes amenable to healthcare.[42] Increases in NHS resources to deprived areas accounted for a reduction in the gap between deprived and affluent areas in male 'mortality amenable to healthcare' of 35 deaths per 100,000 and female mortality of 16 deaths per 100,000. Each additional £10 million of resources allocated to deprived areas was associated with a reduction in 4 male deaths per 100,000 and 2 female deaths per 100,000.[43]

Table 6.2: Infant mortality rates in England, routine and manual socioeconomic group compared with national average (infant deaths per 1,000 live births)[44]

Time Period	Routine and Manual	English Average rate	Absolute gap	Relative gap
1997-99	6.3	5.6	0.7	13%
2002-04	5.9	5.0	0.9	18%
2003-05	5.7	4.9	0.8	17%
2004-06	5.6	4.8	0.8	16%
2005-07	5.4	4.7	0.7	16%
2006-08	5.3	4.5	0.7	16%
2007-09	5.0	4.4	0.5	12%
2008-10	4.7	4.3	0.4	10%
Change since 1997-99	-1.6	-1.3	-0.3	-3.0
% change since 1997-99	-1.2	-0.7	-0.5	-8.0

However, when looking beyond these arguably rather minor changes in very specific areas (IMR and mortality amenable to healthcare) and examining the broader social and spatial patterning of death and disease, health inequalities remained high, and indeed grew during this period. This is shown in Figure 6.2, which tracks trends in the size of the gap in death rates between the most and least affluent 10% of neighbourhoods for those aged less than 65 from the 1920s to the mid-2000s.[45] The health divide between the richest and poorest areas had decreased until the late 1970s, but then increased since the 1980s and throughout the post-1997 years of the Labour government.

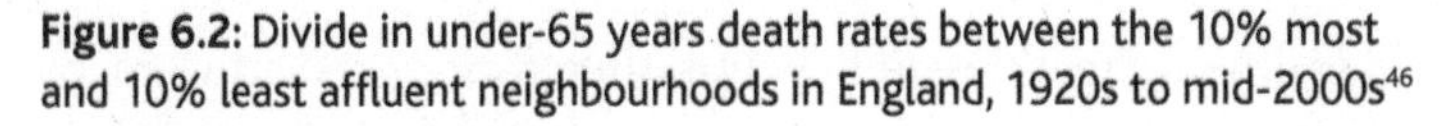
Figure 6.2: Divide in under-65 years death rates between the 10% most and 10% least affluent neighbourhoods in England, 1920s to mid-2000s[46]

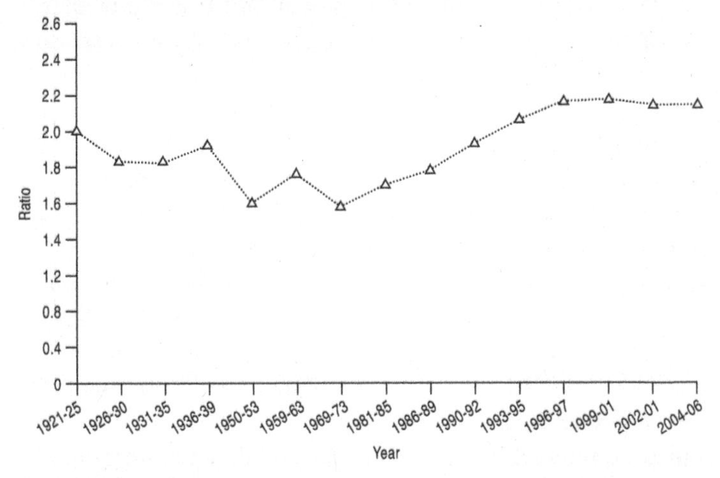

The most important reason for the very limited success of health inequalities policies in the UK since 1997 is the 'lifestyle drift' whereby policy went from thinking about the wider economic and social context to focusing almost exclusively on the individual-level, behavioural, compositional factors.[47] The only very limited success of the English strategy is therefore because there is only so much that can be achieved by focusing on individual behaviour change or the provision of more smoking cessation programmes or by increasing access to healthcare services. While there were policies enacted under the 1997–2010 New Labour governments that focused on the more fundamental determinants (for example, the implementation of a national minimum wage, the minimum pension, and tax credits for working parents, and a reduction in child poverty) as well as significant investment in the NHS, there was, however, little redistribution of income between rich and poor individuals or areas. Nor was there much by way of an economic rebalancing of the country (for example, between North and South). Indeed, a senior Labour government minister claimed at the time that he was 'seriously relaxed' about people getting rich. Further, in wider policy, the New Labour governments continued the neoliberal approach of Thatcherism – including, for example, further marketisation and privatisation of the NHS.

Health inequalities policy was therefore overshadowed by the far more powerful, fundamental and politically driven trends in economic and social policy, both domestically and internationally, as a result of the rise of neoliberalism. As described in Chapter 5, the effects of these neoliberal economic and social policies on health inequalities have been stark (or of 'epidemic' proportions), and have meant that those at the bottom have fallen even further behind.[48] In the face of such substantial (and largely unchallenged by what was previously a social democratic Labour Party) neoliberal structural changes to the fundamental determinants of health, the specialist area of 'health inequalities policy' (as outlined in this chapter) was unable to turn the tide on such longstanding health divides. It was therefore a case of 'too little, too late' – a lot of rhetoric and good intentions, but little in the end by way of meaningful action. The earlier post-war experience – in which smaller health inequalities were achieved through a more extensive welfare state and a different spatial and socioeconomic distribution of national wealth (as described in Chapter 5) – and the results of the various policy reviews examined earlier in this chapter – do, however, provide clear evidence as to *what is actually needed* to really 'turn the tide' on health divides. The likelihood of such substantial change happening became even more remote with the election of the coalition (Conservative–Liberal Democrat) government in 2010 and then another Conservative majority government in 2015, both of which were committed to neoliberal-inspired austerity.

Coalition, (more) Conservatism and health inequalities since 2010

In 2008, a third policy review of health inequalities was commissioned, the Marmot Review.[49, 50] It was commissioned by a Labour government that was coming towards the end of its third term and was not enjoying public or media support. The government had also by this stage moved some way from its initial commitment to tackling the 'upstream' structural determinants of health, and was more focused on 'downstream' individual lifestyle factors. Within three months of being published in February

2010, a Conservative–Liberal Democrat coalition formed a new government. Indeed, the timing of the Marmot Review had 'eerie echoes' of the Black Report in the sense that it was commissioned under a Labour government but the decision to implement (or not) many of its recommendations had fallen to a Conservative-led government.[51] Awareness of this political context may have influenced how the Marmot Review was drafted, possibly informing the decision to make rather vague and diluted recommendations that could be interpreted by, and remain acceptable to, different ideological perspectives, and thus avoid the political marginalisation that befell the Black Report in the 1980s.[52] In addition, the international banking crisis and high levels of debt facing the UK meant that this was once again a period in which the government was committed to reducing public expenditure. It built on the earlier Black and Acheson Reports, although following 13 years of policy efforts to reduce health inequalities it had far more evidence on which to draw. Nevertheless, as Table 6.1 outlines, the Marmot Review's policy recommendations largely mirror those of the earlier Black and Acheson Reports.

The coalition government accepted in principle the majority of the Marmot Review headline recommendations (all except the recommendations under heading 4, on income and poverty), and cited it as the basis for setting out a new public health system – for England – in their 2011 White Paper *Healthy lives, healthy people*. This included the transfer of public health responsibilities from the NHS to local authorities with the establishment of Health and Wellbeing Boards (between local authorities and local clinical commissioning groups [CCGs] of GPs), and the creation of a new organisation, Public Health England (PHE). In 2012, the government also created the Public Health Outcomes Framework, a set of indicators to monitor the new system that includes the aim of 'reduced differences in life expectancy and healthy life expectancy between communities'. Under the new system, local authorities – via the Health and Wellbeing Boards – were tasked with reducing health inequalities via actions on the local contextual and compositional determinants of health. This means that health inequalities and public health can now be 'placed' within broader local policies.

PHE was also created as a national body, and it has some responsibility for reducing health inequalities at the national level and between local communities. Its core mission is to 'protect and improve the nation's health and to address inequalities'. NHS England and CCGs, established under the Health and Social Care Act 2012, were also given a legal duty to reduce inequalities in access to – and outcomes from – NHS care. The Department of Health maintained a role in reducing health inequalities via its mandate with NHS England, and a framework agreement with PHE. The Secretary of State for Health is also required to 'have regard to reducing health inequalities'. So now, in England, central government responsibilities for reducing health inequalities have been devolved to local authorities, the NHS and PHE, all of which have very limited powers to have an impact on the contextual or fundamental determinants of health (that is, the 'rules of the game', as noted in Chapter 5).

In light of the new public health system set up by the coalition government in which local authorities have lead responsibility for reducing health inequalities, in 2014, PHE commissioned an independent inquiry to examine health inequalities specifically affecting the North of England, with a particular focus on how to reduce the North–South health divide in England (and, to a lesser extent, reducing inequalities in health within the towns and cities of the North), the *Due North* report.[53, 54] This concluded that the underlying causes of the North–South health divide in England and local health inequalities within Northern towns and cities were social, economic and political inequalities: differences in poverty, power and the resources needed for health; differences in exposure to health-damaging environments, such as poorer living and working conditions and unemployment; differences in the chronic disease and disability left by the historical legacy of heavy industry and its decline; and differences in opportunities to enjoy positive health factors and protective conditions that help maintain health, such as good quality early years education, economic and food security, control over life decisions, social support and feeling part of society. In order to tackle these root causes, the Inquiry set out four sets of recommendations (supported by evidence and analysis) to target inequalities both within the North and between the North and the rest of

England. They focused on addressing: (1) the economic and employment causes of health inequalities – calling for a regional strategy that 'not only ameliorates the impact of poverty but also seeks to prevent poverty in the future, not least by investing in people, as well as investing in places';[55] (2) the role of unequal early years in the development of health inequalities across the life course – calling for increased welfare support for families with children and for universal childcare; (3) the need to share power over resources and to increase the influence that the public has on how resources are used to improve the determinants of health via the devolution of power within England; and (4) strengthening the role of the health sector in promoting health equity as the NHS can influence health inequalities by providing equitable high quality healthcare, by directly influencing the social determinants of health through procurement and as an employer, and as a champion and facilitator that influences other sectors to take action to reduce inequalities in health.

Scotland, Wales and Northern Ireland maintained the pre-2010 NHS-based system with responsibility for reducing health inequalities lying solely with the healthcare sector – leading to increased divergence across the four UK countries in their approaches to health inequalities.[56] In Labour-run Wales there has been little change, with a continuing focus on health promotion (as opposed to tackling health inequalities). Meanwhile, the restoration of powers to the Northern Ireland Assembly facilitated a fresh concern with public health, and a new Public Health Agency was established in 2009. The most significant developments, however, occurred in Scotland and England, where policies moved in very opposite directions. In SNP-governed Scotland (Scotland was led by a Labour–Liberal Democrat coalition from 1999 to 2007, and then the SNP from 2011), public health policy continued to articulate a social determinants approach to tackling health inequalities and that accepted the need for central government action.[57, 58] In contrast, the UK-wide Conservative and Liberal Democrat coalition government's *Public health* White Paper for England paid little more than lip service to the wider social, economic, environmental and political determinants of health, choosing instead to stress that the causes of premature death are dominated by 'diseases of lifestyle' (compositional factors), for which the government accepts only limited responsibility. The lifestyle, individualised and very partial approach to health inequalities is continuing under the current majority Conservative UK government (elected in 2015).

What is to be done? Evidence-based health inequalities policy[59]

So far this chapter has outlined how the UK governments from the 1980s onwards had an impact on health divides, showing a pattern of increasing inequalities despite (limited) action by the 1997–2010 Labour government. It has also alluded to what policy-makers and governments should do if they want to reduce health inequalities. However, this latter task is not reliant on mere speculation as the health inequalities reports commissioned by government agencies themselves over the last four decades – Black, Acheson, Marmot and *Due North* – provide an evidence base to underpin what could and should be done.

The four reports have much in common in terms of the explanations of the underlying causes of health inequalities: all four clearly state that health inequalities are a result of other societal inequalities and differences, and all take a 'multi-causal' approach to explaining their existence. Furthermore, they all emphasise the importance of considering determinants across the whole life course, not just the point at which health inequalities are most apparent, with emphasis placed on the early years of life. Indeed, the Marmot Review's statement that it is the 'cumulative effects of hazards and disadvantage through life' that produce the social patterning of disease and ill health in the UK echoes almost precisely the Black Report's conclusion that 'inequalities in health tend to arise from the cumulative deprivation of a life-time'. Each places an emphasis on the social and economic (material) drivers of inequalities in health, although Acheson, Marmot and *Due North* – drawing on the wealth of health inequalities research undertaken since the 1980 Black Report – also highlight the complexity of the way in which material factors often interrelate with various other determinants, particularly psychosocial determinants.

The Black Report was published before psychosocial theories had emerged as a credible body of academic work, and hence, unsurprisingly, does not refer to psychosocial determinants. The Marmot Review and *Due North* both place considerable emphasis on psychosocial explanations of health inequalities, giving issues such as isolation, a sense of control and individual and community empowerment far more prominence than in the earlier reports. *Due North*, however, is much more materially (and psychosocially) focused than either Acheson or Marmot in that it overtly rejects the role of behavioural factors.

Despite the existence of some theoretical differences between the reports, as described above, and a gap of almost 35 years, many of the evidence-based policy recommendations are remarkably similar. This section provides a brief thematic comparison of the main recommendations.

- *Early years and young people:* For all four reports, the recommendations relating to early years bear striking similarities. While Black aimed for children to have 'a better start in life', with recommendations relating to increasing child benefits, improving pre-school childcare and providing free school meals, almost two decades later the Acheson Inquiry strongly echoed these recommendations. The Marmot Review is less directive, but as part of a policy objective to 'give every child the best start in life', various recommendations relating to maternal care, pre-school childcare and care within the education system are made. Similarly, the *Due North* report has 'promote healthy development in early childhood' as one of its four strategic recommendations.
- *Education, training and employment:* The Black Report and the Acheson Inquiry both focused largely on pre-school services so the Marmot Review recommendation that reducing inequalities in education outcomes should form a central part of efforts to reduce health inequalities could be said to represent a new focus. The Black Report featured no direct recommendation relating to employment either. In contrast, the Acheson Inquiry highlighted the detrimental effects of unemployment, and suggested increasing opportunities for work and training. The Marmot Review continued the

strong emphasis on employment and training opportunities, but supplemented this with an emphasis on the quality and flexibility of employment. Likewise, the *Due North* report highlighted the need for employment opportunities to be increased within the North, and for good quality early years education proportionate to need.

- *Working conditions/environment:* The Black Report highlighted the need for 'minimally acceptable and desirable conditions of work'. This was expanded by the Acheson Inquiry to include a call to address psychosocial work hazards. The Marmot Review further developed these concerns, placing particular emphasis on psychosocial-related issues such as equality and stress. All three of these national level reports recommend that the workplace be used an arena in which to undertake health-promoting activities. *Due North* does not talk about the work environment beyond a call for the living wage to be implemented.
- *Tackling poverty and redistributing wealth and resources:* The Black Report put forward the ambitious aim of abolishing child poverty as a national goal for the 1980s, although it acknowledged that this was likely to be very costly, and also included a number of other recommendations (particularly around benefits) that were intended to tackle poverty. Fast forward to 1998, and while Acheson did not recommend such an ambitious goal, it, too, emphasised the need to tackle income inequality, specifically recommending that: 'Further steps should be taken to reduce income inequalities and improve living standards of poor households.' This focus is echoed in the Marmot Review, which recommends the implementation of a more progressive taxation system and the introduction of a minimum income for healthy living. The latter is also recommended by the *Due North* report alongside tackling child poverty and introducing a living wage.
- *Housing:* All four reports call for an upgrading of housing stock. The Black Report focused on the quality and availability of local authority housing. The Acheson Inquiry added recommendations on fuel poverty and insulation and reducing accidents in homes, and placed particular emphasis on the housing of older people. The Marmot Review, less

specifically, calls for the creation and development of 'healthy and sustainable places and communities', but in the longer term, it, too, calls for the 'upgrade of housing stock'. *Due North* – reflecting the rising housing crisis in the UK – calls for a licensing scheme to improve private housing stock.

- *The role of the NHS:* All the reports stress the need for cross-departmental working at local and national levels of government. None of the reports suggest that the NHS can (or should) play a prominent role in addressing health inequalities, but the Black Report and Acheson Inquiry both make some recommendations concerning the need to ensure fair and equal access to healthcare services, and the Marmot Review suggests the 'prevention and early detection of those conditions most strongly related to health inequalities' should be prioritised. *Due North* highlights the importance of integrated local services and joint commissioning, and notes the role of higher funding allocations in deprived areas as a way of reducing mortality amenable to healthcare.
- *Empowerment and community control:* As noted earlier, the Black Report pre-dated research into health inequalities that emphasised the role of psychosocial factors. The Acheson Report made recommendations about control at work. However, in the Marmot Review, social capital, described as the 'links that bind and connect people within and between communities', is presented as a 'source of resilience' and 'a buffer against risks of poor health'. Related to this, the phrase 'capabilities' is used throughout the report to help illustrate the importance the review places on enabling individuals to have the opportunity to live fair and healthy lives throughout their life course. *Due North* goes even further in terms of having one of its four strategic recommendations to 'increase the influence that the public has on how resources are used to improve the determinants of health'. It has the devolution of power from central to local government and down to communities as a central theme of the report.
- *Health behaviours:* The first two reports also made some specific recommendations concerning the supply, marketing and consumption of tobacco products, whereas Marmot does not. None of the reports make similar recommendations for

alcohol. In terms of diet and exercise, the Black Report was relatively vague in suggesting that measures were required to 'encourage the desirable changes in people's diet [and] exercise'. In contrast, Acheson made some rather specific recommendations, including increasing the availability of food to ensure the supply of 'an adequate and affordable diet'. The Marmot Review is more similar to Black than Acheson, marking a return to relatively broad and unspecific suggestions such as 'efforts to reduce the social gradient in obesity'. *Due North* is very overt in rejecting the role of behavioural factors as an issue in the North–South health divide, and makes no recommendations in this area.

So these reports provide a clear policy agenda for what *should* be done to reduce health inequalities. However, as is clear in the review of *actual* policies from the 1980s outlined earlier in this chapter, the national policy effects of the reviews were minimal beyond leading to a welcome discourse around health inequalities.[60] This is because good evidence alone does not lead to action – political support is required.[61] The future politics of health divides in the UK and beyond is the subject of the final, concluding, chapter.

CHAPTER 7

Past, present, future

This book has examined how where you live can kill you by looking at health divides at various scales – internationally, nationally, regionally and locally. It has focused on case studies of the US health disadvantage, the 'Scottish health effect', the North–South health divide in England and local health inequalities within the towns and cities of wealthy democracies. It has examined the historical emergence of these divisions, drawing parallels with the 19th century. It has outlined what they are like today, and how place matters in terms of a variety of different health outcomes. It has also explored the determinants of geographical inequalities in health, arguing that while place matters for health, politics matters for place. It has asserted that the fundamental determinants of health are political and arise from the unequal distribution of economic and political power. The role of politics in both increasing and reducing health divides has been examined with a particular focus on the role of neoliberalism. The book has also explored the failure of previous policies to properly tackle these issues in the context of growing social and spatial inequalities during the neoliberal era. It has also reflected on what the evidence suggests should be done to reduce the relationship between health and place. Drawing on the public health research evidence, this concluding chapter focuses on what can be learned about the political geography of life and death from past experience, what dangers the present holds for health divides and what the future might look like.

The case studies examined in this book show that health divides have waxed and waned over time as the importance of place for health has varied. This has important lessons for how health divides can be reduced and what they might be like in the future. In the 19th century, industrialism and the emergence of liberal, laissez-faire capitalism resulted in environmental, living and working conditions in which infectious disease thrived and in which population health was reduced (such as the falling life expectancies of the early- to mid-19th century), and substantial health divides between rural and urban areas, North and South, and rich and poor were produced. The 19th century also provides the first evidence for how politics matters for the geographies of health. The epidemiological shift that occurred in the late 19th and early 20th century, whereby health improved as infectious disease was replaced by chronic disease as the main cause of death, was brought about by political change: it was political change that led to the public health legislation which introduced sanitation, it was the activity of trade union movements that led to higher living standards and improved working conditions, which in turn enabled better nutrition, and ultimately created a population better equipped to withstand infectious disease. It is the first example of how politics has an impact on population health.

The emergence of the US health disadvantage in the 1980s provides a more negative example of the effect of politics on health. The US had been the healthiest and tallest of the rich democracies until the post-war period (1945+). By the late 1970s and certainly from the 1980s onwards, it began to slip down the international league tables for key health outcomes such as infant mortality rates (IMR) or average life expectancy. The reasons for this are complex, involving both compositional (such as higher poverty rates) and contextual factors (a less accessible healthcare system). However, the political dimension cannot be overlooked – the composition of the US population and the wider context within which Americans live differs from those of other wealthy democracies, such as those of Western Europe, as a result of political decisions. The US has always had a less generous welfare state and so it has higher poverty rates. The US does not have universal healthcare and it has less public health regulation. These contextual factors are within the power of national government to change, but the US chose, under Reagan, to pursue neoliberalism from the 1980s onwards, which further eroded its meagre welfare state, resulting in a further decline in the conditions for better population health.

Likewise, the exacerbation of the 'Scottish health effect' that also occurred in the 1980s can be explained by reference to the politics of health. The neoliberal economic and political agenda pursued by the UK Thatcher governments resulted in an increase in the health gap between Scotland and England, with the diseases of despair (violence, drugs etc) replacing heart disease as the driver of the divide. The deindustrialisation, unemployment, welfare reductions and radical reduction of the public sector in this period can be considered as a 'political attack' on the Scottish working class, and one which has had long-term health consequences. The effect of the imposition of such neoliberal 'shock doctrine' policies on population health is also evident in other countries, such as those of the former Eastern bloc. In contrast, the case of East Germany provides an example of the positive role that different political choices can have in reducing health divides. The reunification of East and West Germany was accompanied by an increase in incomes and pensions in the East, alongside large infrastructure investments in healthcare and the wider economy. This was a firm economic commitment made as part of the wider political project of reunification. The investment approach, in complete contrast to a neoliberal approach of cutting public sector investment and welfare, led to a rapid and unprecedented reduction in the health disadvantage of the formerly communist East.

Meanwhile, the North–South divide in England, first noted in the 19th century, continues to persist; in fact, it has increased in recent years, with the North now experiencing the greatest health penalty at any time in the post-war era. The history of local health divides within towns and cities provides both positive and negative lessons on how politics matters for health and place. In the post-war welfare state era, in countries like the UK, the US and New Zealand, local health divides decreased. In contrast, they increased in the neoliberal era from the 1980s onwards. The expansion of the welfare state in the US during the 1960s' 'War on Poverty' resulted in smaller inequalities in health. Likewise, the health gaps between deprived and affluent areas in the UK decreased from the 1940s until the 1970s. However, in the 1980s, with the beginning of the neoliberal era, typified by welfare state cuts, health inequalities increased as the ability of the poorest to live a healthy life decreased.

This book has on the whole been perhaps a rather depressing read for anyone interested in the pursuit of health equity. The depth of our health divides, their historical and international pervasiveness, and the failure of even the 'most systematic strategy in Europe' to address them, all breeds a feeling of despair and hopelessness. It is rather difficult to think positively about the effects of today's politics on health divides as, despite the financial crisis, the neoliberal political economy still dominates – exemplified by the austerity policies pursued in countries such as the UK, Spain and Greece. Austerity has been used to turbo-charge the neoliberal agenda of reducing workers' rights and job security, decreasing wages and welfare, while increasing poverty and working hours. Current politics, especially in Europe, is going against what the evidence suggests is required to reduce health divides, and arguably, neoliberal austerity is creating an environment in which existing health divides will only increase. Indeed, future projections of local geographical health inequalities in England suggest that they will continue to increase.[1] Further, many of the big future challenges for public health – rising income inequalities, obesity and climate change – could all exacerbate existing health divides as their negative effects are unevenly distributed. New health divides may even emerge.

Historical trends and international examples also give reason for hope, however, and suggest political solutions that will reduce the link between health and place: geography does not have to be a matter of life and death. Neoliberalism may increase health divides, but there is also evidence presented in this book that social democratic-style policies of resource redistribution, poverty reduction and public health regulation can reduce them, breaking the link between where you live, who you are and when you die. Health divides may be ubiquitous, but past lessons suggest that their magnitude varies, and it is therefore possible to reduce – if not eliminate – them, although this is only possible if radical steps are taken. Further, there are evidence-based solutions to health divides and real world examples of how they work in practice, ranging from the epidemiological transition, to German reunification, to the decline in local health divides in the post-war period. This gives credence to the fact that health inequalities are not inevitable or insurmountable: they can be reduced. There is plenty of evidence from public health researchers to show what sorts of policies are required to reduce the key health divides examined in this book.

Reducing the US health disadvantage

Drawing on their overview of the evidence, the 2013 US National Academies report into the US health disadvantage concluded that the following areas of action should be undertaken to improve the relative epidemiological standing of the US:[2]

- *Develop healthy and safe community environments*: This can be achieved by improving the quality of air, land and water, and developing affordable, accessible, safe and healthy housing. The powers of public health departments should be strengthened to increase the provision of essential services; health should be incorporated into policy decision-making across multiple sectors; and cross-sector collaboration in community planning and design should be increased to promote health and safety.
- *Improve community-based preventive health services*: This could include: a focus on improving cardiovascular health; using payment and reimbursement mechanisms to encourage the delivery of clinical preventive services; making better use of health information technology; linking community-based preventive services with clinical care; and reducing barriers to accessing clinical and community preventive services, especially among populations at greatest risk.
- *Empower people*: Provide people with the tools and information to make healthy choices; support positive social interactions and healthy decision-making; engage and empower people and communities to plan and implement prevention policies and programmes; and improve education and employment opportunities.
- *Eliminate health disparities (inequalities)*: Make a strategic focus on communities at greatest risk; reduce disparities in access

to quality healthcare; increase the capacity of the prevention workforce to identify and address disparities; support research to identify effective strategies to eliminate health disparities; and collect standardised data to better identify and address disparities.

- *Promote tobacco-free living*: Support comprehensive tobacco-free policies and other evidence-based tobacco control policies; bring in full implementation of the Family Smoking Prevention and Tobacco Control Act (2009); expand the use of the tobacco cessation service; and use the media to educate and encourage people to live tobacco-free lives.
- *Prevent drug abuse and excessive alcohol use*: Support the implementation and enforcement of alcohol control policies; create environments that empower young people not to drink or use other drugs; identify alcohol and other drug abuse disorders early and provide intervention, referral and treatment; and reduce inappropriate access to, and use of, prescription drugs.
- *Promote healthy eating*: Increase access to healthy and affordable foods in communities; implement organisational and programmatic nutrition standards and policies; improve nutritional quality of the food supply; help people recognise and make healthy food and beverage choices; support policies and programmes that promote breastfeeding; and enhance food safety.
- *Support active living*: Encourage community design and development that supports physical activity; promote and strengthen school and early learning policies and programmes that increase physical activity; facilitate access to safe, accessible and affordable places for physical activity; support workplace policies and programmes that increase physical activity; and assess physical activity levels, providing education, counselling and referrals.
- *Enable injury and violence-free living*: Implement and strengthen policies and programmes to enhance transportation safety; support community and streetscape design that promotes safety and prevents injuries; promote and strengthen policies and programmes to prevent falls, especially among older adults; promote and enhance policies and programmes to increase

safety and prevent injury in the workplace; strengthen policies and programmes to prevent violence; and provide individuals and families with the knowledge, skills and tools to make safe choices that prevent violence and injuries.

- *Improve reproductive and sexual health*: Increase the use of preconception and prenatal care; support reproductive and sexual health services and support services for pregnant and parenting women; provide effective sexual health education, especially for adolescents; and enhance the early detection of HIV, viral hepatitis and other sexually transmitted infections and improve linkage to care.
- *Promote better mental and emotional wellbeing*: Support positive early childhood development, including positive parenting and violence-free homes; facilitate social connectedness and community engagement across the lifespan; provide individuals and families with the support necessary to maintain positive mental wellbeing; and promote early identification of mental health needs and access to quality services.
- *Explore innovative policy options*: Undertake an analytic review of the available evidence on: (1) the effects of policies (including social, economic, educational, urban and rural development and transportation, healthcare financing and delivery) on the areas in which the US has an established health disadvantage; (2) how these policies have varied over time across high-income countries; and (3) the extent to which those policy differences may explain cross-national health differences in one or more health domains. This review should be followed by a series of issue-focused investigative studies to explore why the US experiences poorer outcomes.

Diffusing the 'Scottish health effect'

In 2016, the Glasgow Centre for Population Health[3] released a comprehensive review and analysis of the 'Scottish health effect', its causes and potential remedies. Their report put forward the following evidence-based policy recommendations for the national Scottish government and Scottish local authorities:[4]

- *National economic strategy:* Make the reduction of income and wealth inequalities the central objective of Scotland's economic policy, thereby achieving 'inclusive growth'. This can be done by reducing inequalities in the ownership of capital (land, housing or shares) by promoting cooperative ownership models (for example, of companies or land); increasing the tax take and implementing greater progressivity in taxation, providing greater resources for redistribution and public services; a reduction in wage inequality through the introduction of a Scottish living wage reducing the gap between the highest and lowest earners; diversifying the economy and reducing reliance on the financial services sector and oil industry; removing barriers to worker organisation and ownership to ensure there is a rebalancing of power between the owners of wealth and those who work to create it (for example, through greater collective bargaining); the social security system should offer increased levels of protection and less conditionality, thereby ensuring the provision of a more effective 'safety net' for the most vulnerable in society; reduce costs that have an impact on most of the poorest groups (including childcare, housing, heating, transport and food); and the Scottish government should adopt a 'poverty proofing' approach to all policies and major spending decisions by adopting the WHO's principle of 'Health in All' policies
- *National housing and the physical environment policy:* There is a need to improve housing and the physical environment, particularly in deindustrialised areas such as Glasgow and the West of Scotland. This could include a substantial expansion of the social house building programme of high-quality, low-rent, sustainable, social housing; an extension of the housing quality standards to the private rented sector and tied housing; targeting cold and damp housing and people who struggle to afford fuel by implementing affordable heating, ventilation and quality energy efficiency measures in all housing, both new and existing properties, with a focus on the private rented and owner-occupied sectors; improving greenspace access and quality in deprived areas; improving the maintenance of streets and open, green and public spaces, ensuring that

environmental incivilities, crime and anti-social behaviour do not act as disincentives to their use and enjoyment; and improving road safety for pedestrians and cyclists by establishing 20 mph zones, area-wide traffic calming schemes and segregation of pedestrians, cyclists and traffic, as the norm for residential and urban areas.

- *Local authorities (including Glasgow in particular):* There are also policy actions that can be taken at a local level, such as recognising, understanding and acting on the impact of local decision-making on population health; the need to avoid repeating historical mistakes, ensuring that viable and supportive communities are created and kept together; and building further affordable public sector housing. Local government also has a part to play in distributing income, with progressive use of proceeds from a fairer system of local taxation; the boundaries and/or the funding allocation system for local government should be reviewed with the explicit objective of ascertaining whether any potential changes could more effectively facilitate resource distribution across Scotland; a 'poverty proofing' approach to local government (and partner organisation) policy-making should be adopted, alongside the WHO's 'Health in All' policies; and actions to narrow local inequalities should also be enacted, such as the full implementation of the living wage, adoption of 20 mph speed limits and taking 'health first' approaches to tackling worklessness.
- *Understanding deprivation:* There is an urgent need to prioritise further research on the true nature of deprivation in Scotland that is not captured by existing data and measurements. The 'lived reality' of living in socially and materially deprived circumstances in Scotland differs from elsewhere in Britain, and it is imperative that new research, perhaps based on ethnographic methodologies and involving a comparative approach, is undertaken to better understand those differences, and to formulate appropriate policy responses.

Closing the North–South health divide

The 2014 *Due North* report examined how to reduce inequalities both within the North and between the North and the rest of England. The recommendations each had two aspects:

1. What can the North of England do itself to reduce the gap with the South? And
2. What can only central government do to reduce health inequalities?[5]

The Inquiry set out four sets of recommendations, supported by evidence and analysis:[6]

- *Tackle poverty and economic inequality within the North and between the North and the rest of England:* Agencies in the North should/can work together to embed health-focused approaches into the local economic development strategy and delivery; work together across the public sector to adopt a common progressive procurement approach to promote health; implement and regulate the living wage at the local authority level; assess the impact in the North of changes in national economic and welfare policies; and implement the actions in Recommendation 2 on child poverty reduction. Northern agencies should/can lobby central government to extend the national measurement of the wellbeing programme to better monitor progress and influence policy on inequalities; develop a national industrial strategy that reduces inequalities between the regions; assess the impact of changes in national policies on health inequalities in general and regional inequalities in particular; expand the role of Credit Unions and take measures to end the poverty premium; introduce a licensing scheme to improve private housing stock; end in-work poverty by implementing and regulating a living wage; ensure that welfare systems provide a minimum income for healthy living; advocate for city and county regions to be given greater control over the use of the skills budget and to make the Work Programme more equitable and responsive to differing local labour markets; and develop a new deal between local partners and national government that more fairly allocates the total public resources for local populations.

- *Promote healthy development in early childhood:* Agencies in the North should/can work together to monitor and incrementally increase the proportion of overall expenditure allocated to giving every child the best possible start in life, and ensure that the level of expenditure on early years development reflects levels of need; provide good quality universal early years education and childcare with greater emphasis on those with the greatest needs to ensure that all children achieve an acceptable level of school readiness; and maintain and protect universal integrated neighbourhood support for early child development, with a central role for health visitors and children's centres that clearly articulates the proportionate universalism approach. Agencies in the North should/can lobby central government to embed a rights-based approach to children's health; reduce child poverty through the measures advocated by the Child Poverty Commission, which includes investment in action on the social determinants of all parents' ability to properly care for children, such as paid parental leave, flexible work schedules, the living wage, secure and promising educational futures for young women, and affordable high-quality childcare; reverse recent falls in the living standards of less advantaged families; commit to carrying out a cumulative impact assessment of any future welfare changes to ensure a better understanding of their impacts on poverty and to allow negative impacts to be more effectively mitigated; invest in raising the qualifications of staff working in early years childcare and education; increase the proportion of overall expenditure, allocated to early years and ensure expenditure on early years development is focused according to need; provide universal support to families through parenting programmes, children's centres and key workers, delivered to meet social needs; and provide good quality early years education and childcare proportionately, according to need.
- *Share power over resources and increase the influence that the public has on how resources are used to improve the determinants of health:* Agencies in the North should/can work together to develop

community-led systems for health equity monitoring and accountability; expand the involvement of citizens in shaping how local budgets are used; increase the provision of services by participative and representative organisations that are based on 'mutual' models of public ownership; develop the capacity of communities to participate in local decision-making and develop solutions that inform policies and investments at local and national levels; develop deep collaboration between combined authorities in the North to develop a pan-Northern approach to economic development and health inequalities; and revitalise Health and Wellbeing Boards to become stronger advocates for health, both locally and nationally. Agencies in the North should/can lobby central government to give local government a greater role in deciding how public resources are used to improve the health and wellbeing of the communities they serve; and revise national policy to give greater flexibility to local government to raise funds for investment and use assets to improve the health and wellbeing of their communities.

- *Strengthen the role of the health sector in promoting health equity:* PHE should conduct a cumulative assessment of the impact of welfare reform and cuts to local and national public services; support local authorities to produce a Health Inequalities Risk Mitigation Strategy; establish a cross-departmental system of health impact assessment; support the involvement of Health and Wellbeing Boards and public health teams in the governance of Local Enterprise Partnerships and combined authorities; contribute to a review of current systems for the central allocation of public resources to local areas; develop a network of Health and Wellbeing Boards across the North of England with a special focus on health equity; lead the development of a charter to protect the rights of children; and work with HealthWatch and Health and Wellbeing Boards across the North of England to develop community-led systems for health equity monitoring and accountability. CCGs and other NHS agencies in the North should work together to lead the way in using the Social Value Act to ensure that procurement and commissioning maximises opportunities for high-quality local employment, high-quality care and reductions in economic and health inequalities; pool resources with other partners to ensure that universal integrated neighbourhood support for early childhood development is developed and maintained; CCGs and the local area teams of NHS England should develop a community-orientated model of primary care; work with the Department for Work and Pensions (DWP) to develop 'health first' employment support programmes for people with chronic health conditions; work more effectively with local authority directors of public health and PHE to address the risk conditions (social and economic determinants of health) that drive health and social care system demand; support Health and Wellbeing Boards to integrate budgets and jointly direct health and wellbeing spending plans for the NHS and local authorities; and provide leadership to support health services and clinical teams to reduce children's exposure to poverty, and its consequences.

Tackling local inequalities in health

The *Strategic review of health inequalities in England* (Marmot Review) was commissioned by the UK national government in 2008, and it reported in 2010.[7] Its remit was to identify, for the health inequalities challenge facing England, the evidence most relevant to underpinning future policy and action; show how this evidence could be translated into practice; advise on possible objectives and measures; and publish a report that would contribute to the development of a post-2010 health inequalities strategy. The following broad recommendations were made:[8]

- *Give every child the best start in life:*
  - *Priority objectives*: to reduce inequalities in the early development of physical and emotional health, and cognitive, linguistic and social skills; to ensure high-quality maternity services, parenting programmes, childcare and early years education to meet need across the social gradient; and to build the resilience and wellbeing of young children across the social gradient.

  - *Policy recommendations:* to increase the proportion of overall expenditure allocated to early years, and ensure expenditure on early years development is focused progressively across the social gradient; to support families to achieve progressive improvements in early child development (including giving priority to pre- and post-natal interventions that reduce adverse outcomes of pregnancy and infancy; providing paid parental leave in the first year of life with a minimum income for healthy living; provide routine support to families through parenting programmes, children's centres and key workers, delivered to meet social need via outreach to families; and developing programmes for the transition to school); and to provide good quality early years education and childcare proportionately across the gradient (this provision should be combined with outreach to increase the take-up by children from disadvantaged families, provided on the basis of evaluated models and to meet quality standards).

- *Enable all children young people and adults to maximise their capabilities and have control over their lives:*
  - *Priority objectives:* to reduce the social gradient in skills and qualifications; to ensure that schools, families and communities work in partnership to reduce the gradient in the health, wellbeing and resilience of children and young people; and to improve the access and use of quality lifelong learning across the social gradient.
  - *Policy recommendations:* to ensure that reducing social inequalities in pupils' educational outcomes is a sustained priority; to prioritise reducing social inequalities in life skills (by extending the role of schools in supporting families and communities and taking a 'whole child' approach to education; consistently implementing 'full service' extended school approaches; and developing the school-

based workforce to build their skills in working across school–home boundaries and addressing social and emotional development, physical and mental health and wellbeing); and to increase access and use of quality lifelong learning opportunities across the social gradient (by providing easily accessible support and advice for 16- to 25-year-olds on life skills, training and employment opportunities; providing work-based learning, including apprenticeships, for young people and those changing jobs/careers; and increasing the availability of non-vocational lifelong learning across the life course).

- *Create fair employment and good work for all:*
  - *Priority objectives:* to improve access to good jobs and reduce long-term unemployment across the social gradient; to make it easier for people who are disadvantaged in the labour market to obtain and keep work; and to improve the quality of jobs across the social gradient.
  - *Policy recommendations:* to prioritise active labour market programmes to achieve timely interventions to reduce long-term unemployment; to encourage, incentivise and, where appropriate, enforce the implementation of measures to improve the quality of jobs across the social gradient (by ensuring public and private sector employers adhere to equality guidance and legislation; implementing guidance on stress management; and the effective promotion of wellbeing and physical and mental health at work); and to develop greater security and flexibility in employment (by prioritising greater flexibility of retirement age; and encouraging and incentivising employers to create or adapt jobs that are suitable for lone parents, carers and people with mental and physical health problems).

- *Ensure a healthy standard of living for all:*
  - *Priority objectives:* to establish a minimum income for healthy living for people of all ages; to reduce the social gradient in the standard of living through progressive taxation and other fiscal policies; and to reduce the cliff edges faced by people moving between benefits and work.
  - *Policy recommendations:* to develop and implement standards for a minimum income for healthy living; to remove 'cliff edges' for those moving in and out of work and improve flexibility of employment; and to review and implement systems of taxation, benefits, pensions and tax credits to provide a minimum income for healthy living standards and pathways for moving upwards.

- *Create and develop healthy and sustainable places and communities:*
  - *Priority objectives:* to develop common policies to reduce the scale and impact of climate change and health inequalities; and to improve community capital and reduce social isolation across the social gradient.
  - *Policy recommendations:* to prioritise policies and interventions that reduce both health inequalities and mitigate climate change (by improving active travel across the social gradient; improving the availability of good quality open and green spaces across the social gradient; improving the food environment in local areas across the social gradient; and improving the energy efficiency of housing across the social gradient); to fully integrate the planning, transport, housing, environmental and health systems to address the social determinants of health in each locality; and to support locally developed and evidence-based community regeneration programmes (that remove barriers to community participation and action and reduce social isolation).

- *Strengthen the role and impact of ill health prevention:*
  - *Priority objectives:* to prioritise prevention and early detection of those conditions most strongly related to health inequalities; and to increase the availability of long-term and sustainable funding in ill health prevention across the social gradient.
  - *Policy recommendations:* to prioritise investment in ill health prevention and health promotion across government departments to reduce the social gradient; to implement an evidence-based programme of ill health preventive interventions that are effective across the social gradient (by increasing and improving the scale and quality of medical drug treatment programmes; focusing public health interventions such as smoking cessation programmes and alcohol reduction on the social gradient; and improving programmes to address the causes of obesity across the social gradient); and to focus core efforts of public health departments on interventions related to the social determinants of health proportionately across the gradient.

Concluding thoughts

So, as these varying and extensive recommendations show, health divides can be reduced, and we *do* have the tools with which to do the job, operating at different scales – from the individual to the local, the national and international. In fact, we perhaps have rather too many tools and policy ideas listed above! Looking across each of the international, national, regional and local health divides examined in this book, it is clear, however, that while many things contribute to the relationship between health and place, some aspects are more important and more fundamental than others. It is therefore possible to put forward three key things that would make the most difference to health divides, particularly in the UK:

- *Income redistribution*: by taxing higher earners and businesses more than is currently the case, and using the money to fund better public services, healthcare and social security payments;
- *Devolution of power*: devolving decision-making from corporate and political elites to local democratic institutions, communities and individuals, so that local people have a say over the shaping of their neighbourhoods;
- *Resourcing the regions*: developing and implementing an industrial policy that takes into account the fact that places matter to people, promoting economic growth in all parts of the country.

However, even when reducing the policy shopping list to just three things, it is clear that implementation in the real world, and not just in an academic book or in the pages of dusty government reports, requires considerable political impetus. Health inequalities can be reduced, but there needs to be a real *desire* to do so, and ultimately a political *choice* must be made to do so. There needs to be the will and the accompanying action to radically change the political and economic priorities and structures of wealthy democracies, away from neoliberal individualism and towards a more collective (social democratic) approach, so that the conditions of life, work and play are to the benefit of the health of all people and places, not just those with power and resources. This requires the right political choices to be made, not just by politicians, but also by electorates: we can vote for and support political parties and movements that offer programmes that will reduce health divides, or not. But if we don't, geography will remain a matter of life and death, and where you live may well continue to kill you.

Notes

Chapter 1

[1] Schrecker, T. and Bambra, C. (2015) *How politics makes us sick: Neoliberal epidemics*, Basingstoke: Palgrave Macmillan.

[2] Woolf, S. and Aron, L. (2013) *US health in international perspective: Shorter lives, poorer health*, Washington, DC: The National Academies Press.

[3] Woolf and Aron (2013).

[4] Data from OECD (Organisation for Economic Co-operation and Development) (2013) *Health at a Glance 2013: OECD indicators*, http://dx.doi.org/10.1787/health_glance-2013-en

[5] WHO (World Health Organization) (2013) *Life expectancy at birth*, Geneva: WHO, www.who.int/gho/mortality_burden_disease/life_tables/situation_trends/en/

[6] ONS (Office for National Statistics) (2015) *Life expectancy at birth for England, Wales and Northern Ireland, 2012-14*, Newport: ONS.

[7] Smith, K.E. and Bambra, C. (2012) 'British and Northern Irish experiences', in D. Raphael (ed) *Tackling health inequalities: Lessons from international experiences*, Toronto: Canadian Scholars' Press Inc, p 93.

[8] Hunter, D.J. (2011) 'Change of government: one more big bang health care reform in England's National Health Service', *International Journal of Health Services*, vol 41, no 1, pp 159-74.

[9] Data from BBC News (2015) 'General Election results', www.bbc.co.uk/news/election/2015/results

[10] ONS (Office for National Statistics) (2014) 'Adult health in Great Britain', *Statistical Bulletin*, Newport: ONS.

[11] National Records of Scotland (2014) *Life expectancy for administrative areas within Scotland 2011-2013*, Edinburgh: National Records of Scotland (www.nrscotland.gov.uk/statistics-and-data/statistics/statistics-by-theme/life-expectancy/life-expectancy-in-scottish-areas/2011-2013).

[12] Scott-Samuel, A., Bambra, C., Collins, C., Hunter, D.J., McCartney, G. and Smith, K. (2014) 'The impact of Thatcherism on health and well-being in Britain', *International Journal of Health Services*, vol 44, no 1, pp 53-71.

[13] Hanlon, P., Lawder, R.S., Buchanan, D., Redpath, A., Walsh, D., Wood, R. et al (2005) 'Why is mortality higher in Scotland than in England and Wales? Decreasing influence of socioeconomic deprivation between 1981

and 2001 supports the existence of a "Scottish Effect"', *Journal of Public Health*, vol 27, no 2, pp 199-204.

[14] ONS (2015).

[15] National Records of Scotland (2014).

[16] ONS (Office for National Statistics) (2014) *Disability-free life expectancy (DFLE) and life expectancy (LE) at birth by upper tier local authority at birth, England 2012-14,* Newport: ONS.

[17] Hacking, J.M., Muller, S. and Buchan, I.E. (2011) 'Trends in mortality from 1965 to 2008 across the English north-south divide: comparative observational study', *British Medical Journal*, vol 342, d508.

[18] Bambra, C., Barr, B. and Milne, E. (2014) 'North and South: Addressing the English health divide', *Journal of Public Health*, vol 36, no 2, pp 183-6.

[19] Dorling, D. and Thomas, B. (2009) 'Geographical inequalities in health over the last century', in H. Graham (ed) *Understanding health inequalities*, Maidenhead: Open University Press, p 66.

[20] Dorling, D. (2013) *Unequal health: The scandal of our times*, Bristol: Policy Press.

[21] Reproduced from Bambra et al (2014) , with permission of Oxford University Press.

[22] Whitehead, M. and Doran, T. (2011) 'The North-South health divide', *British Medical Journal*, vol 342, no 7794, d584.

[23] Bambra et al (2014).

[24] Dorling, D. (2010) 'Persistent North-South divides', in N. Coe and A. Jones (eds) *The economic geography of the UK*, London: Sage, pp 12-28.

[25] Bambra, C. and Orton, C. (2015) 'A train journey through the English health divide: topological map', *Environment and Planning A*, December.

[26] Data from ONS (Office for National Statistics) (2014) *Life expectancy at birth and at age 65 by local areas in England and Wales: 2011 to 13*, Newport: ONS.

[27] Data from ONS (2014) ibid.

[28] Reproduced under Creative Commons licence from Bambra and Orton (2016) ibid.

[29] Reproduced under Creative Commons licence from Bambra and Orton (2016) ibid.

[30] Dorling (2010).

[31] Milne, E. and Schrecker, T. (2014) 'Lots of planets have a North...', *Journal of Public Health*, vol 36, no 2, pp 181-2.

[32] Data from Eurostat (2013) *Life expectancy*, http://ec.europa.eu/eurostat/statistics-explained/index.php/Mortality_and_life_expectancy_statistics

[33] National Records of Scotland (2014).

[34] Cook, I., Chaolin, G.U. and Halsall, J. (2013) 'China's growing urban health inequalities: The challenges ahead', *Journal of Management and Sustainability*, vol 3, no 2, p 10.

[35] Data from Social Science Research Council (2014) *Measure of America report 2013-14*, Brooklyn, NY: Social Science Research Council, http://www.measureofamerica.org/measure_of_america2013-2014/

[36] DCLG (Department for Communities and Local Government) (2011) *English indices of deprivation 2010*, London: DCLG.

[37] Data from ONS (Office for National Statistics) (2015) *Inequality in healthy life expectancy at birth by national deciles of area deprivation: England, 2011 to 2013*, Newport: ONS.

[38] Marmot, M. (2010) *Fair society, healthy lives: The Marmot Review*, London: University College London.

[39] LHO (London Health Observatory) (2012) *Health inequalities*, London: LHO, www.lho.org.uk/LHO_Topics/National_Lead_Areas/HealthInequalitiesOverview.aspx

[40] Adapted from LHO (2012) ibid.

[41] Reid, M. (2011) 'Behind the "Glasgow effect"', *Bulletin of the World Health Organization*, vol 89, no 10, pp 706-7.

[42] Marmot, M. (2004) 'Status syndrome', *Significance*, vol 1, no 4, pp 150-4.

[43] Cook et al (2013).

[44] Bambra et al (2014).

[45] Bambra, C. (2011) *Work, worklessness, and the political economy of health*, Oxford: Oxford University Press.

[46] Gatrell, A. and Elliot, S. (2009) *Geographies of health: An introduction*, London: Wiley.

[47] Agnew, J. (2011) 'Space and place', in J. Agnew and D. Livingstone (eds) *The SAGE handbook of geographical knowledge*, London: Sage, p 317.

[48] Agnew (2011) ibid, p 318.

[49] Cummins, S., Curtis, S., Diez-Roux, A.V. and Macintyre, S. (2007) 'Understanding and representing "place" in health research: A relational approach', *Social Science & Medicine*, vol 65, p 13.

[50] Macintyre, S., Ellaway, A. and Cummins, S. (2002) 'Place effects on health: How can we conceptualise, operationalise and measure them?', *Social Science & Medicine*, vol 55, no 1, pp 1825-38.

[51] Ibid.

[52] Nazroo, J. and Williams, D. (2006) 'The social determination of ethnic/racial inequalities in health', in M. Marmot and R. Wilkinson (eds) *The social determinants of health*, Oxford: Oxford University Press, pp 238-66.

[53] Davey Smith, G., Chaturvedi, N., Harding, S., Nazroo, J. and Williams, R. (2003) 'Ethnic inequalities in health: A review of UK epidemiological evidence', in G. Davey Smith (ed) *Health inequalities: Lifecourse approaches*, Bristol: Policy Press, pp 271-309.

[54] Krieger, N., Kosheleva, A., Waterman, P.D., Chen, J.T., Beckfield, J. and Kiang, M.V. (2014) '50-year trends in US socioeconomic inequalities in health: US-born Black and White Americans, 1959-2008', *International Journal of Epidemiology*, vol 43, no 4, pp 1294-313.

[55] Jarvis, M. and Wardle, J. (2006) 'Social patterning of individual health behaviours: The case of cigarette smoking', in M. Marmot and R. Wilkinson (eds) *The social determinants of health*, Oxford: Oxford University Press, pp 240-55.

[56] Bambra, C., Joyce, K.E., Bellis, M.A., Greatley, A., Greengross, S., Hughes, S. et al (2010) 'Reducing health inequalities in priority public health conditions:

Using rapid review to develop proposals for evidence-based policy', *Journal of Public Health*, vol 32, no 4, pp 496-505.

[57] Bambra (2011).

[58] Marmot (2010).

[59] Marmot, M. (2006) 'Introduction', in M. Marmot and R. Wilkinson (eds) *The social determinants of health*, Oxford: Oxford University Press, p 5.

[60] Bambra (2011).

[61] Macintyre et al (2002).

[62] WHO (World Health Organization) (2008) *Commission on the Social Determinants of Health: Closing the gap in a generation*, Geneva: WHO.

[63] Mitchell, R. and Popham, F. (2007) 'Greenspace, urbanity and health: relationships in England', *Journal of Epidemiology and Community Health*, vol 61, no 8, pp 681-3.

[64] Martuzzi, M., Mitis, F. and Forastiere, F. (2010) 'Inequalities, inequities, environmental justice in waste management and health', *European Journal of Public Health*, vol 20, p 5.

[65] Bambra, C., Robertson, S., Kasim, A., Smith, J., Cairns-Nagi, J., Copeland, A. et al (2014) 'Healthy land? An examination of the area-level association between brownfield land and morbidity and mortality in England', *Environment and Planning A*, vol 46, no 2, pp 433-54.

[66] Stafford, M. and McCarthy, M. (2006) 'Neighbourhoods, housing and health', in M. Marmot and R. Wilkinson (eds) *The social determinants of health*, Oxford: Oxford University Press, pp 78-96.

[67] Walton, H., Dajnak, D., Beevers, S., Williams, M., Watkiss, P. and Hunt, A. (2015) *Understanding the health impacts of air pollution in London*, London: King's College London (www.kcl.ac.uk/lsm/research/divisions/aes/research/ERG/research-projects/HIAinLondonKingsReport14072015final.pdf).

[68] Shortt, N.K., Richardson, E., Mitchell, R. and Pearce, J. (2011) 'Re-engaging with the physical environment: a health-related environmental classification of the UK', *Area*, vol 43, no 1, pp 76-87.

[69] Bambra, C., Fox, D. and Scott-Samuel, A. (2005) 'Towards a politics of health', *Health Promotion International*, vol 20, no 2, pp 187-93.

[70] Krieger, N. (2013) 'Ecosocial theory of disease distribution', YouTube video (www.youtube.com/watch?v=5pBnnDJ9HQY).

[71] Schrecker and Bambra (2015).

[72] Stuckler, D. and Basu, S. (2013) *The body economic: Why austerity kills*, London: Allan Lane.

[73] Bambra et al (2005).

[74] McKinley, J. (1975) 'The case for refocusing upstream: The political economy of illness', in American Heart Association (ed) *Applying behavioral science to cardiovascular risk*, New York: American Heart Association.

[75] Schrecker and Bambra (2015).

[76] Krieger (2013).

Chapter 2

[1] Chadwick, E. (1842) *Report on the sanitary conditions of the labouring classes in Britain*, London: HMSO.
[2] Hacker, J.D. (2010) 'Decennial life tables for the white population of the United States, 1790-1900', *Historical Methods*, vol 43, no 2, pp 45-79.
[3] Hobbes, T. (1651) *Leviathan*.
[4] Tonge, N. and Quiency, M. (1985) *Cholera and public health*, London: Macmillan.
[5] Ibid.
[6] Cheronomas, R. and Hudson, I. (2013) *To live and die in America: Class, power, health and healthcare*, London: Pluto Press.
[7] Doyal, L. (1979) *The political economy of health*, London: Pluto Press.
[8] Engels, F. (1844/2009) *The conditions of the working class in England*, London: Penguin Classics.
[9] Cheronomas and Hudson (2013).
[10] Doyal (1979).
[11] Gaskell, E.C. (1855) *North and South*, London: Wordsworth.
[12] Doyal (1979).
[13] Engels (1844/2009).
[14] Burnett, J. (1991) 'Housing and the decline of mortality', in R. Schofield, D. Reher and A. Bideau (eds) *The decline of mortality in Europe*, Oxford: Clarendon, pp 158-76.
[15] Ibid.
[16] Chadwick (1842).
[17] Cheronomas and Hudson (2013).
[18] Chadwick (1842).
[19] Cartoon from Punch Magazine Archive, reproduced with permission of Punch Ltd.
[20] Mooney, G. (2007) 'Infectious diseases and epidemiologic transition in Victorian Britain? Definitely', *Social History of Medicine*, vol 20, no 3, pp 595-606.
[21] Doyal (1979) , p 54.
[22] Harrison, M. (2004) *Disease and the modern world, 1500 to the present*, London: Polity Press.
[23] Doyal (1979).
[24] NHS Choices (2015) 'Dysentery' (www.nhs.uk/conditions/Dysentery/Pages/Introduction.aspx).
[25] CDC (Centers for Disease Control and Prevention) (2013) 'Typhoid fever' (www.cdc.gov/nczved/divisions/dfbmd/diseases/typhoid_fever/).
[26] NHS Choices (2015) 'Typhoid fever' (www.nhs.uk/Conditions/Typhoid-fever/Pages/Introduction.aspx).
[27] NHS Choices (2015) 'Typhus conditions' (www.nhs.uk/conditions/typhus/Pages/Introduction.aspx).
[28] Ibid.
[29] Peterson, R.K.D. (1995) 'Insects, disease, and military history: The Napoleonic campaigns and historical perception', *American Entomologist*, vol 41, no 3, pp 147-60.

[30] Sweeney, T. (1991) 'Medicine in the bloodiest war', *OzarksWatch*, vol 4, no 4, pp 42-6.
[31] WHO (World Health Organization) (2015) 'Small pox', Geneva: WHO (www.who.int/csr/disease/smallpox/en/).
[32] CDC (Centers for Disease Control and Prevention) (2013) 'Small pox' (www.bt.cdc.gov/agent/smallpox/overview/disease-facts.asp).
[33] Riedel, S. (2005) 'Edward Jenner and the history of smallpox and vaccination', *Baylor University Medical Center Proceedings*, vol 18, no 1, pp 21-5.
[34] Willis, N.J. (1997) 'Edward Jenner and the eradication of smallpox', *Scottish Medical Journal*, vol 42, no 4, pp 118-21.
[35] Doyal (1979).
[36] Harrison (2004).
[37] Ibid.
[38] WHO (World Health Organization) (2015) *Tuberculosis*, Geneva: WHO, http://www.who.int/topics/tuberculosis/en/
[39] Harrison (2004).
[40] Ibid.
[41] Dorling, D. (2013) *Unequal health: The scandal of our times*, Bristol: Policy Press.
[42] Harrison (2004), p 105.
[43] Harrison (2004).
[44] Ibid.
[45] Ibid.
[46] Snow, J. (1855) *On the mode of communication of Cholera*, London: John Churchill.
[47] Dorling (2013).
[48] Redrawn from Snow (1855).
[49] Russell, D. (2004) *Looking North: Northern England and the national imagination*, Manchester: Manchester University Press.
[50] Dickens, C. (1854/1999) *Hard times*, London: Wordsworth.
[51] Dickens, C. (1859/1999) *A tale of two cities*, London: Wordsworth Classics.
[52] Gaskell (1855).
[53] Chadwick (1842).
[54] Ibid.
[55] Hacker (2010).
[56] Szreter, S. and Mooney, G. (1998) 'Urbanization, mortality, and the standard of living debate: new estimates of the expectation of life at birth in nineteenth-century British cities', *Economic History Review*, vol 51, no 1, p 84.
[57] Dorling (2013).
[58] Mackenbach, J. (2006) *Health inequalities: Europe in profile*, European Commission, Public Health, Rotterdam: University Medical Center (www.who.int/social_determinants/resources/european_inequalities.pdf).
[59] Kesztenbaum, L. and Rosenthal, J. (2012) *The democratization of longevity: How the poor became old in Paris, 1870-1940*, Paris: Paris School of Economics.
[60] Dorling, D. (2011) *So you think you know about Britain?*, London: Constable.
[61] Costa, D. and Steckel, R. (1997) 'Long-term trends in health, welfare, and economic growth in the United States', in R. Steckel and R. Floud (eds)

Health and welfare during industrialization, Chicago, IL: University of Chicago Press, pp 47-90.

[62] Szreter and Mooney (1998).

[63] Dorling (2011).

[64] Szreter and Mooney (1998).

[65] Chadwick (1842).

[66] Dorling (2013).

[67] Kesztenbaum and Rosenthal (2012).

[68] Slater, T. (2013) 'Your life chances affect where you live: A critique of the "cottage industry" of neighbourhood effects research', *International Journal of Urban and Regional Research*, vol 137, p 20.

[69] Cheronomas and Hudson (2013).

[70] Ibid.

[71] Ibid.

[72] Mooney (2007).

[73] Cheronomas and Hudson (2013).

[74] Harrison (2004).

[75] Ibid.

[76] Cheronomas and Hudson (2013).

[77] Harrison (2004).

[78] Cheronomas and Hudson (2013).

[79] McKeown, T. (1976) *The role of medicine*, London: Nuffield.

[80] Ibid.

[81] Cheronomas and Hudson (2013).

[82] Cutler, D., Deaton, A. and Lleras-Muney, A. (2006) 'The determinants of mortality', *Journal of Economic Perspectives*, vol 20, no 3, pp 97-120.

[83] McKeown (1976).

[84] Doyal (1979).

[85] Polanyi, K. (1944) *The great transformation*, Boston, MA: Beacon Press.

[86] Cheronomas and Hudson (2013).

[87] Ibid.

[88] M'Gonigle, G. and Kirby, J. (1936) *Poverty and public health*, London: Victor Gollancz.

[89] Wilkinson, E. (1939) *The town that was murdered*, London: Victor Gollancz.

[90] Cheronomas and Hudson (2013).

Chapter 3

[1] WHO (World Health Organization) (2013) *Global Burden of Disease*, Geneva: WHO.

[2] Data from WHO (2013) ibid.

[3] NHS Choices (2015) 'Cardiovascular disease' (www.nhs.uk/conditions/cardiovascular-disease/Pages/Introduction.aspx).

[4] Capewell, S. et al (2008) *Modelling the UK burden of disease to 2020*, London: British Heart Foundation.

[5] Scarborough, P., Wickramasinghe, K., Bhatnagar, P. and Rayner, M. (2011) *Trends in coronary heart disease, 1961-2011*, London: British Heart Foundation.

[6] Cancer Research UK (2011) 'About cancer' (www.cancerresearchuk.org/about-cancer/).

[7] NHS Choices (2015) 'Cancer' (www.nhs.uk/conditions/Cancer/Pages/Introduction.aspx).

[8] Cancer Research UK (2011).

[9] PHE (Public Health England) (2014) *Adult obesity and type 2 diabetes*, London: PHE.

[10] Ibid.

[11] NHS Choices (2015) 'Diabetes' (www.nhs.uk/conditions/diabetes/pages/diabetes.aspx).

[12] Gregg, E.W., Zhuo, X., Cheng, Y.J., Albright, A.L., Venkat Narayan, K.M. and Thompson, T.J. (2014) 'Trends in lifetime risk and years of life lost due to diabetes in the USA, 1985–2011: A modelling study', *The Lancet: Diabetes & Endocrinology*, vol 2, no 11, pp 867-74.

[13] Reilly, J.J., Methven, E., McDowell, M.E., Hacking, B., Alexander, D., Stewart, L. and Kelnar, C.J. (2003) 'Health consequences of obesity', *Archives of Disease in Childhood*, vol 88, no 9, pp 748-52.

[14] Schrecker, T. and Bambra, C. (2015) *How politics makes us sick: Neoliberal epidemics*, Basingstoke: Palgrave Macmillan.

[15] Rennie, K.L. and Jebb, S.A. (2005) 'Prevalence of obesity in Great Britain', *Obesity Reviews*, vol 6, no 1, pp 11-12.

[16] HSCIC (Health & Social Care Information Centre) (2014) *Statistics on obesity, physical activity and diet, England 2014*, London: HSCIC.

[17] WHO (World Health Organization) (2014) 'Suicide', Geneva: WHO (www.who.int/mediacentre/factsheets/fs398/en/).

[18] ONS (Office for National Statistics) (2013) *Measuring national well-being, Health, 2013*, Newport: ONS (http://webarchive.nationalarchives.gov.uk/20160105160709/http://www.ons.gov.uk/ons/rel/wellbeing/measuring-national-well-being/health--2013/index.html).

[19] WHO (World Health Organization) (2008) *Commission on the Social Determinants of Health: Closing the gap in a generation*, Geneva: WHO.

[20] Ibid.

[21] Bambra, C., Joyce, K.E., Bellis, M.A., Greatley, A., Greengross, S., Hughes, S. et al (2010) 'Reducing health inequalities in priority public health conditions: Using rapid review to develop proposals for evidence-based policy', *Journal of Public Health*, vol 32, no 4, pp 496-505.

[22] WHO (2014).

[23] Mental Health Foundation (2015) *Suicide*, London: Mental Health Foundation (www.mentalhealth.org.uk/help-information/mental-health-a-z/s/suicide).

[24] Punnett, L. and Wegman, D.H. (2004) 'Work-related musculoskeletal disorders: the epidemiologic evidence and the debate', *Journal of Electromyography and Kinesiology*, vol 14, no 1, p 13.

[25] Luttman, A., Jäger, M. and Griefahn, B. (2003) *Preventing musculoskeletal disorders in the workplace*, Protecting Workers' Health Series No 5, Geneva: WHO (www.who.int/occupational_health/publications/muscdisorders/en/).
[26] Woolf, S. and Aron, L. (2013) *US health in international perspective: Shorter lives, poorer health*, Washington, DC: The National Academies Press.
[27] Stevens, G.A., Singh, G.M., Lu, Y., Danaei, G., Lin, J.K., Finucane, M.M. et al (2012) 'National, regional, and global trends in adult overweight and obesity prevalences', *Population Health Metrics*, vol 10, no 1, p 22.
[28] International Diabetes Federation (2013) *IDF diabetes atlas* (6th edn), Brussels: International Diabetes Federation.
[29] Bromet, E., Andrade, L.H., Hwang, I., Sampson, N.A., Alonso, J., de Girolamo, G. et al (2011) 'Cross-national epidemiology of DSM-IV major depressive episode', *BMC Medicine*, vol 9.
[30] Woolf and Aron (2013).
[31] Komlos, J. and Baur, M. (2004) 'From the tallest to (one of) the fattest: The enigmatic fate of the American population in the 20th century', *Economics and Human Biology*, vol 2, no 1, pp 57-74.
[32] Ibid.
[33] Stevens et al (2012).
[34] Komlos and Baur (2004).
[35] Stevens et al (2012).
[36] CDC (Centers for Disease Prevention and Control) (2011) *Obesity prevalence maps*, Atlanta, GA: CDC.
[37] Ibid.
[38] RWJF (Robert Wood Johnson Foundation) (2013) *Does where you live affect how long you live?*, Princeton, NJ: RWJF (www.rwjf.org/en/library/features/health-where-you-live.html).
[39] Statistics Canada (2012) *Life expectancy at birth, by sex, by province* (www.statcan.gc.ca/tables-tableaux/sum-som/l01/cst01/health26-eng.htm)
[40] Townsend, N., Williams, J., Bhatnagar, P., Wickramasinghe, K. and Rayner, M. (2014) *Cardiovascular disease statistics 2014*, London: British Heart Foundation, p 114.
[41] ONS (Office for National Statistics) (2012) *Mortality statistics 2013*, Newport: ONS.
[42] ONS (Office for National Statistics) (2013) *General Lifestyle Survey: 2011*, Newport: ONS (www.ons.gov.uk/ons/rel/ghs/general-lifestyle-survey/2011/rpt-chapter-7.html?format=print).
[43] National Records of Scotland (2013) *Suicide rates in Scotland*, Edinburgh: National Records of Scotland.
[44] NISRA (Northern Ireland Statistics and Research Agency) (2013) *Suicide rates in Northern Ireland*, Belfast: NISRA.
[45] ONS (Office for National Statistics) (2011) *Life expectancy and disability free life expectancy*, Newport: ONS.
[46] HSCIC (Health & Social Care Information Centre) (2014) *Health Survey for England – 2013*, Leeds: HSCIC.

[47] Welsh Government (2014) *Welsh Health Survey 2013*, Cardiff: Welsh Government.

[48] Scottish Government (2014) *The Scottish Health Survey 2013*, Edinburgh: Scottish Government.

[49] DHSSPS (Department of Health, Social Services and Public Safety) (2014) *Health Survey Northern Ireland 2012/13*, Belfast: DHSSPS.

[50] Audit Scotland (2012) *Health inequalities in Scotland* (www.audit-scotland.gov.uk/docs/health/2012/nr_121213_health_inequalities.pdf).

[51] Hanlon, P., Lawder, R.S., Buchanan, D., Redpath, A., Walsh, D., Wood, R. et al (2005) 'Why is mortality higher in Scotland than in England and Wales? Decreasing influence of socioeconomic deprivation between 1981 and 2001 supports the existence of a "Scottish effect"', *Journal of Public Health*, vol 27, no 2, pp 199-204.

[52] Foster, J. (2011) 'The Scottish effect: Some comments from a historical perspective', *Scottish 'excess' mortality: Comparing Glasgow with Liverpool and Manchester – Commentaries and synthesis*, Glasgow: Glasgow Centre for Population Health (www.gcph.co.uk/assets/0000/4022/Scottish_excess_mortality_-_commentaries_and_synthesis.pdf).

[53] Reid, M. (2011) 'Behind the "Glasgow effect"', *Bulletin of the World Health Organization*, vol 89, no 10, pp 706-7.

[54] Data from Max Planck Institute for Demographic Research (2014) *The Human Mortality Database* (www.mortality.org/).

[55] Data from Eurostat (2013) *Life expectancy*, http://ec.europa.eu/eurostat/statistics-explained/index.php/Mortality_and_life_expectancy_statistics

[56] Data from Max Planck Institute for Demographic Research (2014).

[57] Martin, G.R.R. (2011) *A song of ice and fire*, London: Harper Voyager.

[58] Russell, D. (2004) *Looking North: Northern England and the national imagination*, Manchester: Manchester University Press.

[59] Data from ONS (2011).

[60] Priestley, J.B. (1934) *An English journey*, London: Victor Gollancz.

[61] Russell (2004).

[62] Ibid.

[63] Dorling, D. (2010) 'Persistent North-South divides', in N. Coe and A. Jones (eds) *The economic geography of the UK*, London: Sage, pp 12-28.

[64] Russell (2004) , p 15.

[65] Hill, J. and Williams, J. (1996) *Sport and identity in the North of England*, Keele: Keele University Press.

[66] Green, A.E. (1988) 'The North-South divide in Great Britain: an examination of the evidence', *Transactions of the Institute of British Geographers*, pp 179-98.

[67] Russell (2004).

[68] Ibid.

[69] Popham, F. and Bambra, C. (2010) 'Evidence from the 2001 English Census on the contribution of employment status to the social gradient in self-rated health', *Journal of Epidemiology and Community Health*, vol 64, no 3, pp 277-80.

[70] Data from ONS (2013).

[71] Data from PHE (Public Health England) (2015) *Public Health Outcomes Framework*, London: PHE (www.phoutcomes.info/).

[72] Ibid.

[73] Ibid.

[74] Ibid.

[75] Ibid.

[76] Whitehead, M. and Doran, T. (2011) 'The North-South health divide', *British Medical Journal*, vol 342, no 7794, d584.

[77] Hacking, J.M., Muller, S. and Buchan, I.E. (2011) 'Trends in mortality from 1965 to 2008 across the English north-south divide: comparative observational study', *British Medical Journal*, vol 342, d508.

[78] Ibid.

[79] Data from PHE (2015).

[80] Reproduced, with permission of the Centre for Local Economic Strategies and the University of Liverpool, from Whitehead, M.C. et al (2014) *Due North: Report of the Inquiry on Health Equity for the North*, Liverpool and Manchester: University of Liverpool and Centre for Local Economic Strategies (www.cles.org.uk/wp-content/uploads/2014/09/Due-North-Report-of-the-Inquiry-on-Health-Equity-in-the-North-final.pdf).

[81] Reproduced under Creative Commons licence, from Bambra, C. (2015) 'Who are the top teams in the health league?', Conversation.com (http://theconversation.com/who-are-the-top-football-teams-in-the-health-league-42002).

[82] Dorling, D. (2013) *Unequal health: The scandal of our times*, Bristol: Policy Press.

[83] Data from PHE (2015).

[84] Ibid.

[85] Audit Scotland (2012).

[86] Scottish Government (2011) *Scottish Health Survey: Topic report; Obesity*, Edinburgh: Scottish Government (www.gov.scot/Publications/2011/10/1138).

[87] Scottish Government (2013) *Trends in mortality by SIMD quintile 2004-2013*, Edinburgh: Scottish Government.

[88] Scottish Public Health Observatory (2014) *Life expectancy and healthy life expectancy: Deprivation quintiles*, Edinburgh: Scottish Public Health Observatory.

[89] Scottish Government (2014) *Scotland: Age-standardised incidence and mortality rates by SIMD*, Edinburgh: Scottish Government.

[90] Grundmann, N., Mielck, A., Siegel, M. and Maier, W. (2014) 'Area deprivation and the prevalence of type 2 diabetes and obesity: Analysis at the municipality level in Germany', *BMC Public Health*, vol 14.

[91] Sundquist, K., Malmstrom, M. and Johansson, S.E. (2004) 'Neighbourhood deprivation and incidence of coronary heart disease: a multilevel study of 2.6 million women and men in Sweden', *Journal of Epidemiology and Community Health*, vol 58, no 1, pp 71-7.

[92] Stimpson, J.P., Ju, H., Raji, M.A. and Eschbach, K. (2007) 'Neighborhood deprivation and health risk behaviors in NHANES III', *American Journal of Health Behavior*, vol 31, no 2, pp 215-22.

[93] White, H.L., Matheson, F.I., Moineddin, R., Dunn, J.R. and Glazier, R.H. (2011) 'Neighbourhood deprivation and regional inequalities in self-reported health among Canadians: Are we equally at risk?', *Health & Place*, vol 17, no 1, pp 361-9.

[94] Debrand, T., Pierre, A., Allonier, C. and Lucas-Gabrielli, V. (2012) 'Critical urban areas, deprived areas and neighbourhood effects on health in France', *Health Policy*, vol 105, no 1, pp 92-101.

[95] Riva, M., Gauvin, L. and Barnett, T.A. (2007) 'Toward the next generation of research into small area effects on health: a synthesis of multilevel investigations published since July 1998', *Journal of Epidemiology and Community Health*, vol 61, no 10, pp 853-61.

[96] PHE (2015).

[97] Redrawn, with permission from the Centre for Local Economic Strategies, the University of Liverpool, from (2014) *Due North: Report of the Inquiry on Health Equity for the North, Liverpool and Manchester*, University of Liverpool and Centre for Local Economic Strategies (www.cles.org.uk/wp-content/uploads/2014/09/Due-North-Report-of-the-Inquiry-on-Health-Equity-in-the-Northfinal.pdf).

[98] Data from PHE (Public Health England) (2013) *Local health* (www.localhealth.org.uk).

[99] Rydin, Y., Bleahu, A., Davies, M., Dávila, J.D., Friel, S., de Grandis, G. et al (2012) 'Shaping cities for health: complexity and the planning of urban environments in the 21st century', *The Lancet*, vol 379, no 9831, pp 2079-108.

[100] Reproduced with permission of Newcastle University and Nexus (2014) *Healthy Life Simulation* (www.ncl.ac.uk/ageing/partners/simulation/).

[101] Bambra, C. (2013) *Local health inequalities in an age of austerity: The Stockton on Tees Study*, Durham: University of Durham (https://www.dur.ac.uk/health.inequalities/).

[102] Marmot, M. (2004) 'Status syndrome', *Significance*, vol 1, no 4, pp 150-4.

[103] Bambra (2013).

[105] Rydin et al (2012).

[104] For readers in the US, the Robert Wood Johnson Foundation has a website where you can enter your zip code and see the average life expectancy of people living in your neighbourhood. This is available here: www.rwjf.org/en/library/features/health-where-you-live.html

Chapter 4

[1] ONS (Office for National Statistics) (2014) *Disability-free life expectancy (DFLE) and life expectancy (LE) at birth by upper tier local authority at birth, England 2012-14*, Newport: ONS.

[2] Doyal, L. (1995) 'What makes women sick: Gender and the political economy of health', *British Medical Journal*, vol 311, p 577.

[3] Jones, M. and Daykin, N. (2015) 'Sociology and health', in J. Naidoo and J. Wills (eds) *Health studies: An introduction*, London: Palgrave, pp 155-95.

[4] Hill, S. (2015) 'Axes of health inequalities and intersectionality', in K.E. Smith and C. Bambra (eds) *Health inequalities: Critical perspectives*, Oxford: Oxford University Press.

[5] Stanistreet, D., Bambra, C. and Scott-Samuel, A. (2005) 'Is patriarchy the source of male mortality?', *Journal of Epidemiology and Community Health* vol 59, pp 873-6.

[6] Nazroo, J. and Williams, D. (2006) 'The social determination of ethnic/racial inequalities in health', in M. Marmot and R. Wilkinson (eds) *The social determinants of health*, Oxford: Oxford University Press, pp 238-66.

[7] Davey Smith, G., Chaturvedi, N., Harding, S., Nazroo, J. and Williams, R. (2003) 'Ethnic inequalities in health: A review of UK epidemiological evidence', in G. Davey Smith (ed) *Health inequalities: Lifecourse approaches*, Bristol: Policy Press, pp 271-309.

[8] Arias, E., Rostron, B. and Tejada-Vera, B. (2010) 'United States life tables, 2005', *National Vital Statistics Reports*, vol 58, no 10, pp 1-132.

[9] Hill (2015).

[10] Ibid.

[11] Jarvis, M. and Wardle, J. (2006) 'Social patterning of individual health behaviours: The case of cigarette smoking', in M. Marmot and R. Wilkinson (eds) *The social determinants of health*, Oxford: Oxford University Press, pp 240-55.

[12] Bambra, C., Joyce, K. and Maryon-Davies, A. (2009) *Priority health conditions – Task Group 8 Report to the Strategic Review of Health Inequalities in England post-2010 (Marmot Review)*, London: University College London.

[13] Khaw, K.-T., Wareham, N., Bingham, S., Welch, A., Luben, R. et al (2008) 'Combined impact of health behaviours and mortality in men and women: The EPIC-Norfolk prospective population study', *Plos Medicine*, vol 5, no 1, pp 39-47.

[14] Bambra, C. (2011) *Work, worklessness, and the political economy of health*, Oxford: Oxford University Press.

[15] Marmot, M. (2010) *Fair society, healthy lives: The Marmot Review*, London: University College London.

[16] Bambra et al (2009).

[17] Coleman, M.P., Rachet, B., Woods, L.M., Mitry, E., Riga, M., Cooper, N. et al (2004) 'Trends and socioeconomic inequalities in cancer survival in England and Wales up to 2001', *British Journal of Cancer*, vol 90, no 7, pp 1367-73.

[18] Capewell, S. et al (2008) *Modelling the UK burden of disease to 2020*, London: British Heart Foundation.

[19] Ibid.

[20] Menvielle, G., Boshuizen, H., Kunst, A.E., Dalton, S.O., Vineis, P., Bergmann, M.M. et al (2009) 'The role of smoking and diet in explaining educational inequalities in lung cancer incidence', *Journal of the National Cancer Institute*, vol 101, no 5, pp 321-30.

[21] White, M., Adamson, A., Chadwick, T., Dezateux, C., Griffiths, L., Howel, D. et al (2007) *The changing social patterning of obesity: an analysis to inform practice and policy development*, Newcastle: Public Health Research Consortium.

[22] Bambra, C., Joyce, K. and Maryon-Davis, A. (2009) *Strategic review of health inequalities in England post-2010 (Marmot Review): Task Group 8 Priority public health conditions – Final report* (www.instituteofhealthequity.org/projects/marmot-review-task-groups).

[23] White et al (2007).

[24] Melzer, D., Fryers, T. and Jenkins, R. (2004) *Social inequalities and the distribution of the common mental disorders*, Hove: Psychology Press.

[25] McManus, S., Meltzer, H., Brugha, T., Bebbington, P. and Jenkins, R. (2009) *Adult psychiatric morbidity in England, 2007: Results of a household survey*, Leeds: NHS Information Centre.

[26] McManus et al (2009).

[27] Wood, J., Hennell, T., Jones, A., Hooper, J., Tocque, K. and Bellis, M.A. (2006) *Where wealth means health: Illustrating inequality in the North West*, Liverpool: North West Public Health Observatory.

[28] Marmot, M. (2006) 'Introduction', in M. Marmot and R. Wilkinson (eds) *The social determinants of health*, Oxford: Oxford University Press, p 5.

[29] Marmot (2010).

[30] Cancer Research UK (2008) 'Socioeconomic inequalities in cancer', Policy Statement, April (www.cancerresearchuk.org/prod_consump/groups/cr_common/@nre/@pol/documents/generalcontent/crukmig_1000ast-3347.pdf).

[31] Marmot (2006).

[32] Data from Eikemo, T., Huisman, M., Bambra, C. and Kunst, A. (2008) 'Health inequalities according to educational level in different welfare regimes: a comparison of 23 European countries', *Sociology of Health & Illness*, vol 30, no 4, pp 565-82.

[33] Dahlgren, G. and Whitehead, M. (1991) *Policies and strategies to promote social in health*, Stockholm: Institute for Future Studies.

[34] Bambra (2011).

[35] Ibid.

[36] Harrington, J.M., Gill, F., Aw, T.-C. and Gardiner, K. (1998) *Occupational health* (4th revised edn), London: Blackwell.

[37] Bambra (2011).

[38] Ibid.

[39] Gillen, M., Yen, I.H., Trupin, L., Swig, L., Rugulies, R. and Mullen, K. (2007) 'The association of socioeconomic status and psychosocial and physical workplace factors with musculoskeletal injury in hospital workers', *American Journal of Industrial Medicine*, vol 50, no 4, pp 245-60.

[40] Lahelma, E., Laaksonen, M. and Aittomäki, A. (2009) 'Occupational class inequalities in health across employment sectors: the contribution of working conditions', *International Archives of Occupational and Environmental Health*, vol 82, no 2, pp 185-90.

[41] Bambra (2011).

[42] Ibid.

[43] Karasek, R.A. and Theorell, T. (1990) *Healthy work: Stress, productivity, and the reconstruction of working life*, New York: Basic Books.

[44] Hemingway, H. and Marmot, M. (1999) 'Psychosocial factors in the aetiology and prognosis of coronary heart disease: Systematic review of prospective cohort studies', *British Medical Journal*, vol 318, no 7196, pp 1460-7.
[45] Marmot, M., Siegrist, J. and Theorell, T. (2006) 'Health and the psychosocial work environment', in M. Marmot and R. Wilkinson (eds) *The social determinants of health*, Oxford: Oxford University Press, pp 97-130.
[46] Brunner, E.J., Chandola, T. and Marmot, M.G. (2007) 'Prospective effect of job strain on general and central obesity in the Whitehall II Study', *American Journal of Epidemiology*, vol 165, no 7, pp 828-37.
[47] Bongers, P.M., de Winter, C.R., Kompier, M.A. and Hildebrandt, V.H. (1993) 'Psychosocial factors at work and musculoskeletal disease', *Scandinavian Journal of Work, Environment & Health*, pp 297-312.
[48] Stansfeld, S. (2002) 'Work, personality and mental health', *The British Journal of Psychiatry*, vol 181, no 2, pp 96-8.
[49] Bambra (2011).
[50] Ibid.
[51] Marmot, M.G., Bosma, H., Hemingway, H., Brunner, E. and Stansfield, S. (1997) 'Contribution of job control and other risk factors to social variations in coronary heart disease incidence', *The Lancet*, vol 350, no 9073, pp 235-9.
[52] Bambra, C. and Eikemo, T. (2009) 'Welfare state regimes, unemployment and health: A comparative study of the relationship between unemployment and self-reported health in 23 European countries', *Journal of Epidemiology and Community Health*, vol 63, no 2, pp 92-8.
[53] Bartley, M., Ferrie, J. and Montgomery, S. (2006) 'Health and labour market disadvantage: Unemployment, non-employment, and job insecurity', in M. Marmot and R. Wilkinson (eds) *The social determinants of health*, Oxford: Oxford University Press.
[54] Platt, S. (1986) 'Parasuicide and unemployment', *British Journal of Psychiatry*, vol 149, pp 401-5.
[55] Bartley, M. and Plewis, I. (2002) 'Accumulated labour market disadvantage and limiting long-term illness: data from the 1971-1991 Office for National Statistics' Longitudinal Study', *International Journal of Epidemiology*, vol 31, no 2, pp 336-41.
[56] Montgomery, S.M., Cook, D.G., Bartley, M. and Wadsworth, M.E.J. (1998) 'Unemployment, cigarette smoking, alcohol consumption and body weight in young British men', *European Journal of Public Health*, vol 8, no 1, pp 21-7.
[57] Moser, K.A., Fox, A.J. and Jones, D.R. (1984) 'Unemployment and mortality in the OPCS longitudinal study', *The Lancet*, vol 324, no 8415, pp 1324-9.
[58] Bambra (2011).
[59] Arber, S. (1987) 'Social class, non-employment, and chronic illness: Continuing the inequalities in health debate', *British Medical Journal*, vol 294, no 6579, pp 1069-73.
[60] Popham, F. and Bambra, C. (2010) 'Evidence from the 2001 English Census on the contribution of employment status to the social gradient in self-rated health', *Journal of Epidemiology and Community Health*, vol 64, no 3, pp 277-80.
[61] Ibid.

[62] Bartley, M. and Owen, C. (1996) 'Relation between socioeconomic status, employment, and health during economic change, 1973-93', *British Medical Journal*, vol 313, no 7055, pp 445-9.
[63] Bambra (2011).
[64] Schuring, M., Burdorf, A., Voorham, A.J., der Weduwe, K. and Mackenbach, J.P. (2009) 'Effectiveness of a health promotion programme for long-term unemployed subjects with health problems: a randomised controlled trial', *Journal of Epidemiology and Community Health*, vol 63, no 11, pp 893-9.
[65] Ibid.
[66] Pope, D. and Bambra, C. (2005) 'Has the disability discrimination act closed the employment gap?', *Disability and Rehabilitation*, vol 27, no 20, pp 1261-6.
[67] McDonough, P. and Amick III, B.C. (2001) 'The social context of health selection: a longitudinal study of health and employment', *Social Science & Medicine*, vol 53, no 1, pp 135-45.
[68] Whitehead, M., Clayton, S., Holland, P., Drever, F. et al (2009) *Helping chronically ill or disabled people into work: What can we learn from international comparative analyses?*, London: Public Health Research Consortium.
[69] Ibid.
[70] Dahlgren, G., Nordgren, P. and Whitehead, M. (1996) *Health impact assessment of the EU Common Agricultural Policy*, Solna: Sweden's National Institute of Public Health.
[71] Garthwaite, K.A., Collins, P.J. and Bambra, C. (2015) 'Food for thought: An ethnographic study of negotiating ill health and food insecurity in a UK foodbank', *Social Science & Medicine*, vol 132, pp 38-44.
[72] Trussell Trust, The (2014) 'Biggest ever increase in UK food bank use: 170% rise in numbers turning to foodbanks in last 12 months', Salisbury: The Trussell Trust.
[73] Garthwaite et al (2015).
[74] Department of Energy and Climate Change (2013) *Fuel poverty report – Updated August 2013*, London: Department of Energy and Climate Change.
[75] Levell, P. and Oldfield, Z. (2011) 'The spending patterns and inflation experience of low-income households over the past decade', *IFS Commentary C119*, London: Institute for Fiscal Studies.
[76] Dorling, D. (2013) *Unequal health: The scandal of our times*, Bristol: Policy Press.
[77] Stafford, M. and McCarthy, M. (2006) 'Neighbourhoods, housing and health', in M. Marmot and R. Wilkinson (eds) *The social determinants of health*, Oxford: Oxford University Press, pp 78-96.
[78] Smith, S.J., Searle, B.A. and Cook, N. (2009) 'Rethinking the risks of home ownership', *Journal of Social Policy*, vol 38, no 1, pp 83-102.
[79] Gibson, M., Petticrew, M., Bambra, C., Sowden, A.J., Wright, K.E. and Whitehead, M. (2011) 'Housing and health inequalities: A synthesis of systematic reviews of interventions aimed at different pathways linking housing and health', *Health & Place*, vol 17, no 1, pp 175-84.
[80] Shaw, M. (2004) 'Housing and public health', *Annual Review of Public Health*, vol 25, no 1, pp 397-418.
[81] Gibson et al (2011).

[82] Bambra, C. (2005) 'Cash versus services: "worlds of welfare" and the decommodification of cash benefits and health care services', *Journal of Social Policy*, vol 34, no 2, pp 195-213.

[83] Gelormino, E., Bambra, C., Spadea, T. et al (2011) 'The effects of health care reforms on health inequalities: a review and analysis of the European evidence base', *International Journal of Health Services*, vol 41, no 2, pp 209-30.

[84] Ibid.

[85] Tudor-Hart, J. (1971) 'The inverse care law', *The Lancet*, vol 297, no 7696, pp 405-12.

[86] Bartley, M. (2004) *Health inequality: An introduction to theories, concepts and methods*, Cambridge: Polity Press.

[87] Skalická, V., van Lenthe, F., Bambra, C., Krokstad, S. and Mackenbach, J. (2009) 'Material, psychosocial, behavioural and biomedical factors in the explanation of relative socio-economic inequalities in mortality: evidence from the HUNT study', *International Journal of Epidemiology*, vol 38, no 5, pp 1272-84.

[88] Phelan, J.C., Link, B.G., Diez-Roux, A., Kawachi, I. and Levin, B. (2004) '"Fundamental causes" of social inequalities in mortality: A test of the theory', *Journal of Health and Social Behavior*, vol 45, no 3, pp 265-85.

[89] Link, B. and Phelan, J. (1995) 'Social conditions as fundamental causes of disease', *Journal of Health and Social Behavior*, vol X, p 14.

[90] Hill (2015).

[91] Ibid.

[92] Ibid.

[93] Macintyre, S., Ellaway, A. and Cummins, S. (2002) 'Place effects on health: How can we conceptualise, operationalise and measure them?', *Social Science & Medicine*, vol 55, no 1, pp 1825-38.

[94] Diez-Roux, A.V., Merkin, S.S., Arnett, D., Chambless, L., Massing, M., Nieto, F.J. et al (2001) 'Neighborhood of residence and incidence of coronary heart disease', *The New England Journal of Medicine*, vol 345, no 2, pp 99-106.

[95] Shaw, M., Dorling, D., Gordon, D. and Davey Smith, G. (1999) *The widening gap: Health inequalities and policy in Britain*, Bristol: Policy Press.

[96] Lakshman, R., McConville, A., How, S., Flowers, J., Wareham, J. and Cosford, P. (2011) 'Association between area-level socioeconomic deprivation and a cluster of behavioural risk factors: cross-sectional, population-based study', *Journal of Public Health*, vol 33, no 2, pp 234-45.

[97] Data from Lakshman et al (2011) ibid, with permission from Oxford University Press.

[98] Diez-Roux et al (2001).

[99] McCartney, G., Walsh, D., Whyte, B. and Collins, C. (2012) 'Has Scotland always been the "sick man" of Europe? An observational study from 1855 to 2006', *European Journal of Public Health*, vol 22, no 6, pp 756-60.

[100] Webster, D. (2000) 'The geographical concentration of labour-market disadvantage', *Oxford Review of Economic Policy*, vol 16, no 1, p 124.

[101] Fletcher, D. (2007) 'A culture of worklessness? Historical insights from the Manor and Park areas of Sheffield', *Policy & Politics*, vol 35, p 20.

[102] Walkerdine, V. and Jimenez, L. (2012) *Gender, work and community after de-industrialisation: A psychosocial approach to affect*, Identity Studies in the Social Sciences, Basingstoke: Palgrave Macmillan.

[103] Harvey, D. (2014) *Seventeen contradictions and the end of capitalism*, London: Pluto Press.

[104] Data reproduced under open access licence from Taulbut, M., Walsh, D., McCartney, G., Parcell, S., Hartmann, A., Poirier, G. et al (2014) 'Spatial inequalities in life expectancy within postindustrial regions of Europe: a cross-sectional observational study', *BMJ Open*, vol 4, no 6, e004711.

[105] Riva, M. and Curtis, S.E. (2012) 'Long-term local area employment rates as predictors of individual mortality and morbidity: a prospective study in England, spanning more than two decades', *Journal of Epidemiology and Community Health*, vol 66, no 10, pp 919-26.

[106] Taulbut et al (2014).

[107] Macintyre et al (2002).

[108] Beaulac, J., Kristjansson, E. and Cummins, S. (2009) 'A systematic review of food deserts, 1966-2007', *Preventing Chronic Disease*, vol 6, no 3, A105.

[109] Breyer, B. and Voss-Andreae, A. (2013) 'Food mirages: Geographic and economic barriers to healthful food access in Portland, Oregon', *Health & Place*, vol 24, p 8.

[110] Pearce, J., Blakely, T., Witten, K. and Bartie, P. (2007) 'Neighborhood deprivation and access to fast-food retailing – A national study', *American Journal of Preventive Medicine*, vol 32, no 5, pp 375-82.

[111] Burgoine, T., Alvanides, S. and Lake, A.A. (2011) 'Assessing the obesogenic environment of North East England', *Health & Place*, vol 17, no 3, pp 738-47.

[112] Richardson, E.A., Hill, S.E., Mitchell, R., Pearce, J. and Shortt, N.K. (2015) 'Is local alcohol outlet density related to alcohol-related morbidity and mortality in Scottish cities?', *Health & Place*, vol 33, pp 172-80.

[113] Pearce, J., Rind, E., Shortt, N., Tisch, C. and Mitchell, R. (2015) 'Tobacco retail environments and social inequalities in individual-level smoking and cessation among Scottish adults', *Nicotine & Tobacco Research*, pp 1-9.

[114] Tudor Hart (1971).

[115] Todd, A., Copeland, A., Husband, A., Kasim, A. and Bambra, C. (2015) 'Access all areas? An area-level analysis of the relationship between community pharmacy and primary care distribution, urbanity and social deprivation in England', *BMJ Open*, 5:e007328.

[116] Todd, A., Copeland, A., Husband, A., Kasim, A. and Bambra, C. (2014) 'The positive pharmacy care law: an area-level analysis of the relationship between community pharmacy distribution, urbanity and social deprivation in England', *BMJ Open*, vol 4, no 8.

[117] Todd et al (2015).

[118] Gatrell, A. and Elliot, S. (2009) *Geographies of health: An introduction*, London: Wiley.

[119] Thompson, L., Pearce, J. and Barnett, J.R. (2007) 'Moralising geographies: stigma, smoking islands and responsible subjects', *Area*, vol 39, no 4, pp 508-17.

[120] Putnam, R. (1993) *Making democracy work: Civic traditions in modern Italy*, Princeton, NJ: Princeton University Press, p 167.

[121] Whitehead, M. and Diderichsen, F. (2001) 'Social capital and health: tip-toeing through the minefield of evidence', *The Lancet*, vol 358, no 9277, pp 165-6.

[122] Ibid.

[123] Hawe, P. and Shiell, A. (2000) 'Social capital and health promotion: a review', *Social Science & Medicine*, vol 51, no 6, pp 871-85.

[124] Ibid.

[125] Cairns-Nagi, J.M. and Bambra, C. (2013) 'Defying the odds: A mixed-methods study of health resilience in deprived areas of England', *Social Science & Medicine*, vol 91, pp 229-37.

[126] Curtis, S. (2010) *Space, place and mental health*, Farnham: Ashgate.

[127] Greiner, K.A., Chaoyang, L., Kawachi, I., Hunt, D.C. and Ahluwalia, J.S. (2004) 'The relationships of social participation and community ratings to health and health behaviors in areas with high and low population density', *Social Science & Medicine*, vol 59, no 11, pp 2303-12.

[128] Ellaway, A. and Macintyre, S. (2007) 'Is social participation associated with cardiovascular disease risk factors?', *Social Science & Medicine*, vol 64, no 7, pp 1384-91.

[129] Goffman, E. (1963) *Stigma: Notes on the management of spoiled identity*, Harmondsworth: Penguin.

[130] Bush, J., Moffatt, S. and Dunn, C. (2001) '"Even the birds round here cough": Stigma, air pollution and health in Teesside', *Health & Place*, vol 7, no 1, pp 47-56.

[131] Ibid.

[132] Airey, L. (2003) '"Nae as nice a scheme as it used to be": lay accounts of neighbourhood incivilities and well-being', *Health & Place*, vol 9, no 2, pp 129-37.

[133] WHO (World Health Organization) (2008) *Commission on the Social Determinants of Health: Closing the gap in a generation*, Geneva: WHO.

[134] Mitchell, R. and Popham, F. (2007) 'Greenspace, urbanity and health: relationships in England', *Journal of Epidemiology and Community Health*, vol 61, no 8, pp 681-3.

[135] Martuzzi, M., Mitis, F. and Forastiere, F. (2010) 'Inequalities, inequities, environmental justice in waste management and health', *European Journal of Public Health*, vol 20, p 5.

[136] Bambra, C., Robertson, S., Kasim, A., Smith, J., Cairns-Nagi, J., Copeland, A. et al (2014) 'Healthy land? An examination of the area-level association between brownfield land and morbidity and mortality in England', *Environment and Planning A*, vol 46, no 2, pp 433-54.

[137] Stafford, M. and McCarthy, M. (2006) 'Neighbourhoods, housing and health', in M. Marmot and R. Wilkinson (eds) *The social determinants of health*, Oxford: Oxford University Press, pp 78-96.

[138] Markowitz, G. and Rosner, D. (2003) *Deceit and denial: The deadly politics of industrial pollution*, New York: University of California Press.

[139] Shortt, N.K., Richardson, E., Mitchell, R. and Pearce, J. (2011) 'Re-engaging with the physical environment: a health-related environmental classification of the UK', *Area*, vol 43, no 1, pp 76-87.

[140] Pearce, J.R., Richardson, E.A., Mitchell, R.J. and Shortt, N.K. (2010) 'Environmental justice and health: the implications of the socio-spatial distribution of multiple environmental deprivation for health inequalities in the United Kingdom', *Transactions of the Institute of British Geographers*, vol 35, no 4, pp 522-39.

[141] Richardson, E.A., Mitchell, R., Shortt, N.K., Pearce, J. and Dawson, T.P. (2010) 'Developing summary measures of health-related multiple physical environmental deprivation for epidemiological research', *Environment and Planning A*, vol 42, no 7, pp 1650-8.

[142] Ibid.

[143] Pearce et al (2010).

[144] Shortt et al (2011).

[145] Hartig, T., Evans, G.W., Jamner, L.D., Davis, D.S. and Gärling, T. (2003) 'Tracking restoration in natural and urban field settings', *Journal of Environmental Psychology*, vol 23, no 2, pp 109-23.

[146] Maas, J., Verheij, R.A., Groenewegen, P.P., de Vries, S. and Spreeuwenberg, P. (2005) 'Green space, urbanity, and health: how strong is the relation?', *Journal of Epidemiology & Community Health*, vol 60, no 7, pp 587-92.

[147] Abraham, A., Sommerhalder, K. and Abel, T. (2010) 'Landscape and well-being: a scoping study on the health-promoting impact of outdoor environments', *International Journal of Public Health*, vol 55, no 1, pp 59-69.

[148] Curtis (2010) , p 38.

[149] Curtis (2010).

[150] Gesler, W. (2003) *Healing places*, London: Rowman & Littlefield.

[151] Richardson, E.A. and Mitchell, R. (2010) 'Gender differences in relationships between urban green space and health in the United Kingdom', *Social Science & Medicine*, vol 71, no 3, pp 568-75.

[152] Bambra et al (2014).

[153] Catney, P., Eiser, D., Henneberry, J. and Stafford, T. (2007) 'Democracy, trust and risk related to contaminated sites in the UK', in T. Dixon, M. Raco, P. Catney and D.N. Lerner (eds) *Sustainable brownfield regeneration: Liveable places from problem spaces*, Oxford: Blackwell, pp 35-66.

[154] Lin, J.L., Lin-Tan, D.-T., Hsu, K.-H. and Yu, C.-C. (2003) 'Environmental lead exposure and progression of chronic renal diseases in patients without diabetes', *New England Journal of Medicine*, vol 348, no 4, pp 277-86.

[155] Mitchell and Popham (2007).

[156] Bambra et al (2014).

[157] Litt, J.S., Tran, N.L. and Burke, T.A. (2002) 'Examining urban brownfields through the public health "macroscope"', *Environmental Health Perspectives*, vol 110, pp 183-93.

[158] Bambra et al (2014).

[159] Bambra, C., Cairns, J.M., Kasim, A., Smith, J., Robertson, S., Copeland, A. and Johnson, K. (2015) 'This divided land: An examination of regional

inequalities in exposure to brownfield land and the association with morbidity and mortality in England', *Health & Place*, vol 34, pp 257-69.

[160] Reproduced from Bambra et al (2015) , under open access licence.

[161] Macintyre et al (2002).

[162] Cummins, S., Curtis, S., Diez-Roux, A. and Macintyre, S. (2007) 'Understanding and representing "place" in health research: A relational approach', *Social Science & Medicine*, vol 65, p 13.

[163] Macintyre et al (2002).

[164] Cummins et al (2007).

[165] Macintyre, S. (2007) 'Deprivation amplification revisited; or, is it always true that poorer places have poorer access to resources for healthy diets and physical activity?', *International Journal of Behavioral Nutrition and Physical Activity*, vol 4, no 1, p 32.

[166] Whitehead, M.C. et al (2014) *Due North: Report of the Inquiry on Health Equity for the North*, Liverpool and Manchester: University of Liverpool and Centre for Local Economic Strategies (www.cles.org.uk/wp-content/uploads/2014/09/Due-North-Report-of-the-Inquiry-on-Health-Equity-in-the-North-final.pdf).

[167] Bambra and Eikemo (2009).

[168] Cummins et al (2007).

[169] Ibid.

[170] Woolf, S. and Aron, L. (2013) *US health in international perspective: Shorter lives, poorer health*, Washington, DC: The National Academies Press.

[171] Disclaimer: I co-authored a commissioned background paper as part of this study, Bambra, C. and Beckfield, J. (2012) 'Institutional arrangements as candidate explanations of the US health disadvantage' (http://scholar.harvard.edu/files/jbeckfield/files/bambra_and_beckfield_2012.pdf).

[172] Woolf and Aron (2013).

[173] Preston, S., Glei, D. and Wilmouth, J. (2010) 'Contributions of smoking to international differences in life expectancy', in E. Crimmins, S. Preston and B. Cohen (eds) *International differences in mortality at older ages*, Washington, DC: The National Academies Press.

[174] Woolf and Aron (2013).

[175] Ibid.

[176] Preston, S.H. and Stokes, A. (2011) 'Contribution of obesity to international differences in life expectancy', *American Journal of Public Health*, vol 101, no 11, pp 2137-43.

[177] Woolf and Aron (2013).

[178] Ibid.

[179] Ibid.

[180] Ibid, p 186.

[181] Ibid, p 187.

[182] Ibid.

[183] Gottschalk, M. (2004) *Caught: The prison state and the lockdown of American politics*, Princeton, NJ: Princeton University Press.

[184] Woolf and Aron (2013).

[185] OECD (Organisation for Economic Co-operation and Development) (2011) *Society at a glance 2011: OECD Social indicators*, Paris: OECD.

[186] Woolf and Aron (2013).

[187] Anjum Hajat, A., Diez-Roux, A.V., Adar, S.D., Auchincloss, A.H., Lovasi, G.S., O'Neill, M.S. et al (2013) 'Air pollution and individual and neighborhood socioeconomic status: Evidence from the Multi-Ethnic Study of Atherosclerosis (MESA)', *Environmental Health Perspectives*, DOI:10.1289/ehp.1206337.

[188] Foster, J. (2011) 'The Scottish effect: Some comments from a historical perspective', *Scottish 'excess' mortality: Comparing Glasgow with Liverpool and Manchester – Commentaries and synthesis*, Glasgow: Glasgow Centre for Population Health (www.gcph.co.uk/assets/0000/4022/Scottish_excess_mortality_-_commentaries_and_synthesis.pdf).

[189] Collins, C. and McCartney, G. (2011) 'The impact of neoliberal political attack on health: the case of the Scottish effect', *International Journal of Health Services*, vol 41, p 22.

[190] Foster (2011).

[191] Walsh, D., Taulbut, M. and Hanlon, P. (2010) 'The aftershock of deindustrialization-trends in mortality in Scotland and other parts of post-industrial Europe', *European Journal of Public Health*, vol 20, no 1, pp 58-64.

[192] Foster (2011).

[193] Hanlon, P., Lawder, R.S., Buchanan, D., Redpath, A., Walsh, D., Wood, R. et al (2005) 'Why is mortality higher in Scotland than in England and Wales? Decreasing influence of socioeconomic deprivation between 1981 and 2001 supports the existence of a "Scottish effect"', *Journal of Public Health*, vol 27, no 2, pp 199-204.

[194] McCartney et al (2012).

[195] Walsh et al (2010).

[196] Nomis (2015) *Labour market profile* (www.nomisweb.co.uk/).

[197] Bambra, C. and Garthwaite, K. (2014) *Welfare and austerity, Report to the Independent Inquiry on Health Equity in the North*, Manchester: Centre for Local Economic Strategies.

[198] PHE (Public Health England) (2015) *Public Health Outcomes Framework*, London: PHE (www.phoutcomes.info/).

[199] Bambra, C. et al (2017, in press) *The North or Northerners? An exploration of the contextual and compositional determinants of the North South health divide.*

[200] Nomis (2015).

[201] Ibid.

[202] Cox, E. and Schmuecker, K. (2011) 'On the wrong track: An analysis of the autumn statement announcements on transport infrastructure', Briefing, *IPPR North*, London: Institute for Public Policy Research.

[203] Todd, A., Akhter, N., Copeland, A., Husband, A., Kasim, A, Walton, N. and Bambra, C. (2016, in press) *A North South health care divide? A regional analysis of geographical access to community pharmacy and primary care services in England.* .

[204] Bambra et al (2015).

[205] Bambra et al (2017, in press).

[206] Calculated by N.Akhter and A.Kasim from data collected as part of Bambra, C. (2013) *Local health inequalities in an age of austerity: The Stockton-on-Tees Study*, Leverhulme Trust Research Leadership Award, Durham: Durham University.

Chapter 5

[1] Bambra, C., Fox, D. and Scott-Samuel, A. (2005) 'Towards a politics of health', *Health Promotion International*, vol 20, no 2, pp 187-93.
[2] Slater, T. (2013) 'Your life chances affect where you live: A critique of the "cottage industry" of neighbourhood effects research', *International Journal of Urban and Regional Research*, vol 137, p 20.
[3] Bambra, C. (2011) *Work, worklessness, and the political economy of health*, Oxford: Oxford University Press.
[4] Schrecker, T. and Bambra, C. (2015) *How politics makes us sick: Neoliberal epidemics*, Basingstoke: Palgrave Macmillan.
[5] Krieger, N. (2013) 'Ecosocial theory of disease distribution', YouTube video (www.youtube.com/watch?v=5pBnnDJ9HQY).
[6] Bambra et al (2005).
[7] Schrecker and Bambra (2015).
[8] Krieger (2013).
[9] Schrecker and Bambra (2015).
[10] Bambra (2011).
[11] Heywood, A. (2000) *Key concepts in politics*, London: Macmillan.
[12] Millett, K. (1969) *Sexual politics*, London: Virago.
[13] Heywood, A. (1992) *Political ideologies*, London: Palgrave Macmillan.
[14] Gallie, W.B. (1955) 'Essentially contested concepts', *Proceedings of the Aristotelian Society*, JSTOR.
[15] Heywood, A. (1994) *Political ideas and concepts*, London: Macmillan.
[16] Millett (1969).
[17] Based on Heywood (1992, 1994, 2000).
[18] Althusser, L. (1971) *Lenin and philosophy and other essays*, New York: Monthly Review Press, pp 127-86.
[19] Bambra et al (2005).
[20] Blane, D., Brunner, E. and Wilkinson, R.G. (1996) *Health and social organization: Towards a health policy for the twenty-first century*, London: Routledge.
[21] Bambra et al (2005).
[22] Secretary of State for Social Services (1988) *Public health in England. The report of the Committee of Inquiry into the future development of the public health function*, Cmnd 289, London: HMSO.
[23] Winslow, C.E. (1920) 'The untilled fields of public health', *Science*, vol 51, no 1306, pp 23-33.
[24] Bambra et al (2005).
[25] Ibid.
[26] UN (United Nations) (1948) *Universal declaration of human rights*, New York: UN General Assembly.

[27] Marshall, T.H. (1963) *Sociology at the crossroads: And other essays*, London: Hutchinson.
[28] Schrecker, T. (2014) 'Health equity in a globalising world: The importance of human rights', in A. Robertson (ed) *Commonwealth health partnerships 2014*, London: The Commonwealth, pp 18-21.
[29] Ibid.
[30] Smith, J.C. and Medalia, C. (2015) *Health insurance coverage in the United States: 2014*, Current Population Reports, Washington, DC: US Census Bureau (www.census.gov/content/dam/Census/library/publications/2015/demo/p60-253.pdf).
[31] This section is adapted, with permission from the authors, from Bambra, C., Smith, K. and Kennedy, L. (2008) 'Politics and health', in J. Naidoo and J. Wills (eds) *Health studies* (2nd edn), Basingstoke: Palgrave Macmillan.
[32] Bambra, C., Fox, D. and Scott-Samuel, A. (2007) 'A politics of health glossary', *Journal of Epidemiology and Community Health*, vol 61, no 7, pp 571-4.
[33] Ledwith, M. (2001) 'Community work as critical pedagogy: re-envisioning Freire and Gramsci', *Community Development Journal*, vol 36, no 3, pp 171-82.
[34] Bambra et al (2005).
[35] Gramsci, A. (1971) *Prison notebooks*, New York: International Publishers.
[36] Eccleshall, R. (1994) 'Conservatism', in R. Eccleshall, A. Finlayson, V. Geoghegan, M. Kenny, M. Lloyd, I. MacKenzie and R. Wilford (eds) *Political ideologies: An introduction*, London: Taylor & Francis, pp 47-68.
[37] Dearlove, J. and Saunders, P. (1991) *Introduction to British politics* (2nd edn), Cambridge: Polity Press.
[38] Fukuyama, F. (1989) 'The end of history?', *The National Interest*, pp 3-18.
[39] Heywood (1992).
[40] Ibid.
[41] Giddens, A. (1998) *The third way: The renewal of social democracy*, Cambridge: Polity Press.
[42] Giddens (1998).
[43] Bambra (2011).
[44] Schrecker and Bambra (2015).
[45] Navarro, V., Muntaner, C., Borrell, C., Benach, J., Quiroga, A., Rodriguez-Sanz, M. et al (2006) 'Politics and health outcomes', *The Lancet*, vol 368, no 9540, pp 1033-7.
[46] Chung, H. and Muntaner, C. (2006) 'Political and welfare state determinants of infant and child health indicators: An analysis of wealthy countries', *Social Science & Medicine*, vol 63, no 3, pp 829-42.
[47] Woolf, S. and Aron, L. (2013) *US health in international perspective: Shorter lives, poorer health*, Washington, DC: The National Academies Press.
[48] Bambra, C. and Beckfield, J. (2012) *Institutional arrangements as candidate explanations for the US mortality disadvantage*, Cambridge, MA: Harvard University.
[49] Beckfield, J. and Bambra, C. (2016, in press) *Shorter lives, stingier states: Welfare shortcomings help explain the US mortality disadvantage*.

[50] Beckfield, J., Bambra, C., Eikemo, T.A., Huijts, T., McNamara, C. and Wendt, C. (2015) 'An institutional theory of welfare state effects on the distribution of population health', *Social Theory & Health*, vol 13, no 3-4, pp 227-44.
[51] Esping-Andersen, G. (1990) *The three worlds of welfare capitalism*, London: Polity Press.
[52] Bambra (2011).
[53] Ibid.
[54] Esping Andersen (1990).
[55] Schrecker and Bambra (2015).
[56] Esping Andersen (1990).
[57] Bambra (2007).
[58] Esping Andersen (1990).
[59] Bambra, C., Netuveli, G. and Eikemo, T. (2010) 'Welfare state regime life courses: The development of Western European welfare state regimes and age-related patterns of educational inequalities in self-reported health', *International Journal of Health Services*, vol 40, no 3, pp 399-420.
[60] Jessop, B. (1991) 'The welfare state in transition from Fordism to post-Fordism', in B. Jessop, K. Nielsen, H. Kastendiek and O.K. Pederson (eds) *The politics of flexibility: Restructuring state and industry in Britain, Germany and Scandinavia*, Aldershot: Edward Elgar, pp 82-105.
[61] Ibid.
[62] Ibid.
[63] Beckfield et al (2015).
[64] Navarro et al (2006).
[65] Coburn, D. (2000) 'Income inequality, social cohesion and the health status of populations: the role of neo-liberalism', *Social Science & Medicine*, vol 51, no 1, pp 135-46.
[66] Chung and Muntaner (2006).
[67] Lundberg, O., Yngwe, M.A., Stjärne, M.K., Elstad, J.I. Ferrarini, T., Kangas, O. et al (2008) 'The role of welfare state principles and generosity in social policy programmes for public health: an international comparative study', *The Lancet*, vol 372, p 7.
[68] Beckfield and Brambra (2016).
[69] Schrecker and Bambra (2015).
[70] Woolf and Aron (2013).
[71] Smith and Medalia (2015).
[72] Woolf and Aron (2013).
[73] Bambra, C. (2005) 'Cash versus services: "Worlds of Welfare" and the decommodification of cash benefits and health care services', *Journal of Social Policy*, vol 34, no 2, pp 195-213.
[74] Woolf and Aron (2013).
[75] Wilkinson, R. and Pickett, K. (2010) *The spirit level: Why equality is better for everyone*, London: Penguin.
[76] Schrecker and Bambra (2015).
[77] OECD (Organisation for Economic Co-operation and Development) (2014) *Trade union density*, Paris: OECD.

[78] Bambra and Beckfield (2012).

[79] Krieger, N., Chen, J.T., Coull, B., Waterman, P.D. and Beckfield, J. (2013) 'The unique impact of abolition of Jim Crow laws on reducing inequities in infant death rates and implications for choice of comparison groups in analyzing societal determinants of health', *American Journal of Public Health*, vol 103, no 12, pp 2234-44.

[80] Mackenbach, J.P. and McKee, M. (2013) 'Social-democratic government and health policy in Europe: a quantitative analysis', *International Journal of Health Services*, vol 43, no 3, pp 389-413.

[81] Schrecker and Bambra (2015).

[82] de Vogli, R., Kouvonen, A. and Gimeno, D. (2014) 'The influence of market deregulation on fast food consumption and body mass index: a cross-national time series analysis', *Bulletin of the World Health Organization*, vol 92, no 2, pp 99-107.

[83] Mackenbach and McKee (2013).

[84] This section is adapted, with permission from the authors, from Schrecker and Bambra (2015).

[85] Schrecker and Bambra (2015).

[86] Ward, K. and England, K. (2007) 'Introduction: Reading neoliberalization', in K. England and K. Ward (eds) *Neoliberalization: States, networks, people*, Oxford: Blackwell.

[87] Harvey, D. (2005) *A brief history of neoliberalism*, Oxford: Oxford University Press.

[88] Fourcade-Gourinchas, M. and Babb, S.L. (2002) 'The rebirth of the liberal creed: Paths to neoliberalism in four countries', *American Journal of Sociology*, vol 108, no 3, pp 533-79.

[89] Harvey (2005).

[90] Ward and England (2007).

[91] Bambra et al (2010).

[92] Fraser Institute (2013) *Economic freedom of the world annual report 2013*, Vancouver: Fraser Institute.

[93] Data from the Fraser Institute (2013).

[94] Benach, J., Amable, M., Muntaner, C. and Benavides, F.G. (2002) 'The consequences of flexible work for health: are we looking at the right place?', *Journal of Epidemiology and Community Health*, vol 56, no 6, pp 405-6.

[95] Virtanen, P., Vahtera, J., Kivimäki, M., Pentti, J. and Ferrie, J. (2002) 'Employment security and health', *Journal of Epidemiology and Community Health*, vol 56, no 8, pp 569-74.

[96] Shildrick, T., MacDonald, R., Webster, C. and Garthwaite, K. (2012) *Poverty and insecurity: Life in low-pay, no-pay Britain*, Bristol: Policy Press, p 59.

[97] Standing, G. (2014) *The precariat: The new dangerous class* (revised edn), London: Bloomsbury.

[98] Seymour, R. (2014) 'Zero-hours contracts, and the sharp whip of insecurity that controls us all', *The Guardian*, 1 May.

[99] House of Commons (1991) *Hansard debate, 16 May 1991.*

[100] BBC News (1998) 'Business: The economy - Governor tries to douse North's fire', 22 October.

[101] Scruggs, L., Detlef, J. and Kuitto, K. (2014) 'Comparative welfare entitlements dataset 2, Version 2014-03' (http://cwed2.org/).

[102] Saez, E. and Zucman, G. (2014) *Wealth inequality in the United States since 1913: Evidence from capitalized income tax data*, NBER Working Paper, Cambridge: National Bureau of Economic Research.

[103] Dorling, D. (2012) *Fair play*, Bristol: Policy Press.

[104] Schrecker and Bambra (2015).

[105] Reproduced with permission of Policy Press from Dorling, D. (2012) *Fair play*, Bristol: Policy Press.

[106] Collins, C. and McCartney, G. (2011) 'The impact of neoliberal political attack on health: the case of the Scottish effect', *International Journal of Health Services*, vol 41, p 22.

[107] Stuckler, D. and Basu, S. (2013) *The body economic: Why austerity kills*, London: Allan Lane.

[108] Collins and McCartney (2011).

[109] Ibid.

[110] Ibid.

[111] Bambra, C., Barr, B. and Milne, E. (2014) 'North and South: Addressing the English health divide', *Journal of Public Health*, vol 36, no 2, pp 183-6.

[112] Reproduced with permission from Oxford University Press from Bambra et al (2014).

[113] Fulbrook, M. (2005) *The people's state: East German society from Hitler to Honecker*, New Haven, CT: Yale University Press.

[114] CIA (Central Intelligence Agency) (2003) *CIA world factbook 1990*, Fairfax, CA: CIA.

[115] Krueger, A. and Pischke, J. (1995) 'A comparative analysis of East and West German labor markets: Before and after unification', in R. Freeman and L. Katz (eds) *Differences and changes in wage structures*, Chicago, IL: University of Chicago Press, pp 405-46.

[116] Ibid.

[117] Gjonça, A., Brockmann, H. and Maier, H. (2000) 'Old-age mortality in Germany prior to and after reunification', *Demographic Research*, vol 3.

[118] Fulbrook (2005).

[119] Kibele, E.U.B., Kluesener, S. and Scholz, R.D. (2015) 'Regional mortality disparities in Germany: Long-term dynamics and possible determinants', *Kolner Zeitschrift fur Soziologie und Sozialpsychologie*, vol 67, pp 241-70.

[120] Data from Max Planck Institute for Demographic Research (2014) *The Human Mortality Database* (www.mortality.org/).

[121] Ibid.

[122] Data from Senatsverwaltung für Gesundheit und Soziales (2014) *Handlungsorientierter Sozialstrukturatlas Berlin 2013*.

[123] Parkes, K.S. (1997) *Understanding contemporary Germany*, London: Taylor & Francis.

[124] Gjonça et al (2000).

[125] Ibid.

[126] Ibid.

[127] Ibid.

[128] Gokhale, J., Raffelhuschen, B. and Walliser, J. (1994) *The burden of German unification: A generational accounting approach*, Cleveland, OH: Federal Reserve Bank of Cleveland, pp 141-65.

[129] Nolte, E., Scholz, R., Shkolnikov, V. and McKee, M. (2002) 'The contribution of medical care to changing life expectancy in Germany and Poland', *Social Science & Medicine*, vol 55, no 11, pp 1905-21.

[130] Nolte, E., Brand, A., Koupilová, I. and McKee, M. (2000) 'Neonatal and postneonatal mortality in Germany since unification', *Journal of Epidemiology and Community Health*, vol 54, no 2, pp 84-90.

[131] Nolte et al (2002).

[132] Ibid.

[133] Ibid.

[134] Ibid.

[135] PHE (Public Health England) (2013) *Local health* (www.localhealth.org.uk).

[136] This section, reproduced under Creative Commons licence, draws on Bambra, C. (2013) '"All in it together?" Health inequalities, austerity and the "great recession"', in C. Woods (ed) *Health and austerity*, London: Demos; and Bambra, C. and Garthwaite, K. (2015) 'Austerity, welfare reform and the English health divide', *Area*, vol 47, pp 341-3.

[137] Gamble, A. (2009) *The spectre at the feast: Capitalist crisis and the politics of recession*, Basingstoke: Palgrave.

[138] Updated from Bambra, C. and Garthwaite, K. (2014) *Welfare and austerity, Report to the Independent Inquiry on Health Equity in the North*, Manchester: Centre for Local Economic Strategies.

[139] Beatty, C. and Fothergill, S. (2014) 'The local and regional impact of the UK's welfare reforms', *Cambridge Journal of Regions Economy and Society*, vol 7, no 1, pp 63-79.

[140] Ibid.

[141] Ibid.

[142] Redrawn, with permission from the Centre for Local Economic Strategies and the University of Liverpool, from (2014) *Due North: Report of the Inquiry on Health Equity for the North*, Liverpool and Manchester: University of Liverpool and Centre for Local Economic Strategies (www.cles.org.uk/wp-content/uploads/2014/09/Due-North-Report-of-the-Inquiry-on-Health-Equity-in-the-North-final.pdf).

[143] Beatty and Fothergill (2014).

[144] Hastings, A., Bailey, N., Besemer, K., Bramley, G., Gannon, M. and Watkins, D. (2015) 'Coping with the cuts? The management of the worst financial settlement in living memory', *Local Government Studies*, vol 41, no 4, pp 601-21.

[145] Redrawn, with permission from the Centre for Local Economic Strategies and the University of Liverpool, from (2014) *Due North: Report of the Inquiry on Health Equity for the North*, Liverpool and Manchester: University of

Liverpool and Centre for Local Economic Strategies (www.cles.org.uk/wp-content/uploads/2014/09/Due-North-Report-of-the-Inquiry-on-Health-Equity-in-the-North-final.pdf).

[146] Pearce, J. (2013) 'Financial crisis, austerity policies, and geographical inequalities in health: Introduction commentary', *Environment and Planning A*, vol 45, no 9, pp 2030-45.

[147] End Child Poverty (2013) *Child poverty map of the UK* (www.endchildpoverty.org.uk/images/ecp/Report_on_child_poverty_map_2014.pdf).

[148] Trussell Trust, The (2014) 'Biggest ever increase in UK food bank use: 170% rise in numbers turning to foodbanks in last 12 months', Salisbury: The Trussell Trust.

[149] Bambra and Garthwaite (2014).

[150] Department of Energy and Climate Change (2013).

[151] Stuckler and Basu (2013).

[152] MacLeavy, J. (2011) 'A "new politics" of austerity, workfare and gender? The UK coalition government's welfare reform proposals', *Cambridge Journal of Regions Economy and Society*, vol 4, no 3, pp 355-67.

[153] Pearce (2013).

[154] ONS (Office for National Statistics) (2014) *Suicides in the United Kingdom: 2012 registrations*, Newport: ONS.

[155] Spence, R., Roberts, A., Ariti, C. and Bardsley, M. (2014) *Focus on: Antidepressant prescribing. Trends in the prescribing of antidepressants in primary care*, QualityWatch, London: The Health Foundation and the Nuffield Trust (www.qualitywatch.org.uk/sites/files/qualitywatch/field/field_document/140218_QualityWatch_Focus_on_distance_emergency_care_0.pdf).

[156] The Trussell Trust (2014).

[157] ONS (Office for National Statistics) (2015) *Life expectancy at birth for England, Wales and Northern Ireland, 2012–14*, Newport: ONS.

[158] Möller, H., Haigh, F., Harwood, C., Kinsella, T. and Pope, D. (2013) 'Rising unemployment and increasing spatial health inequalities in England: further extension of the North–South divide', *Journal of Public Health*, vol 35, no 2, pp 313-21.

[159] Pearce (2013).

[160] Ibid, p 2031.

[161] Schrecker and Bambra (2015).

[162] Krieger, N., Rehkopf, D.H., Chen, J.T., Waterman, P.D., Marcelli, E. and Kennedy, M. (2008) 'The fall and rise of US inequities in premature mortality: 1960-2002', *Plos Medicine*, vol 5, no 2, pp 227-41.

[163] Shaw, C., Blakely, T., Atkinson, J. and Crampton, P. (2005) 'Do social and economic reforms change socioeconomic inequalities in child mortality? A case study: New Zealand 1981-1999', *Journal of Epidemiology and Community Health*, vol 59, no 8, pp 638-44.

[164] Blakely, T., Tobias, M. and Atkinson, J. (2008) 'Inequalities in mortality during and after restructuring of the New Zealand economy: repeated cohort studies', *British Medical Journal*, vol 336, no 7640, pp 371-5.

[165] Pearce, J. and Dorling, D. (2006) 'Increasing geographical inequalities in health in New Zealand, 1980-2001', *International Journal of Epidemiology*, vol 35, no 3, pp 597-603.
[166] Pearce, J., Dorling, D., Wheeler, B., Barnett, R. and Rigby, J. (2006) 'Geographical inequalities in health in New Zealand, 1980-2001: the gap widens', *Australian and New Zealand Journal of Public Health*, vol 30, no 5, pp 461-6.
[167] Scott-Samuel, A., Bambra, C., Collins, C., Hunter, D.J., McCartney, G. and Smith, K. (2014) 'The impact of Thatcherism on health and well-being in Britain', *International Journal of Health Services*, vol 44, no 1, pp 53-71.
[168] Scott-Samuel et al (2014).
[169] Thomas, B., Dorling, D. and Davey Smith, G. (2010) 'Inequalities in premature mortality in Britain: observational study from 1921 to 2007', *British Medical Journal*, vol 341.
[170] Hacking, J.M., Muller, S. and Buchan, I.E. (2011) 'Trends in mortality from 1965 to 2008 across the English north-south divide: comparative observational study', *British Medical Journal*, vol 342, d508.

Chapter 6

[1] Mackenbach, J.P. (2011) 'Can we reduce health inequalities? An analysis of the English strategy (1997-2010)', *Journal of Epidemiology and Community Health*, vol 65, no 7.
[2] This section is adapted, with permission from the Sage Publishing Group, from Scott-Samuel, A., Bambra, C., Collins, C., Hunter, D.J., McCartney, G. and Smith, K. (2014) 'The impact of Thatcherism on health and wellbeing in Britain', *International Journal of Health Services*, vol 44, pp 53-72.
[3] Berridge, V. and Blume, S. (2003) *Poor health: Social inequality before and after the Black Report*, London: Frank Cass.
[4] Black, D. (Chair) (1980) *Inequalities in health: Report of a research working group*, London: Department of Health and Social Security.
[5] Berridge and Blume (2003).
[6] Adapted, with permission from the BMJ Publishing Group, from Bambra, C., Smith, K.E., Garthwaite, K., Joyce, K.E. and Hunter, D.J. (2011) 'A labour of Sisyphus? Public policy and health inequalities research from the Black and Acheson reports to the Marmot Review', *Journal of Epidemiology and Community Health*, vol 65, no 5, pp 399-406.
[7] Gamble, A. (1994) *The free economy and the strong state*, London: Macmillan.
[8] Hall, S. and Jacques, M. (1983) *The politics of Thatcherism*, London: Lawrence & Wishart.
[9] Moran, M. (1999) *Governing the healthcare state: A comparative study of the UK, the USA and Germany*, Manchester: Manchester University Press.
[10] Ginsburg, N. (1992) *Divisions of welfare: A critical introduction to comparative social policy*, London: Sage.
[11] Ibid.
[12] McVicar, D. (2008) 'Why have UK disability benefit rolls grown so much?', *Journal of Economic Surveys*, vol 22, no 1, pp 114-39.

[13] Davis, J. and Tallis, R. (eds) (2013) *NHS SOS: How the NHS was betrayed and how we can save it*, London: Oneworld.

[14] Scott-Samuel, A., Bambra, C., Collins, C., Hunter, D.J., McCartney, G. and Smith, K. (2014) 'The impact of Thatcherism on health and well-being in Britain', *International Journal of Health Services*, vol 44, no 1, pp 53-71.

[15] Dorling, D. (2014) *All that is solid: How the great housing disaster defines our times, and what we can do about it*, London: Penguin.

[16] Loveland, I. (1993) 'The politics, law and practice of "intentional homelessness": 2-Abandonment of existing housing', *Journal of Social Welfare and Family Law*, vol 15, no 3, pp 185-99.

[17] Bobbitt, P. (2003) *The shield of Achilles: War, peace and the course of history*, London: Penguin.

[18] Hunter, D. (2008) *The health debate*, Bristol: Policy Press.

[19] Davies, S. (2010) 'Fragmented management, hospital contract cleaning and infection control', *Policy & Politics*, vol 38, no 3, pp 445-63.

[20] McCartney, G., Walsh, D., Whyte, B. and Collins, C. (2012) 'Has Scotland always been the "sick man" of Europe? An observational study from 1855 to 2006', *European Journal of Public Health*, vol 22, no 6, pp 756-60.

[21] WHO (World Health Organization) (2012) *Health for All database*, Geneva: WHO.

[22] Hacking, J.M., Muller, S. and Buchan, I.E. (2011) 'Trends in mortality from 1965 to 2008 across the English north-south divide: comparative observational study', *British Medical Journal*, vol 342, d508.

[23] Norman, P., Boyle, P., Exeter, D., Feng, Z. and Popham, F. (2011) 'Rising premature mortality in the UK's persistently deprived areas: Only a Scottish phenomenon?', *Social Science & Medicine*, vol 73, no 11, pp 1575-84.

[24] Whyte, B. and Ajetunmobi, T. (2012) *Still the 'sick man of Europe'? Scottish mortality in a European context 1950-2010. An analysis of comparative mortality trends*, Glasgow: Glasgow Centre for Population Health.

[25] Reproduced with permission of the Sage Publishing Group from Scott-Samuel et al (2014).

[26] Leyland, A.H. (2004) 'Increasing inequalities in premature mortality in Great Britain', *Journal of Epidemiology and Community Health*, vol 58, no 4, pp 296-302.

[27] Mackenbach, J.P., Stirbu, I., Roskam, A.J., Schaap, M.M., Menvielle, G., Leinsalu, M. et al (2008) 'Socioeconomic inequalities in health in 22 European countries', *New England Journal of Medicine*, vol 358, no 23, pp 2468-81.

[28] This section is adapted, with permission of the BMJ Publishing Group, from Bambra et al (2011).

[29] DH (Department of Health) (1997) 'Public health strategy launched to tackle the root causes of ill-health', Press Release, London: DH.

[30] Ibid.

[31] Acheson, D. (1999) *Independent inquiry into inequalities in health: Report*, London: The Stationery Office.

[32] Birch, S. (1999) 'The 39 steps: the mystery of health inequalities in the UK', *Health Economics*, vol 8, no 4, pp 301-8.

[33] Smith, G.D., Morris, J.N. and Shaw, M. (1998) 'The independent inquiry into inequalities in health: Is welcome, but its recommendations are too cautious and vague', *British Medical Journal*, vol 317, no 7171, p 1465.

[34] Smith, K.E., Hunter, D.J., Blackman, T., Elliott, E., Greene, A., Harrington, B.E. et al (2009) 'Divergence or convergence? Health inequalities and policy in a devolved Britain', *Critical Social Policy*, vol 29, no 2, pp 216-42.

[35] Ibid.

[36] Whitehead, M. and Popay, J. (2010) 'Swimming upstream? Taking action on the social determinants of health inequalities', *Social Science & Medicine*, vol 71, no 7, pp 1234-6.

[37] Adapted, with permission from Oxford University Press, from Smith, K.E., Bambra, C., Joyce, K.E., Perkins, N., Hunter, D.J. and Blenkinsopp, E.A. (2009) 'Partners in health? A systematic review of the impact of organizational partnerships on public health outcomes in England between 1997 and 2008', *Journal of Public Health*, vol 31, no 2, pp 210-21.

[38] Mackenbach (2011).

[39] Ibid.

[40] Bambra (2012).

[41] Nolte, E. and McKee, M. (2011) 'Variations in amenable mortality-trends in 16 high-income nations', *Health Policy*, vol 103, no 1, pp 47-52.

[42] Barr, B., Bambra, C. and Whitehead, M. (2014) 'The impact of NHS resource allocation policy on health inequalities in England 2001-11: Longitudinal ecological study', *British Medical Journal*, vol 348.

[43] Ibid.

[44] Reproduced, with permission from the BMJ Publishing Group, from Bambra, C. (2012) 'Reducing health inequalities: New data suggest that the English strategy was partially successful', *Journal of Epidemiology and Community Health*, vol 66, no 7, p 662.

[45] Dorling, D. and Thomas, B. (2009) 'Geographical inequalities in health over the last century', in H. Graham (ed) *Understanding health inequalities*, Maidenhead: Open University Press.

[46] Drawn from data from Dorling and Thomas (2009).

[47] Whitehead and Popay (2010).

[48] Schrecker, T. and Bambra, C. (2015) *How politics makes us sick: Neoliberal epidemics*, Basingstoke: Palgrave Macmillan.

[49] Disclaimer: I was involved in one of the nine Marmot Review Task groups on priority public health conditions.

[50] Marmot, M. (2010) *Fair society, healthy lives: The Marmot Review*, London: University College London.

[51] Hunter, D.J., Popay, J., Tannahill, C., Whitehead, M. and Duncan, W.H. (2010) 'Getting to grips with health inequalities at last?', *British Medical Journal*, vol 340, doi: http://dx.doi.org/10.1136/bmj.c684.

[52] Bambra et al (2012).

[53] Whitehead, M.C. et al (2014) *Due North: Report of the Inquiry on Health Equity for the North*, Liverpool and Manchester: University of Liverpool and Centre for Local Economic Strategies (www.cles.org.uk/wp-content/uploads/2014/09/Due-North-Report-of-the-Inquiry-on-Health-Equity-in-the-North-final.pdf).

[54] Disclaimer: I was a panel member for the *Due North* Inquiry.

[55] Whitehead et al (2014), p 9.

[56] Smith, K. and Hellowell, M. (2012) 'Beyond rhetorical differences: A cohesive account of post-devolution developments in UK health policy', *Social Policy & Administration*, vol 46, no 2, pp 178-98.

[57] Scottish Government (2008) *Equally well: Report of the Ministerial Task Force on health inequalities*, Edinburgh: Scottish Government.

[58] Scottish Government (2010) *Equally well review*, Edinburgh: Scottish Government.

[59] This section is adapted, with permission from the BMJ Publishing Group, from Bambra et al (2011).

[60] Bambra et al (2011).

[61] Bambra, C. (2013) 'The primacy of politics: The rise and fall of evidence-based public health policy?', *Journal of Public Health*, vol 35, no 4, pp 486-7.

Chapter 7

[1] Bennett, J.E., Guangquang, L., Foreman, K. Best, N., Kontis, V., Pearson, C. et al (2015) 'The future of life expectancy and life expectancy inequalities in England and Wales: Bayesian spatiotemporal forecasting', *The Lancet*, vol 386, no 9989, pp 163-70.

[2] Adapted from Woolf, S. and Aron, L. (2013) *US health in international perspective: Shorter lives, poorer health*, Washington, DC: The National Academies Press.

[3] Walsh, D., McCartney, G., Collins, C., Taulbut, M. and Batty, D. (2016) *History, politics and vulnerability: Explaining excess mortality in Scotland and Glasgow*, Glasgow: Glasgow Centre for Population Health.

[4] Text adapted from Walsh et al (2016) ibid.

[5] Whitehead, M.C. et al (2014) *Due North: Report of the Inquiry on Health Equity for the North*, Liverpool and Manchester: University of Liverpool and Centre for Local Economic Strategies (www.cles.org.uk/wp-content/uploads/2014/09/Due-North-Report-of-the-Inquiry-on-Health-Equity-in-the-North-final.pdf).

[6] Text adapted from Whitehead et al (2014) ibid.

[7] Marmot, M. (2010) *Fair society, healthy lives: The Marmot Review*, London: University College London.

[8] Text adapted from Marmot (2010) ibid.

References

Abraham, A., Sommerhalder, K. and Abel, T. (2010) 'Landscape and well-being: a scoping study on the health-promoting impact of outdoor environments', *International Journal of Public Health*, vol 55, no 1, pp 59-69.

Acheson, D. (1999) *Independent inquiry into inequalities in health: Report*, London: The Stationery Office.

Agnew, J. (2011) 'Space and place', in J. Agnew and D. Livingstone (eds) *The SAGE handbook of geographical knowledge*, London: Sage, pp 316-30.

Airey, L. (2003) '"Nae as nice a scheme as it used to be": lay accounts of neighbourhood incivilities and well-being', *Health & Place*, vol 9, no 2, pp 129-37.

Althusser, L. (1971) *Lenin and philosophy and other essays (ss 127-86)*, New York: Monthly Review Press.

Anjum Hajat, A., Diez-Roux, A.V., Adar, S.D., Auchincloss, A.H., Lovasi, G.S., O'Neill, M.S. et al (2013) 'Air pollution and individual and neighborhood socioeconomic status: Evidence from the Multi-Ethnic Study of Atherosclerosis (MESA)', *Environmental Health Perspectives*, DOI:10.1289/ehp.1206337.

Arber, S. (1987) 'Social class, non-employment, and chronic illness: Continuing the inequalities in health debate', *British Medical Journal*, vol 294, no 6579, pp 1069-73.

Arias, E., Rostron, B. and Tejada-Vera, B. (2010) 'United States life tables, 2005', *National Vital Statistics Reports*, vol 58, no 10, pp 1-132.

Audit Scotland (2012) *Health inequalities in Scotland* (www.audit-scotland.gov.uk/docs/health/2012/nr_121213_health_inequalities.pdf).

Bambra, C. (2005) 'Cash versus services: "Worlds of Welfare" and the decommodification of cash benefits and health care services', *Journal of Social Policy*, vol 34, no 2, pp 195-213.

Bambra, C. (2007) 'Going beyond The three worlds of welfare capitalism: regime theory and public health research', *Journal of Epidemiology and Community Health*, vol 61, no 12, pp 1098-102.

Bambra, C. (2011) *Work, worklessness, and the political economy of health*, Oxford: Oxford University Press.

Bambra, C. (2012) 'Reducing health inequalities: New data suggest that the English strategy was partially successful', *Journal of Epidemiology and Community Health*, vol 66, no 7, p 662.

Bambra, C. (2013) *Local health inequalities in an age of austerity: The Stockton-on-Tees Study*, Leverhulme Trust Research Leadership Award, Durham: Durham University.

Bambra, C. (2013) 'The primacy of politics: The rise and fall of evidence-based public health policy?', *Journal of Public Health*, vol 35, no 4, pp 486-7.

Bambra, C. (2015) 'Who are the top teams in the health league?', Conversation.com (http://theconversation.com/who-are-the-top-football-teams-in-the-health-league-42002).

Bambra, C. and Beckfield, J. (2012) *Institutional arrangements as candidate explanations for the US mortality disadvantage*, Cambridge, MA: Harvard University.

Bambra, C. and Eikemo, T. (2009) 'Welfare state regimes, unemployment and health: A comparative study of the relationship between unemployment and self-reported health in 23 European countries', *Journal of Epidemiology and Community Health*, vol 63, no 2, pp 92-8.

Bambra, C. and Garthwaite, K. (2014) *Welfare and austerity, Report to the Independent Inquiry on Health Equity in the North*, Manchester: Centre for Local Economic Strategies.

Bambra, C. and Orton, C. (2015) 'A train journey through the English health divide: topological map', *Environment and Planning A*, December.

Bambra, C., Barr, B. and Milne, E. (2014) 'North and South: Addressing the English health divide', *Journal of Public Health*, vol 36, no 2, pp 183-6.

Bambra, C., Fox, D. and Scott-Samuel, A. (2005) 'Towards a politics of health', *Health Promotion International*, vol 20, no 2, pp 187-93.

Bambra, C., Fox, D. and Scott-Samuel, A. (2007) 'A politics of health glossary', *Journal of Epidemiology and Community Health*, vol 61, no 7, pp 571-4.

Bambra, C., Joyce, K. and Maryon-Davies, A. (2009) *Priority health conditions – Task Group 8 Report to the Strategic Review of Health Inequalities in England post-2010 (Marmot Review)*, London: University College London.

Bambra, C., Joyce, K. and Maryon-Davis, A. (2009) *Strategic review of health inequalities in England post-2010 (Marmot Review): Task Group 8 Priority public health conditions – Final report* (www.instituteofhealthequity.org/projects/marmot-review-task-groups).

Bambra, C., Netuveli, G. and Eikemo, T. (2010) 'Welfare state regime life courses: The development of Western European welfare state regimes and age-related patterns of educational inequalities in self-reported health', *International Journal of Health Services*, vol 40, no 3, pp 399-420.

Bambra, C., Cairns, J.M., Kasim, A., Smith, J., Robertson, S., Copeland, A. and Johnson, K. (2015) 'This divided land: An examination of regional inequalities in exposure to brownfield land and the association with morbidity and mortality in England', *Health & Place*, vol 34, pp 257-69.

Bambra, C., Joyce, K.E., Bellis, M.A., Greatley, A., Greengross, S., Hughes, S. et al (2010) 'Reducing health inequalities in priority public health conditions: Using rapid review to develop proposals for evidence-based policy', *Journal of Public Health*, vol 32, no 4, pp 496-505.

Bambra, C., Smith, K.E., Garthwaite, K., Joyce, K.E. and Hunter, D.J. (2011) 'A labour of Sisyphus? Public policy and health inequalities research from the Black and Acheson reports to the Marmot Review', *Journal of Epidemiology and Community Health*, vol 65, no 5, pp 399-406.

Bambra, C., Robertson, S., Kasim, A., Smith, J., Cairns-Nagi, J., Copeland, A. et al (2014) 'Healthy land? An examination of the area-level association between brownfield land and morbidity and mortality in England', *Environment and Planning A*, vol 46, no 2, pp 433-54.

Bambra, C. et al (2016, in press) *The North or Northerners? An exploration of the contextual and compositional determinants of the North South health divide.*

Barr, B., Bambra, C. and Whitehead, M. (2014) 'The impact of NHS resource allocation policy on health inequalities in England 2001-11: Longitudinal ecological study', *British Medical Journal*, vol 348.

Barr, D., Fenton, L. and Edwards, D. (2004) 'Politics and health', *QJM*, vol 97, no 2, pp 61-2.

Bartley, M. (2004) *Health inequality: An introduction to theories, concepts and methods*, Cambridge: Polity Press.

Bartley, M. and Owen, C. (1996) 'Relation between socioeconomic status, employment, and health during economic change, 1973-93', *British Medical Journal*, vol 313, no 7055, pp 445-9.

Bartley, M. and Plewis, I. (2002) 'Accumulated labour market disadvantage and limiting long-term illness: data from the 1971-1991 Office for National Statistics' Longitudinal Study', *International Journal of Epidemiology*, vol 31, no 2, pp 336-41.

Bartley, M., Ferrie, J. and Montgomery, S. (2006) 'Health and labour market disadvantage: Unemployment, non-employment, and job insecurity', in M. Marmot and R. Wilkinson (eds) *The social determinants of health*, Oxford: Oxford University Press.

BBC News (1998) 'Business: The economy – Governor tries to douse North's fire'.

BBC News (2015) 'General Election results' (www.bbc.co.uk/news/election/2015/results).

Beatty, C. and Fothergill, S. (2014) 'The local and regional impact of the UK's welfare reforms', *Cambridge Journal of Regions Economy and Society*, vol 7, no 1, pp 63-79.

Beaulac, J., Kristjansson, E. and Cummins, S. (2009) 'A systematic review of food deserts, 1966-2007', *Preventing Chronic Disease*, vol 6, no 3, A105.

Beckfield, J. and Bambra, C. (2016, in press) *Shorter lives, stingier states: Welfare shortcomings help explain the US mortality disadvantage.*

Beckfield, J., Bambra, C., Eikemo, T.A., Huijts, T., McNamara, C. and Wendt, C. (2015) 'An institutional theory of welfare state effects on the distribution of population health', *Social Theory & Health*, vol 13, no 3-4, pp 227-44.

Benach, J., Amable, M., Muntaner, C. and Benavides, F.G. (2002) 'The consequences of flexible work for health: are we looking at the right place?', *Journal of Epidemiology and Community Health*, vol 56, no 6, pp 405-6.

Bennett, J.E., Guangquang, L., Foreman, K. Best, N., Kontis, V., Pearson, C. et al (2015) 'The future of life expectancy and life expectancy inequalities in England and Wales: Bayesian spatiotemporal forecasting', *The Lancet*, vol 386, no 9989, pp 163-70.

Berridge, V. and Blume, S. (2003) *Poor health: Social inequality before and after the Black Report*, London: Frank Cass.

Birch, S. (1999) 'The 39 steps: the mystery of health inequalities in the UK', *Health Economics*, vol 8, no 4, pp 301-8.

Black, D. (Chair) (1980) *Inequalities in health: Report of a research working group*, London: Department of Health and Social Security.

Blakely, T., Tobias, M. and Atkinson, J. (2008) 'Inequalities in mortality during and after restructuring of the New Zealand economy: repeated cohort studies', *British Medical Journal*, vol 336, no 7640, pp 371-5.

Blane, D., Brunner, E. and Wilkinson, R.G. (1996) *Health and social organization: Towards a health policy for the twenty-first century*, London: Routledge.

Bobbitt, P. (2003) *The shield of Achilles: War, peace and the course of history*, London: Penguin.

Bongers, P.M., de Winter, C.R., Kompier, M.A. and Hildebrandt, V.H. (1993) 'Psychosocial factors at work and musculoskeletal disease', *Scandinavian Journal of Work, Environment & Health*, pp 297-312.

Breyer, B. and Voss-Andreae, A. (2013) 'Food mirages: Geographic and economic barriers to healthful food access in Portland, Oregon', *Health & Place*, vol 24, p 8.

Bromet, E., Andrade, L.H., Hwang, I., Sampson, N.A., Alonso, J., de Girolamo, G. et al (2011) 'Cross-national epidemiology of DSM-IV major depressive episode', *BMC Medicine*, vol 9.

Brunner, E.J., Chandola, T. and Marmot, M.G. (2007) 'Prospective effect of job strain on general and central obesity in the Whitehall II Study', *American Journal of Epidemiology*, vol 165, no 7, pp 828-37.

Burgoine, T., Alvanides, S. and Lake, A.A. (2011) 'Assessing the obesogenic environment of North East England', *Health & Place*, vol 17, no 3, pp 738-47.

Burnett, J. (1991) 'Housing and the decline of mortality', in R. Schofield, D. Reher and A. Bideau (eds) *The decline of mortality In Europe*, Oxford: Clarendon, pp 158-76.

Bush, J., Moffatt, S. and Dunn, C. (2001) '"Even the birds round here cough": Stigma, air pollution and health in Teesside', *Health & Place*, vol 7, no 1, pp 47-56.

Cairns-Nagi, J.M. and Bambra, C. (2013) 'Defying the odds: A mixed-methods study of health resilience in deprived areas of England', *Social Science & Medicine*, vol 91, pp 229-37.

Cancer Research UK (2008) 'Socioeconomic inequalities in cancer', Policy Statement, April (www.cancerresearchuk.org/prod_consump/groups/cr_common/@nre/@pol/documents/generalcontent/crukmig_1000ast-3347.pdf).

Cancer Research UK (2011) 'About cancer' (www.cancerresearchuk.org/about-cancer/).

Capewell, S. et al (2008) *Modelling the UK burden of disease to 2020*, London: British Heart Foundation.

Catney, P., Eiser, D., Henneberry, J. and Stafford, T. (2007) 'Democracy, trust and risk related to contaminated sites in the UK', in T. Dixon, M. Raco, P. Catney and D.N. Lerner (eds) *Sustainable brownfield regeneration: Liveable places from problem spaces*, Oxford: Blackwell, pp 35-66.

CDC (Center for Disease Prevention and Control) (2011) *Obesity prevalence maps*, Atlanta, GA: CDC.

CDC (Centers for Disease Control and Prevention) (2013) 'Typhoid fever' (www.cdc.gov/nczved/divisions/dfbmd/diseases/typhoid_fever/).

CDC (Centers for Disease Control and Prevention) (2013) 'Small pox' (www.bt.cdc.gov/agent/smallpox/overview/disease-facts.asp).

Chadwick, E. (1842) *Report on the sanitary conditions of the labouring population of Great Britain*, London: HMSO.

Cheronomas, R. and Hudson, I. (2013) *To live and die in America: Class, power, health and healthcare*, London: Pluto Press.

Chung, H. and Muntaner, C. (2006) 'Political and welfare state determinants of infant and child health indicators: An analysis of wealthy countries', *Social Science & Medicine*, vol 63, no 3, pp 829-42.

CIA (Central Intelligence Agency) (2003) *CIA world factbook 1990*, Fairfax, CA: CIA.

Coburn, D. (2000) 'Income inequality, social cohesion and the health status of populations: the role of neo-liberalism', *Social Science & Medicine*, vol 51, no 1, pp 135-46.

Coleman, M.P., Rachet, B., Woods, L.M., Mitry, E., Riga, M., Cooper, N. et al (2004) 'Trends and socioeconomic inequalities in cancer survival in England and Wales up to 2001', *British Journal of Cancer*, vol 90, no 7, pp 1367-73.

Collins, C. and McCartney, G. (2011) 'The impact of neoliberal political attack on health: the case of the Scottish effect', *International Journal of Health Services*, vol 41, p 22.

Cook, I., Chaolin, G.U. and Halsall, J. (2013) 'China's growing urban health inequalities: The challenges ahead', *Journal of Management and Sustainability*, vol 3, no 2, p 10.

Costa, D. and Steckel, R. (1997) 'Long-term trends in health, welfare, and economic growth in the United States', in R. Steckel and R. Floud (eds) *Health and welfare during industrialization*, Chicago, IL: University of Chicago Press, pp 47-90.

Cox, E. and Schmuecker, K. (2011) 'On the wrong track: An analysis of the autumn statement announcements on transport infrastructure', Briefing, *IPPR North*, London: Institute for Public Policy Research.

Cummins, S., Curtis, S., Diez-Roux, A. and Macintyre, S. (2007) 'Understanding and representing "place" in health research: A relational approach', *Social Science & Medicine*, vol 65, p 13.

Curtis, S. (2010) *Space, place and mental health*, Farnham: Ashgate.

Cutler, D., Deaton, A. and Lleras-Muney, A. (2006) 'The determinants of mortality', *Journal of Economic Perspectives*, vol 20, no 3, pp 97-120.

Dahlgren, G. and Whitehead, M. (1991) *Policies and strategies to promote social in health*, Stockholm: Institute for Future Studies.

Dahlgren, G., Nordgren, P. and Whitehead, M. (1996) *Health impact assessment of the EU Common Agricultural Policy*, Solna: Sweden's National Institute of Public Health.

Davey Smith, G., Chaturvedi, N., Harding, S., Nazroo, J. and Williams, R. (2003) 'Ethnic inequalities in health: A review of UK epidemiological evidence', in G. Davey Smith (ed) *Health inequalities: Lifecourse approaches*, Bristol: Policy Press, pp 271-309.

Davies, S. (2010) 'Fragmented management, hospital contract cleaning and infection control', *Policy & Politics*, vol 38, no 3, pp 445-63.

Davis, J. and Tallis, R. (eds) (2013) *NHS SOS: How the NHS was betrayed and how we can save it*, London: Oneworld.

DCLG (Department for Communities and Local Government) (2011) *English indices of deprivation 2010*, London: DCLG.

Dearlove, J. and Saunders, P. (1991) *Introduction to British politics* (2nd edn), Cambridge: Polity Press.

Debrand, T., Pierre, A., Allonier, C. and Lucas-Gabrielli, V. (2012) 'Critical urban areas, deprived areas and neighbourhood effects on health in France', *Health Policy*, vol 105, no 1, pp 92-101.

Department of Energy and Climate Change (2013) *Fuel poverty report – Updated August 2013*, London: Department of Energy and Climate Change.

DHSSPS (Department of Health, Social Services and Public Safety) (2014) *Health Survey Northern Ireland 2012/13*, Belfast: DHSSPS.

de Vogli, R., Kouvonen, A. and Gimeno, D. (2014) 'The influence of market deregulation on fast food consumption and body mass index: a cross-national time series analysis', *Bulletin of the World Health Organization*, vol 92, no 2, pp 99-107.

DH (Department of Health) (1997) 'Public health strategy launched to tackle the root causes of ill-health', Press Release, London: DH.

Dickens, C. (1855) *Hard times*, London: Wordsworth.

Dickens, C. (1999 [1859]) *A tale of two cities*, London: Wordsworth Classics.

Dorling, D. (2010) 'Persistent North-South divides', in N. Coe and A. Jones (eds) *The economic geography of the UK*, London: Sage, pp 12-28.

Diez-Roux, A.V., Merkin, S.S., Arnett, D., Chambless, L., Massing, M., Nieto, F.J. et al (2001) 'Neighborhood of residence and incidence of coronary heart disease', *The New England Journal of Medicine*, vol 345, no 2, pp 99-106.

Dorling, D. (2011) *So you think you know about Britain?*, London: Constable.

Dorling, D. (2012) *Fair play*, Bristol: Policy Press.

Dorling, D. (2013) *Unequal health: The scandal of our times*, Bristol: Policy Press.

Dorling, D. (2014) *All that is solid: How the great housing disaster defines our times, and what we can do about it*, London: Penguin.

Dorling, D. and Thomas, B. (2009) 'Geographical inequalities in health over the last century', in H. Graham (ed) *Understanding health inequalities*, Maidenhead: Open University Press, p 66.

Doyal, L. (1979) *The political economy of health*, London: Pluto Press.

Doyal, L. (1995) 'What makes women sick: Gender and the political economy of health', *British Medical Journal*, vol 311, p 577.

Eccleshall, R. (1994) 'Conservatism', in R. Eccleshall, A. Finlayson, V. Geoghegan, M. Kenny, M. Lloyd, I. MacKenzie and R. Wilford (eds) *Political ideologies: An introduction*, London: Taylor & Francis, pp 47-68.

Eikemo, T., Huisman, M., Bambra, C. and Kunst, A. (2008) 'Health inequalities according to educational level in different welfare regimes: a comparison of 23 European countries', *Sociology of Health & Illness*, vol 30, no 4, pp 565-82.

Ellaway, A. and Macintyre, S. (2007) 'Is social participation associated with cardiovascular disease risk factors?', *Social Science & Medicine*, vol 64, no 7, pp 1384-91.

End Child Poverty (2013) *Child poverty map of the UK* (www.endchildpoverty.org.uk/images/ecp/Report_on_child_poverty_map_2014.pdf).

Engels, F. (2009) *The conditions of the working class in England*, London: Penguin Classics.

Eurostat (2013) *Life expectancy* (http://ec.europa.eu/eurostat/statistics-explained/index.php/Mortality_and_life_expectancy_statistics).

Esping-Andersen, G. (1990) *The three worlds of welfare capitalism*, London: Polity Press.

Fletcher, D. (2007) 'A culture of worklessness? Historical insights from the Manor and Park areas of Sheffield', *Policy & Politics*, vol 35, p 20.

Foster, J. (2011) 'The Scottish fffect: Some comments from a historical perspective', *Scottish 'excess' mortality: Comparing Glasgow with Liverpool and Manchester – Commentaries and synthesis*, Glasgow: Glasgow Centre for Population Health (www.gcph.co.uk/assets/0000/4022/Scottish_excess_mortality_-_commentaries_and_synthesis.pdf).

Fourcade-Gourinchas, M. and Babb, S.L. (2002) 'The rebirth of the liberal creed: Paths to neoliberalism in four countries', *American Journal of Sociology*, vol 108, no 3, pp 533-79.

Fraser Institute (2013) *Economic freedom of the world annual report 2013*, Vancouver: Fraser Institute.

Fukuyama, F. (1989) 'The end of history?', *The National Interest*, pp 3-18.

Fulbrook, M. (2005) *The people's state: East German society from Hitler to Honecker*, New Haven, CT: Yale University Press.

Gallie, W.B. (1955) 'Essentially contested concepts', in *Proceedings of the Aristotelian Society*, JSTOR.

Gamble, A. (1994) *The free economy and the strong state*, London: Macmillan.

Gamble, A. (2009) *The spectre at the feast: Capitalist crisis and the politics of recession*, Basingstoke: Palgrave.

Garthwaite, K.A., Collins, P.J. and Bambra, C. (2015) 'Food for thought: An ethnographic study of negotiating ill health and food insecurity in a UK foodbank', *Social Science & Medicine*, vol 132, pp 38-44.

Gaskell, E.C. (1855) *North and South*, London: Wordsworth.

Gatrell, A. and Elliot, S. (2009) *Geographies of health: An introduction*, London: Wiley.

Gelormino, E., Bambra, C., Spadea, T. et al (2011) 'The effects of health care reforms on health inequalities: a review and analysis of the European evidence base', *International Journal of Health Services*, vol 41, no 2, pp 209-30.

Gesler, W. (2003) *Healing places*, London: Rowman & Littlefield.

Gibson, M., Petticrew, M., Bambra, C., Sowden, A.J., Wright, K.E. and Whitehead, M. (2011) 'Housing and health inequalities: A synthesis of systematic reviews of interventions aimed at different pathways linking housing and health', *Health & Place*, vol 17, no 1, pp 175-84.

Giddens, A. (1998) *The third way: The renewal of social democracy*, Cambridge: Polity Press.

Giddens, A. (2002) *Where now for New Labour?*, Cambridge: Polity Press.

Gillen, M., Yen, I.H., Trupin, L., Swig, L., Rugulies, R. and Mullen, K. (2007) 'The association of socioeconomic status and psychosocial and physical workplace factors with musculoskeletal injury in hospital workers', *American Journal of Industrial Medicine*, vol 50, no 4, pp 245-60.

Ginsburg, N. (1992) *Divisions of welfare: A critical introduction to comparative social policy*, London: Sage.

Gjonça, A., Brockmann, H. and Maier, H. (2000) 'Old-age mortality in Germany prior to and after reunification', *Demographic Research*, vol 3.

Goffman, E. (1963) *Stigma: Notes on the management of spoiled identity*, Harmondsworth: Penguin.

Gokhale, J., Raffelhuschen, B. and Walliser, J. (1994) *The burden of German unification: A generational accounting approach*, Cleveland, OH: Federal Reserve Bank of Cleveland, pp 141-65.

Gottschalk, M. (2004) *Caught: The prison state and the lockdown of American politics*, Princeton, NJ: Princeton University Press.

Gramsci, A. (1971) *Prison notebooks*, New York: International Publishers.

Green, A.E. (1988) 'The North-South divide in Great Britain: an examination of the evidence', *Transactions of the Institute of British Geographers*, pp 179-98.

Gregg, E.W., Zhuo, X., Cheng, Y.J., Albright, A.L., Venkat Narayan, K.M. and Thompson, T.J. (2014) 'Trends in lifetime risk and years of life lost due to diabetes in the USA, 1985–2011: A modelling study', *The Lancet: Diabetes & Endocrinology*, vol 2, no 11, pp 867-74.

Greiner, K.A., Chaoyang, L., Kawachi, I., Hunt, D.C. and Ahluwalia, J.S. (2004) 'The relationships of social participation and community ratings to health and health behaviors in areas with high and low population density', *Social Science & Medicine*, vol 59,no 11, pp 2303-12.

Grundmann, N., Mielck, A., Siegel, M. and Maier, W. (2014) 'Area deprivation and the prevalence of type 2 diabetes and obesity: Analysis at the municipality level in Germany', *BMC Public Health*, vol 14.

Hacker, J.D. (2010) 'Decennial life tables for the white population of the United States, 1790-1900', *Historical Methods*, vol 43, no 2, pp 45-79.

Hacking, J.M., Muller, S. and Buchan, I.E. (2011) 'Trends in mortality from 1965 to 2008 across the English north-south divide: comparative observational study', *British Medical Journal*, vol 342, d508.

Hall, S. and Jacques, M. (1983) *The politics of Thatcherism*, London: Lawrence & Wishart.

Hanlon, P., Lawder, R.S., Buchanan, D., Redpath, A., Walsh, D., Wood, R. et al (2005) 'Why is mortality higher in Scotland than in England and Wales? Decreasing influence of socioeconomic deprivation between 1981 and 2001 supports the existence of a "Scottish effect"', *Journal of Public Health*, vol 27, no 2, pp 199-204.

Harrington, J.M., Gill, F., Aw, T.-C. and Gardiner, K. (1998) *Occupational health* (4th revised edn), London: Blackwell.

Harrison, M. (2004) *Disease and the modern world, 1500 to the present*, London: Polity Press.

Hartig, T., Evans, G.W., Jamner, L.D., Davis, D.S. and Gärling, T. (2003) 'Tracking restoration in natural and urban field settings', *Journal of Environmental Psychology*, vol 23, no 2, pp 109-23.

Harvey, D. (2005) *A brief history of neoliberalism*, Oxford: Oxford University Press.

Harvey, D. (2014) *Seventeen contradictions and the end of capitalism*, London: Pluto Press.

Hastings, A. et al (2015) 'Coping with the cuts? The management of the worst financial settlement in living memory', *Local Government Studies*, vol 41, no 4, pp 601-21.

Hawe, P. and Shiell, A. (2000) 'Social capital and health promotion: a review', *Social Science & Medicine*, vol 51, no 6, pp 871-85.

Hemingway, H. and Marmot, M. (1999) 'Psychosocial factors in the aetiology and prognosis of coronary heart disease: Systematic review of prospective cohort studies', *British Medical Journal*, vol 318, no 7196, pp 1460-7.

Heywood, A. (1992) *Political ideologies*, London: Palgrave Macmillan.

Heywood, A. (1994) *Political ideas and concepts*, London: Macmillan.

Heywood, A. (2000) *Key concepts in politics*, London: Macmillan.

Hill, J. and Williams, J. (1996) *Sport and identity in the North of England*, Keele: Keele University Press.

Hill, S. (2015) 'Axes of health inequalities and intersectionality', in K.E. Smith and C. Bambra (eds) *Health inequalities: Critical perspectives*, Oxford: Oxford University Press.

House of Commons (1991) *Hansard debate, 16 May 1991.*

HSCIC (Health & Social Care Information Centre) (2014) *Statistics on obesity, physical activity and diet, England 2014*, London: HSCIC.

HSCIC (Health & Social Care Information Centre) (2014) *Health Survey for England – 2013*, Leeds: HSCIC.

Hunter, D. (2008) *The health debate*, Bristol: Policy Press.

Hunter, D.J. (2011) 'Change of government: one more big bang health care reform in England's National Health Service', *International Journal of Health Services*, vol 41, no 1, pp 159-74.

Hunter, D.J., Popay, J., Tannahill, C., Whitehead, M. and Duncan, W.H. (2010) 'Getting to grips with health inequalities at last?', *British Medical Journal*, vol 340, doi: http://dx.doi.org/10.1136/bmj.c684.

International Diabetes Federation (2013) *IDF diabetes atlas* (6th edn), Brussels: International Diabetes Federation.

Jarvis, M. and Wardle, J. (2006) 'Social patterning of individual health behaviours: The case of cigarette smoking', in M. Marmot and R. Wilkinson (eds) *The social determinants of health*, Oxford: Oxford University Press, pp 240-55.

Jessop, B. (1991) 'The welfare state in transition from Fordism to post-Fordism', in B. Jessop, K. Nielsen, H. Kastendiek and O.K. Pederson (eds) *The politics of flexibility: Restructuring state and industry in Britain, Germany and Scandinavia*, Aldershot: Edward Elgar, pp 82-105.

Jones, M. and Daykin, N. (2015) 'Sociology and health', in J. Naidoo and J. Wills (eds) *Health studies: An introduction*, London: Palgrave, pp 155-95.

Karasek, R.A. and Theorell, T. (1990) *Healthy work: Stress, productivity, and the reconstruction of working life*, New York: Basic Books.

Kesztenbaum, L. and Rosenthal, J. (2012) *The democratization of longevity: How the poor became old in Paris, 1870-1940*, Paris: Paris School of Economics.

Khaw, K.-T., Wareham, N., Bingham, S., Welch, A., Luben, R. et al (2008) 'Combined impact of health behaviours and mortality in men and women: The EPIC-Norfolk prospective population study', *Plos Medicine*, vol 5, no 1, pp 39-47.

Kibele, E.U.B., Kluesener, S. and Scholz, R.D. (2015) 'Regional mortality disparities in Germany: Long-term dynamics and possible determinants', *Kolner Zeitschrift fur Soziologie und Sozialpsychologie*, vol 67, pp 241-70.

Komlos, J. and Baur, M. (2004) 'From the tallest to (one of) the fattest: The enigmatic fate of the American population in the 20th century', *Economics and Human Biology*, vol 2, no 1, pp 57-74.

Krieger, N. (2013) 'Ecosocial theory of disease distribution', YouTube video (www.youtube.com/watch?v=5pBnnDJ9HQY).

Krieger, N., Chen, J.T., Coull, B., Waterman, P.D. and Beckfield, J. (2013) 'The unique impact of abolition of Jim Crow laws on reducing inequities in infant death rates and implications for choice of cmparison groups in analyzing societal determinants of health', *American Journal of Public Health*, vol 103, no 12, pp 2234-44.

Krieger, N., Kosheleva, A., Waterman, P.D., Chen, J.T., Beckfield, J. and Kiang, M.V. (2014) '50-year trends in US socioeconomic inequalities in health: US-born Black and White Americans, 1959-2008', *International Journal of Epidemiology*, vol 43, no 4, pp 1294-313.

Krieger, N., Rehkopf, D.H., Chen, J.T., Waterman, P.D., Marcelli, E. and Kennedy, M. (2008) 'The fall and rise of US inequities in premature mortality: 1960-2002', *Plos Medicine*, vol 5, no 2, pp 227-41.

Krueger, A. and Pischke, J. (1995) 'A comparative analysis of East and West German labor markets: Before and after unification', in R. Freeman and L. Katz (eds) *Differences and changes in wage structures*, Chicago, IL: University of Chicago Press, pp 405-46.

Lahelma, E., Laaksonen, M. and Aittomäki, A. (2009) 'Occupational class inequalities in health across employment sectors: the contribution of working conditions', *International Archives of Occupational and Environmental Health*, vol 82, no 2, pp 185-90.

Lakshman, R., McConville, A., How, S., Flowers, J., Wareham, J. and Cosford, P. (2011) 'Association between area-level socioeconomic deprivation and a cluster of behavioural risk factors: cross-sectional, population-based study', *Journal of Public Health*, vol 33, no 2, pp 234-45.

Ledwith, M. (2001) 'Community work as critical pedagogy: re-envisioning Freire and Gramsci', *Community Development Journal*, vol 36, no 3, pp 171-82.

Levell, P. and Oldfield, Z. (2011) 'The spending patterns and inflation experience of low-income households over the past decade', *IFS Commentary C119*, London: Institute of Fiscal Studies.

Leyland, A.H. (2004) 'Increasing inequalities in premature mortality in Great Britain', *Journal of Epidemiology and Community Health*, vol 58, no 4, pp 296-302.

LHO (London Health Observatory) (2012) *Health inequalities*, London: LHO (www.lho.org.uk/LHO_Topics/National_Lead_Areas/HealthInequalitiesOverview.aspx).

Lin, J.L., Lin-Tan, D.-T., Hsu, K.-H. and Yu, C.-C. (2003) 'Environmental lead exposure and progression of chronic renal diseases in patients without diabetes', *New England Journal of Medicine*, vol 348, no 4, pp 277-86.

Link, B. and Phelan, J. (1995) 'Social conditions as fundamental causes of disease', *Journal of Health and Social Behavior*, vol X, p 14.

Litt, J.S., Tran, N.L. and Burke, T.A. (2002) 'Examining urban brownfields through the public health "macroscope"', *Environmental Health Perspectives*, vol 110, pp 183-93.

Loveland, I. (1993) 'The politics, law and practice of "intentional homelessness": 2-Abandonment of existing housing', *Journal of Social Welfare and Family Law*, vol 15, no 3, pp 185-99.

Lundberg, O., Yngwe, M.A., Stjärne, M.K., Elstad, J.I. Ferrarini, T., Kangas, O. et al (2008) 'The role of welfare state principles and generosity in social policy programmes for public health: an international comparative study', *The Lancet*, vol 372, p 7.

Luttman, A., Jäger, M. and Griefahn, B. (2003) *Preventing musculoskeletal disorders in the workplace*, Protecting Workers' Health Series No 5, Geneva: WHO (www.who.int/occupational_health/publications/muscdisorders/en/).

McCartney, G., Walsh, D., Whyte, B. and Collins, C. (2012) 'Has Scotland always been the "sick man" of Europe? An observational study from 1855 to 2006', *European Journal of Public Health*, vol 22, no 6, pp 756-60.

McDonough, P. and Amick III, B.C. (2001) 'The social context of health selection: a longitudinal study of health and employment', *Social Science & Medicine*, vol 53, no 1, pp 135-45.

McKeown, T. (1976) *The role of medicine*, London: Nuffield.

McKinley, J. (1975) 'The case for refocusing upstream: The political economy of illness', in American Heart Association (ed) *Applying behavioral science to cardiovascular risk*, Anew York: American Heart Association.

McManus, S., Meltzer, H., Brugha, T., Bebbington, P. and Jenkins, R. (2009) *Adult psychiatric morbidity in England, 2007: Results of a household survey*, Leeds: NHS Information Centre.

McVicar, D. (2008) 'Why have UK disability benefit rolls grown so much?', *Journal of Economic Surveys*, vol 22, no 1, pp 114-39.

Macintyre, S. (2007) 'Deprivation amplification revisited; or, is it always true that poorer places have poorer access to resources for healthy diets and physical activity?', *International Journal of Behavioral Nutrition and Physical Activity*, vol 4, no 1, p 32.

Macintyre, S., Ellaway, A. and Cummins, S. (2002) 'Place effects on health: How can we conceptualise, operationalise and measure them?', *Social Science & Medicine*, vol 55, no 1, pp 1825-38.

MacLeavy, J. (2011) 'A "new politics" of austerity, workfare and gender? The UK coalition government's welfare reform proposals', *Cambridge Journal of Regions Economy and Society*, vol 4, no 3, pp 355-67.

Maas, J., Verheij, R.A., Groenewegen, P.P., de Vries, S. and Spreeuwenberg, P. (2005) 'Green space, urbanity, and health: how strong is the relation?', *Journal of Epidemiology & Community Health*, vol 60, no 7, pp 587-92.

Mackenbach, J. (2006) *Health inequalities: Europe in profile*, European Commission, Public Health, Rotterdam: University Medical Center (www.who.int/social_determinants/resources/european_inequalities.pdf).

Mackenbach, J.P. (2011) 'Can we reduce health inequalities? An analysis of the English strategy (1997-2010)', *Journal of Epidemiology and Community Health*, vol 65, no 7.

Mackenbach, J.P. and McKee, M. (2013) 'Social-democratic government and health policy in Europe: a quantitative analysis', *International Journal of Health Services*, vol 43, no 3, pp 389-413.

Mackenbach, J.P., Stirbu, I., Roskam, A.J., Schaap, M.M., Menvielle, G., Leinsalu, M. et al (2008) 'Socioeconomic inequalities in health in 22 European countries', *New England Journal of Medicine*, vol 358, no 23, pp 2468-81.

Markowitz, G. and Rosner, D. (2003) *Deceit and denial: The deadly politics of industrial pollution*, New York: University of California Press.

Marmot, M. (2004) 'Status syndrome', *Significance*, vol 1, no 4, pp 150-4.

Marmot, M. (2006) 'Introduction', in M. Marmot and R. Wilkinson (eds) *The social determinants of health*, Oxford: Oxford University Press, pp 1-5.

Marmot, M. (2010) *Fair society, healthy lives: The Marmot Review*, London: University College London.

Marmot, M., Siegrist, J. and Theorell, T. (2006) 'Health and the psychosocial work environment', in M. Marmot and R. Wilkinson (eds) *The social determinants of health*, Oxford: Oxford University Press, pp 97-130.

Marmot, M.G., Bosma, H., Hemingway, H., Brunner, E. and Stansfield, S. (1997) 'Contribution of job control and other risk factors to social variations in coronary heart disease incidence', *The Lancet*, vol 350, no 9073, pp 235-9.

Marshall, T.H. (1963) *Sociology at the crossroads: And other essays*, London: Hutchinson.

Martin, G.R.R. (2011) *A song of ice and fire*, London: Harper Voyager.

Martuzzi, M., Mitis, F. and Forastiere, F. (2010) 'Inequalities, inequities, environmental justice in waste management and health', *European Journal of Public Health*, vol 20, p 5.

Max Planck Institute for Demographic Research (2014) *The Human Mortality Database* (www.mortality.org/).

Melzer, D., Fryers, T. and Jenkins, R. (2004) *Social inequalities and the distribution of the common mental disorders*, Hove: Psychology Press.

Mental Health Foundation (2015) *Suicide*, London: Mental Health Foundation (www.mentalhealth.org.uk/help-information/mental-health-a-z/s/suicide).

Menvielle, G., Boshuizen, H., Kunst, A.E., Dalton, S.O., Vineis, P., Bergmann, M.M. et al (2009) 'The role of smoking and diet in explaining educational inequalities in lung cancer incidence', *Journal of the National Cancer Institute*, vol 101, no 5, pp 321-30.

M'Gonigle, G. and Kirby, J. (1936) *Poverty and public health*, London: Victor Gollancz.

Milne, E. and Schrecker, T. (2014) 'Lots of planets have a North...', *Journal of Public Health*, vol 36, no 2, pp 181-2.

Millett, K. (1969) *Sexual politics*, London: Virago.

Mitchell, R. and Popham, F. (2007) 'Greenspace, urbanity and health: relationships in England', *Journal of Epidemiology and Community Health*, vol 61, no 8, pp 681-3.

Möller, H., Haigh, F., Harwood, C., Kinsella, T. and Pope, D. (2013) 'Rising unemployment and increasing spatial health inequalities in England: further extension of the North–South divide', *Journal of Public Health*, vol 35, no 2, pp 313-21.

Montgomery, S.M., Cook, D.G., Bartley, M. and Wadsworth, M.E.J. (1998) 'Unemployment, cigarette smoking, alcohol consumption and body weight in young British men', *European Journal of Public Health*, vol 8, no 1, pp 21-7.

Mooney, G. (2007) 'Infectious diseases and epidemiologic transition in Victorian Britain? Definitely', *Social History of Medicine*, vol 20, no 3, pp 595-606.

Moran, M. (1999) *Governing the healthcare state: A comparative study of the UK, the USA and Germany*, Manchester: Manchester University Press.

Moser, K.A., Fox, A.J. and Jones, D.R. (1984) 'Unemployment and mortality in the OPCS longitudinal study', *The Lancet*, vol 324, no 8415, pp 1324-9.

National Records of Scotland (2013) *Suicide rates in Scotland*, Edinburgh: National Records of Scotland.

National Records of Scotland (2014) *Life expectancy for administrative areas within Scotland 2011-2013*, Edinburgh: National Records of Scotland (www.nrscotland.gov.uk/statistics-and-data/statistics/statistics-by-theme/life-expectancy/life-expectancy-in-scottish-areas/2011-2013).

Navarro, V., Muntaner, C., Borrell, C., Benach, J., Quiroga, A., Rodriguez-Sanz, M. (2006) 'Politics and health outcomes', *The Lancet*, vol 368, no 9540, pp 1033-7.

Nazroo, J. and Williams, D. (2006) 'The social determination of ethnic/racial inequalities in health', in M. Marmot and R. Wilkinson (eds) *The social determinants of health*, Oxford: Oxford University Press, pp 238-66.

Newcastle University and Nexus (2014) *Healthy Life Simulation* (www.ncl.ac.uk/ageing/partners/simulation/).

NHS Choices (2015) 'Dysentery' (www.nhs.uk/conditions/Dysentery/Pages/Introduction.aspx).

NHS Choices (2015) 'Typhoid fever' (www.nhs.uk/Conditions/Typhoid-fever/Pages/Introduction.aspx).

NHS Choices (2015) 'Typhus conditions' (www.nhs.uk/conditions/typhus/Pages/Introduction.aspx).

NHS Choices (2015) 'Cardiovascular disease' (www.nhs.uk/conditions/cardiovascular-disease/Pages/Introduction.aspx).

NHS Choices (2015) 'Cancer' (www.nhs.uk/conditions/Cancer/Pages/Introduction.aspx).

NHS Choices (2015) 'Diabetes' (www.nhs.uk/conditions/diabetes/pages/diabetes.aspx).

NISRA (Northern Ireland Statistics and Research Agency) (2013) *Suicide rates in Northern Ireland*, Belfast: NISRA.

Nolte, E. and McKee, M. (2011) 'Variations in amenable mortality-trends in 16 high-income nations', *Health Policy*, vol 103, no 1, pp 47-52.

Nolte, E., Brand, A., Koupilová, I. and McKee, M. (2000) 'Neonatal and postneonatal mortality in Germany since unification', *Journal of Epidemiology and Community Health*, vol 54, no 2, pp 84-90.

Nolte, E., Scholz, R., Shkolnikov, V. and McKee, M. (2002) 'The contribution of medical care to changing life expectancy in Germany and Poland', *Social Science & Medicine*, vol 55, no 11, pp 1905-21.

Nomis (2015) *Labour market profile* (www.nomisweb.co.uk/).

Norman, P., Boyle, P., Exeter, D., Feng, Z. and Popham, F. (2011) 'Rising premature mortality in the UK's persistently deprived areas: Only a Scottish phenomenon?', *Social Science & Medicine*, vol 73, no 11, pp 1575-84.

OECD (Organisation for Economic Co-operation and Development) (2011) *Society at a glance 2011: OECD Social indicators*, Paris: OECD.

OECD (Organisation for Economic Co-operation and Development) (2013) *Health at a Glance 2013: OECD indicators*, Paris: OECD Publishing (http://dx.doi.org/10.1787/health_glance-2013-en).

OECD (Organisation for Economic Co-operation and Development) (2014) *Trade union density*, Paris: OECD.

ONS (Office for National Statistics) (2011) *Life expectancy and disability free life expectancy*, Newport: ONS.

ONS (Office for National Statistics) (2012) *Mortality statistics 2013*, Newport: ONS.

ONS (Office for National Statistics) (2013) *Measuring national well-being, Health, 2013*, Newport: ONS (http://webarchive.nationalarchives.gov.uk/20160105160709/http://www.ons.gov.uk/ons/rel/wellbeing/measuring-national-well-being/health--2013/index.html).

ONS (Office for National Statistics) (2013) *General Lifestyle Survey: 2011*, Newport: ONS (www.ons.gov.uk/ons/rel/ghs/general-lifestyle-survey/2011/rpt-chapter-7.html?format=print).

ONS (Office for National Statistics) (2014) 'Adult health in Great Britain', *Statistical Bulletin,* Newport: ONS.

ONS (Office for National Statistics) (2014) *Disability-free life expectancy (DFLE) and life expectancy (LE) at birth by upper tier local authority at birth, England 2012–14*, Newport: ONS.

ONS (Office for National Statistics) (2014) *Life expectancy at birth and at age 65 by local areas in England and Wales: 2011 to 13*, Newport: ONS.

ONS (Office for National Statistics) (2014) *Suicides in the United Kingdom: 2012 registrations*, Newport: ONS.

ONS (Office for National Statistics) (2015) *Life expectancy at birth for England, Wales and Northern Ireland, 2012-14*, Newport: ONS.

ONS (Office for National Statistics) (2015) *Inequality in healthy life expectancy at birth by national deciles of area deprivation: England, 2011 to 2013*, Newport: ONS.

Parkes, K.S. (1997) *Understanding contemporary Germany*, London: Taylor & Francis.

Pearce, J. (2013) 'Financial crisis, austerity policies, and geographical inequalities in health: Introduction commentary', *Environment and Planning A*, vol 45, no 9, pp 2030-45.

Pearce, J. and Dorling, D. (2006) 'Increasing geographical inequalities in health in New Zealand, 1980-2001', *International Journal of Epidemiology*, vol 35, no 3, pp 597-603.

Pearce, J., Blakely, T., Witten, K. and Bartie, P. (2007) 'Neighborhood deprivation and access to fast-food retailing – A national study', *American Journal of Preventive Medicine*, vol 32, no 5, pp 375-82.

Pearce, J.R., Richardson, E.A., Mitchell, R.J. and Shortt, N.K. (2010) 'Environmental justice and health: the implications of the socio-spatial distribution of multiple environmental deprivation for health inequalities in the United Kingdom', *Transactions of the Institute of British Geographers*, vol 35, no 4, pp 522-39.

Pearce, J., Dorling, D., Wheeler, B., Barnett, R. and Rigby, J. (2006) 'Geographical inequalities in health in New Zealand, 1980-2001: the gap widens', *Australian and New Zealand Journal of Public Health*, vol 30, no 5, pp 461-6.

Pearce, J., Rind, E., Shortt, N., Tisch, C. and Mitchell, R. (2015) 'Tobacco retail environments and social inequalities in individual-level smoking and cessation among Scottish adults', *Nicotine & Tobacco Research*, pp 1-9.

Peterson, R.K.D. (1995) 'Insects, disease, and military history: The Napoleonic campaigns and historical perception', *American Entomologist*, vol 41, no 3, pp 147-60.

PHE (Public Health England) (2013) *Local health* (www.localhealth.org.uk).

PHE (Public Health England) (2014) *Adult obesity and type 2 diabetes*, London: PHE.

PHE (Public Health England) (2015) *Public Health Outcomes Framework*, London: PHE (www.phoutcomes.info/).

Phelan, J.C., Link, B.G., Diez-Roux, A., Kawachi, I. and Levin, B. (2004) '"Fundamental causes" of social inequalities in mortality: A test of the theory', *Journal of Health and Social Behavior*, vol 45, no 3, pp 265-85.

Platt, S. (1986) 'Parasuicide and unemployment', *British Journal of Psychiatry*, vol 149, pp 401-5.

Polanyi, K. (1944) *The great transformation*, Boston, MA: Beacon Press.

Pope, D. and Bambra, C. (2005) 'Has the disability discrimination act closed the employment gap?', *Disability and Rehabilitation*, vol 27, no 20, pp 1261-6.

Popham, F. and Bambra, C. (2010) 'Evidence from the 2001 English Census on the contribution of employment status to the social gradient in self-rated health', *Journal of Epidemiology and Community Health*, vol 64, no 3, pp 277-80.

Preston, S.H. and Stokes, A. (2011) 'Contribution of obesity to international differences in life expectancy', *American Journal of Public Health*, vol 101, no 11, pp 2137-43.

Preston, S., Glei, D. and Wilmouth, J. (2010) 'Contributions of smoking to international differences in life expectancy', in E. Crimmins, S. Preston and B. Cohen (eds) *International differences in mortality at older ages*, Washington, DC: National Academies Press.

Priestley, J.B. (1934) *An English journey*, London: Victor Gollancz.

Punnett, L. and Wegman, D.H. (2004) 'Work-related musculoskeletal disorders: the epidemiologic evidence and the debate', *Journal of Electromyography and Kinesiology*, vol 14, no 1, pp 13-23.

Putnam, R. (1993) *Making democracy work: Civic traditions in modern Italy*, Princeton, NJ: Princeton University Press.

Reid, M. (2011) 'Behind the "Glasgow effect"', *Bulletin of the World Health Organization*, vol 89, no 10, pp 706-7.

Reilly, J.J., Methven, E., McDowell, M.E., Hacking, B., Alexander, D., Stewart, L. and Kelnar, C.J. (2003) 'Health consequences of obesity', *Archives of Disease in Childhood*, vol 88, no 9, pp 748-52.

Rennie, K.L. and Jebb, S.A. (2005) 'Prevalence of obesity in Great Britain', *Obesity Reviews*, vol 6, no 1, pp 11-12.

Richardson, E.A. and Mitchell, R. (2010) 'Gender differences in relationships between urban green space and health in the United Kingdom', *Social Science & Medicine*, vol 71, no 3, pp 568-75.

Richardson, E.A., Hill, S.E., Mitchell, R., Pearce, J. and Shortt, N.K. (2015) 'Is local alcohol outlet density related to alcohol-related morbidity and mortality in Scottish cities?', *Health & Place*, vol 33, pp 172-80.

Richardson, E.A., Mitchell, R., Shortt, N.K., Pearce, J. and Dawson, T.P. (2010) 'Developing summary measures of health-related multiple physical environmental deprivation for epidemiological research', *Environment and Planning A*, vol 42, no 7, pp 1650-8.

Riedel, S. (2005) 'Edward Jenner and the history of smallpox and vaccination', *Baylor University Medical Center Proceedings*, vol 18, no 1, pp 21-5.

Riva, M. and Curtis, S.E. (2012) 'Long-term local area employment rates as predictors of individual mortality and morbidity: a prospective study in England, spanning more than two decades', *Journal of Epidemiology and Community Health*, vol 66, no 10, pp 919-26.

Riva, M., Gauvin, L. and Barnett, T.A. (2007) 'Toward the next generation of research into small area effects on health: a synthesis of multilevel investigations published since July 1998', *Journal of Epidemiology and Community Health*, vol 61, no 10, pp 853-61.

Russell, D. (2004) *Looking North: Northern England and the national imagination*, Manchester: Manchester University Press.

RWJF (Robert Wood Johnson Foundation) (2013) *Does where you live affect how long you live?*, Princeton, NJ: RWJF (www.rwjf.org/en/library/features/health-where-you-live.html).

Rydin, Y., Bleahu, A., Davies, M., Dávila, J.D., Friel, S., de Grandis, G. et al (2012) 'Shaping cities for health: complexity and the planning of urban environments in the 21st century', *Lancet*, vol 379, no 9831, pp 2079-108.

Saez, E. and Zucman, G. (2014) *Wealth inequality in the United States since 1913: Evidence from capitalized income tax data*, NBER Working Paper, Cambridge: National Bureau of Economic Research.

Scarborough, P., Wickramasinghe, K., Bhatnagar, P. and Rayner, M. (2011) *Trends in coronary heart disease, 1961-2011*, London: British Heart Foundation.

Schrecker, T. (2014) 'Health equity in a globalising world: The importance of human rights', in A. Robertson (ed) *Commonwealth health partnerships 2014*, London: The Commonwealth, pp 18-21.

Schrecker, T. and Bambra, C. (2015) *How politics makes us sick: Neoliberal epidemics*, Basingstoke: Palgrave Macmillan.

Schuring, M., Burdorf, A., Voorham, A.J., der Weduwe, K. and Mackenbach, J.P. (2009) 'Effectiveness of a health promotion programme for long-term unemployed subjects with health problems: a randomised controlled trial', *Journal of Epidemiology and Community Health*, vol 63, no 11, pp 893-9.

Scottish Government (2008) *Equally well: Report of the Ministerial Task Force on health inequalities*, Edinburgh: Scottish Government.

Scottish Government (2010) *Equally well review*, Edinburgh: Scottish Government.

Scottish Government (2011) *Scottish Health Survey: Topic report; Obesity*, Edinburgh: Scottish Government (www.gov.scot/Publications/2011/10/1138).

Scottish Government (2013) *Trends in mortality by SIMD quintile 2004-2013*, Edinburgh: Scottish Government.

Scottish Government (2014) *The Scottish Health Survey 2013*, Edinburgh: Scottish Government.

Scottish Government (2014) *Scotland: Age-standardised incidence and mortality rates by SIMD*, Edinburgh: Scottish Government.

Scottish Public Health Observatory (2014) *Life expectancy and healthy life expectancy: Deprivation quintiles*, Edinburgh: Scottish Public Health Observatory.

Scott-Samuel, A., Bambra, C., Collins, C., Hunter, D.J., McCartney, G. and Smith, K. (2014) 'The impact of Thatcherism on health and well-being in Britain', *International Journal of Health Services*, vol 44, no 1, pp 53-71.

Scruggs, L., Detlef, J. and Kuitto, K. (2014) 'Comparative welfare entitlements dataset 2, Version 2014-03' (http://cwed2.org/).

Secretary of State for Social Services (1988) *Public health in England. The report of the Committee of Inquiry into the future development of the public health function*, C. 289, London: HMSO.

Senatsverwaltung für Gesundheit und Soziales (2014) *Handlungsorientierter Sozialstrukturatlas Berlin 2013*.

Seymour, R. (2014) 'Zero-hours contracts, and the sharp whip of insecurity that controls us all', *The Guardian*.

Shaw, C., Blakely, T., Atkinson, J. and Crampton, P. (2005) 'Do social and economic reforms change socioeconomic inequalities in child mortality? A case study: New Zealand 1981-1999', *Journal of Epidemiology and Community Health*, vol 59, no 8, pp 638-44.

Shaw, M. (2004) 'Housing and public health', *Annual Review of Public Health*, vol 25, no 1, pp 397-418.

Shaw, M., Dorling, D., Gordon, D. and Davey Smith, G. (1999) *The widening gap: Health inequalities and policy in Britain*, Bristol: Policy Press.

Shildrick, T., MacDonald, R., Webster, C. and Garthwaite, K. (2012) *Poverty and insecurity: Life in low-pay, no-pay Britain*, Bristol: Policy Press.

Shortt, N.K., Richardson, E., Mitchell, R. and Pearce, J. (2011) 'Re-engaging with the physical environment: a health-related environmental classification of the UK', *Area*, vol 43, no 1, pp 76-87.

Skalická, V., van Lenthe, F., Bambra, C., Krokstad, S. and Mackenbach, J. (2009) 'Material, psychosocial, behavioural and biomedical factors in the explanation of relative socio-economic inequalities in mortality: evidence from the HUNT study', *International Journal of Epidemiology*, vol 38, no 5, pp 1272-84.

Slater, T. (2013) 'Your life chances affect where you live: A critique of the "cottage industry" of neighbourhood effects research', *International Journal of Urban and Regional Research*, vol 137, p 20.

Smith, G.D., Morris, J.N. and Shaw, M. (1998) 'The independent inquiry into inequalities in health: Is welcome, but its recommendations are too cautious and vague', *British Medical Journal*, vol 317, no 7171, p 1465.

Smith, J.C. and Medalia, C. (2015) *Health insurance coverage in the United States: 2014*, Current Population Reports, Washington, DC: US Census Bureau (www.census.gov/content/dam/Census/library/publications/2015/demo/p60-253.pdf).

Smith, K.E. and Bambra, C. (2012) 'British and Northern Irish experiences', in D. Raphael (ed) *Tackling health inequalities: Lessons from international experiences*, Toronto: Canadian Scholars' Press Inc.

Smith, K. and Hellowell, M. (2012) 'Beyond rhetorical differences: A cohesive account of post-devolution developments in UK health policy', *Social Policy & Administration*, vol 46, no 2, pp 178-98.

Smith, K.E., Bambra, C., Joyce, K.E., Perkins, N., Hunter, D.J. and Blenkinsopp, E.A. (2009) 'Partners in health? A systematic review of the impact of organizational partnerships on public health outcomes in England between 1997 and 2008', *Journal of Public Health*, vol 31, no 2, pp 210-21.

Smith, K.E., Hunter, D.J., Blackman, T., Elliott, E., Greene, A., Harrington, B.E. et al (2009) 'Divergence or convergence? Health inequalities and policy in a devolved Britain', *Critical Social Policy*, vol 29, no 2, pp 216-42.

Smith, S.J., Searle, B.A. and Cook, N. (2009) 'Rethinking the risks of home ownership', *Journal of Social Policy*, vol 38, no 1, pp 83-102.

Snow, J. (1855) *On the mode of communication of Cholera*, London: John Churchill.

Social Science Research Council (2014) *Measure of America report , 2013-14*, Brooklyn, NY: Social Science Research Council (www.measureofamerica.org/measure_of_america2013-2014/).

Spence, R., Roberts, A., Ariti, C. and Bardsley, M. (2014) *Focus on: Antidepressant prescribing. Trends in the prescribing of antidepressants in primary care*, QualityWatch, London: The Health Foundation and the Nuffield Trust (www.qualitywatch.org.uk/sites/files/qualitywatch/field/field_document/140218_QualityWatch_Focus_on_distance_emergency_care_0.pdf).

Stafford, M. and McCarthy, M. (2006) 'Neighbourhoods, housing and health', in M. Marmot and R. Wilkinson (eds) *The social determinants of health*, Oxford: Oxford University Press, pp 78-96.

Standing, G. (2014) *The precariat: The new dangerous class* (revised edn), London: Bloomsbury.

Stansfeld, S. (2002) 'Work, personality and mental health', *The British Journal of Psychiatry*, vol 181, no 2, pp 96-8.

Statistics Canada (2012) *Life expectancy at birth, by sex, by province* (www.statcan.gc.ca/tables-tableaux/sum-som/l01/cst01/health26-eng.htm).

Stevens, G.A., Singh, G.M., Lu, Y., Danaei, G., Lin, J.K., Finucane, M.M. et al (2012) 'National, regional, and global trends in adult overweight and obesity prevalences', *Population Health Metrics*, vol 10, no 1, p 22.

Stimpson, J.P., Ju, H., Raji, M.A. and Eschbach, K. (2007) 'Neighborhood deprivation and health risk behaviors in NHANES III', *American Journal of Health Behavior*, vol 31, no 2, pp 215-22.

Stuckler, D. and Basu, S. (2013) *The body economic: Why austerity kills*, London: Allan Lane.

Sundquist, K., Malmstrom, M. and Johansson, S.E. (2004) 'Neighbourhood deprivation and incidence of coronary heart disease: a multilevel study of 2.6 million women and men in Sweden', *Journal of Epidemiology and Community Health*, vol 58, no 1, pp 71-7.

Sweeney, T. (1991) 'Medicine in the bloodiest war', *Ozarks Watch*, vol 4, no 4, pp 42-6.

Szreter, S. and Mooney, G. (1998) 'Urbanization, mortality, and the standard of living debate: new estimates of the expectation of life at birth in nineteenth-century British cities', *Economic History Review*, vol 51, no 1, p 84.

Taulbut, M., Walsh, D., McCartney, G., Parcell, S., Hartmann, A., Poirier, G. et al (2014) 'Spatial inequalities in life expectancy within postindustrial regions of Europe: a cross-sectional observational study', *British Medical Journal Open*, vol 4, , e004711.

Thomas, B., Dorling, D. and Davey Smith, G. (2010) 'Inequalities in premature mortality in Britain: observational study from 1921 to 2007', *British Medical Journal*, vol 341.

Thompson, L., Pearce, J. and Barnett, J.R. (2007) 'Moralising geographies: stigma, smoking islands and responsible subjects', *Area*, vol 39, no 4, pp 508-17.

Todd, A., Copeland, A., Husband, A., Kasim, A. and Bambra, C. (2014) 'The positive pharmacy care law: an area-level analysis of the relationship between community pharmacy distribution, urbanity and social deprivation in England', *British Medical Journal Open*, vol 4, no 8.

Todd, A., Copeland, A., Husband, A., Kasim, A. and Bambra, C. (2015) 'Access all areas? An area-level analysis of the relationship between community pharmacy and primary care distribution, urbanity and social deprivation in England', *British Medical Journal Open*, 5:e007328.

Todd, A., Akhter, N., Copeland, A.. Husband, A., Kasim, A., Walton, N. and Bambra, C. (2016, in press) *A North South health care divide? A regional analysis of geographical access to community pharmacy and primary care services in England*. .

Tonge, N. and Quiency, M. (1985) *Cholera and public health*, London: Macmillan.

Townsend, N., Williams, J., Bhatnagar, P., Wickramasinghe, K. and Rayner, M. (2014) *Cardiovascular disease statistics 2014*, London: British Heart Foundation, p 114.

Trussell Trust, The (2014) 'Biggest ever increase in UK food bank use: 170% rise in numbers turning to foodbanks in last 12 months', Salisbury: The Trussell Trust.

Tudor-Hart, J. (1971) 'The inverse care law', *The Lancet*, vol 297, no 7696, pp 405-12.

UN (United Nations) (1948) *Universal declaration of human rights*, New York: UN General Assembly.

Virtanen, P., Vahtera, J., Kivimäki, M., Pentti, J. and Ferrie, J. (2002) 'Employment security and health', *Journal of Epidemiology and Community Health*, vol 56, no 8, pp 569-74.

Walkerdine, V. and Jimenez, L. (2012) *Gender, work and community after de-industrialisation: A psychosocial approach to affect*, Identity Studies in the Social Sciences, Basingstoke: Palgrave Macmillan.

Walsh, D., Taulbut, M. and Hanlon, P. (2010) 'The aftershock of deindustrialization-trends in mortality in Scotland and other parts of post-industrial Europe', *European Journal of Public Health*, vol 20, no 1, pp 58-64.

Walsh, D., McCartney, G., Collins, C., Taulbut, M. and Batty, D. (2016) *History, politics and vulnerability: Explaining excess mortality in Scotland and Glasgow*, Glasgow: Glasgow Centre for Population Health.

Walton, H., Dajnak, D., Beevers, S., Williams, M., Watkiss, P. and Hunt, A. (2015) *Understanding the health impacts of air pollution in London*, London: King's College London (www.kcl.ac.uk/lsm/research/divisions/aes/research/ERG/research-projects/HIAinLondonKingsReport14072015final.pdf).

Ward, K. and England, K. (2007) 'Introduction: Reading neoliberalization', in K. England and K. Ward (eds) *Neoliberalization: States, networks, people*, Oxford: Blackwell.

Webster, D. (2000) 'The geographical concentration of labour-market disadvantage', *Oxford Review of Economic Policy*, vol 16, no 1, pp 114-28.

Welsh Government (2014) *Welsh Health Survey 2013*, Cardiff: Welsh Government.

White, M., Adamson, A., Chadwick, T., Dezateux, C., Griffiths, L., Howel, D. et al (2007) *The changing social patterning of obesity: an analysis to inform practice and policy development*, Newcastle: Public Health Research Consortium.

White, H.L., Matheson, F.I., Moineddin, R., Dunn, J.R. and Glazier, R.H. (2011) 'Neighbourhood deprivation and regional inequalities in self-reported health among Canadians: Are we equally at risk?', *Health & Place*, vol 17, no 1, pp 361-9.

Whitehead, M. and Diderichsen, F. (2001) 'Social capital and health: tip-toeing through the minefield of evidence', *The Lancet*, vol 358, no 9277, pp 165-6.

Whitehead, M. and Doran, T. (2011) 'The North-South health divide', *British Medical Journal*, vol 342, no 7794, d584.

Whitehead, M. and Popay, J. (2010) 'Swimming upstream? Taking action on the social determinants of health inequalities', *Social Science & Medicine*, vol 71, no 7, pp 1234-6.

Whitehead, M.C. et al (2014) *Due North: Report of the Inquiry on Health Equity for the North*, Liverpool and Manchester: University of Liverpool and Centre for Local Economic Strategies (www.cles.org.uk/wp-content/uploads/2014/09/Due-North-Report-of-the-Inquiry-on-Health-Equity-in-the-North-final.pdf).

Whitehead, M., Clayton, S., Holland, P., Drever, F. et al (2009) *Helping chronically ill or disabled people into work: What can we learn from international comparative analyses?*, London: Public Health Research Consortium.

WHO (World Health Organization) (2008) *Commission on the Social Determinants of Health: Closing the gap in a generation*, Geneva: WHO.

WHO (World Health Organization) (2012) *Health for All database*, Geneva: WHO.

WHO (World Health Organization) (2013) *Life expectancy at birth*, Geneva: WHO (www.who.int/gho/mortality_burden_disease/life_tables/situation_trends/en/).

WHO (World Health Organization) (2013) *Global Burden of Disease*, Geneva: WHO.

WHO (World Health Organization) (2014) 'Suicide', Geneva: WHO (www.who.int/mediacentre/factsheets/fs398/en/).

WHO (World Health Organization) (2015) 'Small pox', Geneva: WHO (www.who.int/csr/disease/smallpox/en/).

WHO (World Health Organization) (2015) *Tuberculosis*, Geneva: WHO (www.who.int/topics/tuberculosis/en/).

Whyte, B. and Ajetunmobi, T. (2012) *Still the 'sick man of Europe'? Scottish mortality in a European context 1950-2010. An analysis of comparative mortality trends*, Glasgow: Glasgow Centre for Population Health.

Wilkinson, E. (1939) *The town that was murdered*, London: Victor Gollancz.

Wilkinson, R. and Pickett, K. (2010) *The spirit level: Why equality is better for everyone*, London: Penguin.

Willis, N.J. (1997) 'Edward Jenner and the eradication of smallpox', *Scottish Medical Journal*, vol 42, no 4, pp 118-21.

Winslow, C.E. (1920) 'The untilled fields of public health', *Science*, vol 51, no 1306, pp 23-33.

Wood, J., Hennell, T., Jones, A., Hooper, J., Tocque, K. and Bellis, M.A. (2006) *Where wealth means health: Illustrating inequality in the North West*, Liverpool: North West Public Health Observatory.

Woolf, S. and Aron, L. (2013) *US health in international perspective: Shorter lives, poorer health*, Washington, DC: The National Academies Press.

Index

Note: page numbers in *italic* type refer to Figures; those in **bold** type refer to Tables.

N

O

P

Y

Z